Children and Youth with Complex Cerebral Palsy

T0203210

Children and Youth with Complex Cerebral Palsy

Care and Management

Edited by Laurie J. Glader
and Richard D. Stevenson

2019
Mac Keith Press

Managing Director: Ann-Marie Halligan
Project Management: Riverside Publishing Solutions Ltd

First published in this edition in 2019 by Mac Keith Press
2nd Floor, Rankin Building, 139–143 Bermondsey Street, London, SE1 3UW

British Library Cataloguing-in-Publication data
A catalogue record for this book is available from the British Library

Cover design: Hannah Rogers

ISBN: 978-1-909962-98-9

Typeset by Riverside Publishing Solutions Ltd

Printed by Hobbs the Printers Ltd, Totton, Hampshire, UK

From a Parent

When my triplets were born, three teams of medical professionals whisked them away before I could even lay eyes on them. And so in a moment, I had to learn to trust others with the well-being of my children. I had no idea how necessary this lesson would prove in the life of our family. When the boys were nine months old, I asked their occupational therapist why she was working so hard to get them to grab beads rather than working on sitting up – a skill I desperately wanted them to learn. I was crying as I asked, petrified of what her answer would be. I will never forget how, with tears streaming down her own cheeks, she gently told me they had to reach across midline before we could hope for them to reach any further milestones. Her tears were a gift to me that day because I needed to know she cared for my children with a passion and that she valued being on our team. For 21 years, we have had nurses, doctors, therapists and surgeons at birthday parties, theatre performances, and even high school graduations because these professionals, who have so expertly cared for our children, are on our family team, in our circle of supporters. They are our hand-holders and cheerleaders. We are ever grateful.

Yes, you are on the frontlines of your patients' medical care. But more importantly, to the parents of a child with complex cerebral palsy, you are on the frontlines of hope.

Carole Shrader

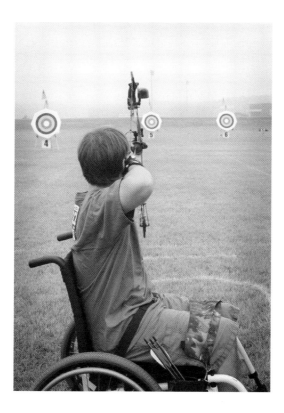

Contents

Author Appointments

Victor Anciano
Resident Physician, Department of Orthopedics, University of Virginia, Charlottesville, VA, USA

Steven J. Bachrach
Professor of Pediatrics, Sidney Kimmel Medical College of Thomas Jefferson University, Philadelphia, PA; Department of Pediatrics, Nemours Alfred I. duPont Hospital for Children, Wilmington, DE, USA

Alisa B. Bahl
Associate Professor of Pediatrics, Division of Developmental Pediatrics, University of Virginia School of Medicine, Charlottesville, VA, USA

Stuart Bauer
Senior Associate in Urology, Boston Children's Hospital; Professor of Surgery (Urology), Harvard Medical School, Boston, MA, USA

Beate Beinvogl
Attending Physician, Pediatric Gastroenterology and Nutrition, Boston Children's Hospital; Instructor of Pediatrics, Harvard Medical School, Boston, MA, USA

Mary C. Bickley
Director, Encouragement Feeding Program, University of Virginia Children's Hospital, Charlottesville, VA, USA

John M. Costello
Director, Augmentative Communication Program, Department of Otolaryngology & Communication Enhancement, Boston Children's Hospital, Boston, MA, USA

Claudio M. de Gusmao
MD, Department of Neurology; Director, Movement Disorders program, Boston Children's Hospital; Attending physician, Brigham and Women's Hospital; Instructor in Neurology, Harvard Medical School, Boston, MA, USA

Eva Delaney
Pediatric Registered Dietitian/Nutritionist and Nutrition Support Specialist, University of Virginia Children's Hospital, Charlottesville, VA, USA

Darcy Fehlings
Professor of Paediatrics, Head of the Division of Developmental Paediatrics, University of Toronto, Holland Bloorview Kids Rehabilitation Hospital, Toronto, ON, Canada

Katheryn F. Frazier
Assistant Professor of Pediatrics, Division of Developmental Pediatrics, Department of Pediatrics, University of Virginia, Charlottesville, VA, USA

Kurt A. Freeman
Fred Fax Professor of Pediatrics; Institute on Development and Disability, Department of Pediatrics, Oregon Health & Science University, Portland, OR, USA

Laurie J. Glader
Associate in Medicine, Co-Director, Cerebral Palsy and Spasticity Center, Director, Complex Care Service Outpatient Program, Boston Children's Hospital; Assistant Professor of Pediatrics, Harvard Medical School, Boston, MA, USA

Howard P. Goodkin
The Shure Professor of Neurology and Pediatrics; Chair, Department of Neurology; Director, Division of Pediatric Neurology; Departments of Neurology and Pediatrics, University of Virginia, Charlottesville, VA, USA

Susan Hayden Gray
Attending Physician, Adolescent and Young Adult Medicine, Boston Children's Hospital; Assistant Professor of Pediatrics, Harvard Medical School, Boston, MA, USA

Jonathan Greenwood
Director, Department of Physical Therapy & Occupational Therapy Services, Boston Children's Hospital, Boston, MA, USA

Richard I. Grossberg
Director, Center for Comprehensive Care, Rainbow Babies and Children's Hospital; Associate Professor of Pediatrics, Case Western Reserve University School of Medicine, Cleveland, OH, USA

Julie Hauer
Medical Director, Seven Hills Pediatric Center, Division of General Pediatrics, Boston Children's Hospital; Assistant Professor of Pediatrics, Harvard Medical School, Boston, MA, USA

Valentina Intagliata
Assistant Professor of Pediatrics, Division of Developmental Pediatrics, University of Virginia, Charlottesville, VA, USA

Umakanth Katwa
Director, Sleep Laboratory, Attending Pulmonary and Sleep Medicine, Boston Children's Sleep Center; Division of Respiratory Diseases, Boston Children's Hospital, Harvard Medical School, Boston, MA, USA

Anne Kawamura
Assistant Professor, Division of Developmental Pediatrics, University of Toronto; Program Director, Developmental Pediatrics Subspecialty Residency Program, University of Toronto, Toronto, ON, Canada

Heidi H. Kecskemethy
Director, Faculty Resources, Nemours Biomedical Research; Clinical Research Scientist, Department of Medical Imaging, Nemours Alfred I. duPont Hospital for Children, Wilmington, DE, USA

Cecilia Lee
Developmental Paediatrician, Holland Bloorview Kids Rehabilitation Hospital; Assistant Professor, Division of Developmental Paediatrics, University of Toronto, Toronto, ON, Canada

Christopher D. Lunsford
Assistant Professor of Pediatric Rehabilitation Medicine, Department of Physical Medicine and Rehabilitation and Department of Pediatrics, University of Virginia School of Medicine, Charlottesville, VA, USA

Jennifer Lyman
Parent of a child with complex cerebral palsy; Therapeutic Recreation Specialist; CP Collaborative Coordinator; Board, CP NOW, New Orleans, LA, USA

Amber Makino
Developmental Paediatrician, Holland Bloorview Kids Rehabilitation Hospital; Lecturer, Division of Developmental Paediatrics, University of Toronto, Toronto, ON, Canada

Munir Mobassaleh
Assistant Clinical Professor of Pediatrics, Harvard Medical School, Boston Children's Hospital, Boston, MA, USA

Kerim M. Munir
Director of Psychiatry, University Center for Excellence in Developmental Disabilities, Division of Developmental Medicine, Boston Children's Hospital; Associate Professor of Psychiatry and Pediatrics, Departments of Psychiatry and Pediatrics, Harvard Medical School, Boston, MA, USA

John R. Mytinger
Assistant Professor, The Ohio State University, Nationwide Children's Hospital, Columbus, OH, USA

Jaylan Norfleet
Baltimore, MD, USA

Garey Noritz
Division and Section Chief, Complex Health Care Program; Medical Director, Cerebral Palsy Program, Nationwide Children's Hospital; Professor, The Ohio State University, Columbus, OH, USA

Kitty O'Hare
Assistant Professor of Medicine, Brigham and Women's Hospital; Assistant Professor of Pediatrics, Boston Children's Hospital; Harvard Medical School, Boston, MA, USA

Andrea L. Paulson
Assistant Professor, Departments of Clinical Pediatrics and Clinical Neurology & Rehabilitation Medicine, Cincinnati Children's Hospital Medical Center, University of Cincinnati College of Medicine, Cincinnati, OH, USA

Jim Plews-Ogan
Associate Professor of Pediatrics, University of Virginia School of Medicine, Charlottesville, VA, USA

Mark J. Romness
Associate Professor of Orthopaedic Surgery, University of Virginia, Charlottesville, VA, USA

Elizabeth N. Rose
Speech Language Pathologist, Boston Children's Hospital, Boston, MA, USA

Ikram Rustamov
Assistant Professor of Psychiatry; Child and Adolescent Mental Health and Development Centre, Department of Psychiatry, Azerbaijan Medical University, Baku, Azerbaijan

Lisa Samson-Fang
Developmental Behavioral Pediatrics, General Pediatrics, Intermountain Medical Group, Bryner Pediatrics at Salt Lake Clinic, Salt Lake City, Utah, USA

Benjamin Shore
Assistant Professor in Orthopaedic Surgery; Associate Program Director, Pediatric Orthopaedic Fellowship, Harvard Medical School; Co-Director, Cerebral Palsy & Spasticity Center; Orthopaedic Surgeon, Child and Young Adult Hip Preservation Program; Boston Children's Hospital, Boston, MA, USA

Benjamin Shrader
Student and advocate, USA

Carol Shrader
Parent of four, two with cerebral palsy; speaker and writer, The Blessing Counter blog, USA

Michele Shusterman
Founder/President, CP NOW nonprofit & CP Daily Living blog, USA

Andrew J. Smith
Author, Heath, OH, USA

Richard D. Stevenson
Professor of Pediatrics; Head, Division of Developmental Pediatrics, University of Virginia School of Medicine, Charlottesville, VA, USA

Chelsea Strawser
Columbus, OH, USA

Jilda N. Vargus-Adams
Associate Professor, Clinical Pediatrics and Clinical Neurology & Rehabilitation Medicine, Cincinnati Children's Hospital Medical Center, University of Cincinnati College of Medicine, Cincinnati, OH, USA

Sebastian K. Welsh
Pediatric Pulmonologist, San Antonio Military Medical Center, TX, USA

Acknowledgments

The opportunity to put together a manual that provides support for general practitioners caring for children with complex cerebral palsy has been deeply meaningful to both of us. We are humbled by the breadth of this field, even more so now that we have lived and breathed it for the last couple of years. In the process of creating this book we have tried to craft something that we wish we had had ourselves many moons ago when we began our own professional journeys.

First and foremost, we want to thank the many children and youth with cerebral palsy and their families whom we have been fortunate enough to work with over the years. In a very real sense, you have been our "continuing education" in the field, helping us to see beyond our sometimes narrow medical view to a perspective that is always broad and meaningful. More than anything else, it is you who have inspired and fuelled the making of this book, but you have also inspired and enriched our careers, both professionally and personally.

We are indebted to our editors, teachers and mentors. We thank Martin Bax for his leadership and vision during his time as Senior Editor for Developmental Medicine and Child Neurology and the book series that has become so fundamental to the work of Mac Keith Press. We extend a special thanks to Hilary Hart and Lewis Rosenbloom who, as members of the Editorial Board, first approached us with the idea for this book. Working with Mac Keith Press has been a pleasure. Thanks to Ann-Marie Halligan and Udoka Ohuonu for the on-going support, gentle reminders and always helpful feedback. We thank all of our professors, teachers and mentors (you know who you are): you have a part in this work through the essential role you have played in our professional development.

The phenomenal contributions of the authors and reviewers must be acknowledged. We have learned tremendously and honed our own skills thanks to your deep expertise, and are greatly indebted to you for sharing that expertise with us. Our external reviewers provided extremely thoughtful and helpful feedback. The project evolved in some very important ways based on that feedback and subsequent conversations with our authors and editors.

We also want to express our thanks to the American Academy for Cerebral Palsy and Developmental Medicine. Every year the Academy supports a wonderful Life Shots event, encouraging families who have children with cerebral palsy to submit photographs of their children delighting in life*. The Academy facilitated our ability to use the beautiful photographs from LifeShots on the cover. Beyond the photos, the Academy has given both of us a professional home in which to develop meaningful and productive relationships in the world of cerebral palsy. Without it, our collaboration would have never occurred.

Finally, both of our families weathered our endless phone calls and emails as this book took shape and for that we are eternally grateful.

Laurie J. Glader and Richard D. Stevenson
Summer, 2018

*Photographer acknowledgments:

Front cover

Photo of girl painting: Gustavo Cisneros Lopez

Photo of girl picking fruit: Ane Lillian Tveit

Photo of boy playing cricket: Gopi Kitnasamy

Photo of boy with chicken: Tricia Potts

Photo of girl cheerleading: Karen Guilbault

Back cover

Photo of boy in beach buggy: Jennifer Lyman

Page v

Photo of boy with bow and arrow: Carol Shrader

Chapter 21

Photo of family: Michele Shusterman

Preface

Children with complex cerebral palsy (CP) are an important group of children within the population of children who have CP and caring for them requires skilled management. What does "complex" really mean in this context? Children with medical complexity are defined as those who have chronic medical conditions often involving multiple systems, who have functional impairment and are often medically fragile or technology dependent. They are frequently high utilizers of medical resources. For the purposes of this book, children with complex CP are those children who have CP and who also have these features. Some might prefer to use the term "severe" rather than "complex" CP, and indeed both terms are utilized in this book. We did not edit out every single use of the term "severe" because it is still in common parlance and the label of "medical complexity" is relatively new. Our point is simply that complexity both encompasses severity and extends beyond it. CP is a common condition of childhood, occurring with a prevalence of approximately 2 per thousand live births. Precise data regarding the prevalence of children with complex CP is not available.

CP is a group of heterogeneous and complex disorders. It is the particular constellation of motor abnormalities, functional limitations, associated cognitive and sensory impairments, and secondary medical conditions belonging to each child that require thoughtful assessment by the clinician. The purpose of this handbook is to provide assistance to practicing physicians and related clinicians in meeting the challenges of assessment, care and management for children with complex manifestations of cerebral palsy.

In general, this book will pertain most to children who cannot walk unaided or independently. In the professional vernacular, this refers to the care of children in Gross Motor Function Classification System (GMFCS) groups III, IV and V. However, it is important to recognize that children with less profound neuromotor impairment at times can be quite complex as well, with significant intertwining needs. This definition of complexity thus encompasses a fairly broad and diverse group of children. The child with normal intelligence, communication, and oral motor skills with fair hand function who can walk indoors with a walker and manage a motorized wheelchair with a joy-stick in the community is quite different from the child with severe intellectual disability, impaired communication, exclusive gastrostomy feeding, and no independent mobility. The latter child is much more likely to have associated medical morbidities and even early mortality. However, all such children are complex and tend to represent outliers to the primary care physician or consulting pediatrician in that they are relatively uncommon in the general pediatric population and thus are not a familiar part of the typical physician's repertoire.

Caring for children with complex forms of CP is a rich and rewarding experience. It also demands breadth of medical knowledge and management of issues that fall outside of the traditional medical box. The former includes many predictable medical, neurologic, orthopedic, and functional concerns. The latter includes things such as helping families through the loss of having a "typical" child, living with the uncertainty of complicating factors, addressing the frustration of accessing much needed services, managing chronic pain, and more. By partnering with families and children, we can anticipate and identify concerns that may require evaluation or management. We can more effectively respond to acute issues if we have a knowledge of risk factors for an individual patient. We can advocate for our patients so that they receive the most robust services to help them achieve their potential. And in playing each of these roles in support of children with complex CP and their families, we get to know them well. The rewards are sharing in their triumphs large and small, and professional moments to savor.

The intent of this handbook is to be comprehensive, but in a practical way. Our aim is to "cover the waterfront" in terms of the issues that regularly face children with complex cerebral palsy, not in an exhaustive, encyclopedic fashion, but in a way that physicians and others will find useful in their practice. More specifically, our intent is to provide clinicians and consultants with the necessary tools to:

1. understand and conceptualize the child with complex CP,

2. evaluate or at least to begin to evaluate the array of secondary conditions and unique concerns common to complex CP,

3. directly treat or refer for treatment primary or secondary issues common to complex CP,

4. explain to families (even when consultants are evaluating or treating) what is happening with their child, and

5. to support families through the ups and downs of evaluation, diagnosis, prognosis, treatment options, decision-making, and outcomes.

The authors in this book are general pediatricians, sub-specialty care providers and therapists who have expertise and experience in caring for children and youth with cerebral palsy and related neurodevelopmental disabilities. Parents of children with CP and youth with CP are also authors. Their voices provide unique and critical wisdom for clinicians providing family-centered care, an essential practice in managing children with complex CP. The topics were chosen and organized to reflect current best practices in the developing world. Each chapter has a summary section of key points at the end for quick reference. Wherever possible, the information presented is supported by published evidence. Where published evidence is limited, the information presented is based on clinical experience and/or consensus of the authors and editors. In addition to the chapters, we have created an Appendix with tools to support clinical care and decision-making that we hope will help guide the practicing clinician in evaluation, management, preventive care, and crisis response.

Laurie J. Glader
Richard D. Stevenson
Summer, 2018

The Care Tools found in Chapter 23 are available to download at http://www.mackeith. co.uk/shop/complex-cerebral-palsy-care-and-management/

Chapter 1

Overview of cerebral palsy: definition, classification and impact

Laurie J. Glader and Richard D. Stevenson

History of CP and definitions

While individuals with cerebral palsy (CP) have been represented in art and literature as far back as ancient times, the scientific study of the condition began in the early 1800s (Morris 2009). The English surgeon John Little (1810–1894) was the first to study the condition extensively and he coined the term spastic diplegia to reflect the particular subtype of CP with which he was most familiar. He initially thought that CP was a result of a problem around the time of birth and he identified preterm birth, difficult delivery and perinatal asphyxia as specific risk factors. Canadian-born William Osler (1849–1919) published his case series of 151 patients in 1889 as "The Cerebral Palsies of Children" and used the term to refer to a broader range of subtypes of the condition and he concluded that problems causing hemorrhage inside the brain were likely the prime cause. Before his career in psychiatry, the Austrian neurologist Sigmund Freud contributed the idea that in addition to peri- and post-natal causes, CP might reflect conditions present before birth.

Despite these evolving concepts regarding the etiology of CP, the medical community largely ignored the condition until the middle of the 20th century, when American orthopedic surgeon Winthrop Phelps began treating the disorder from a musculoskeletal perspective. He developed surgical techniques for operating on the secondary musculoskeletal sequelae of CP. Phelps was extremely influential and in 1947, along with five other colleagues from the fields of neurology, internal medicine, rehabilitation medicine, pediatrics, and neurosurgery, established what has become the American

Academy for Cerebral Palsy and Developmental Medicine, the first and now a leading multidisciplinary scientific organization focused on CP and related neurodevelopmental disorders of childhood.

The definition of CP continued to evolve. In 1964, British Child Neurologist Martin Bax contributed the most widely quoted definition of CP as a 'non-progressive disorder of movement and posture due to a defect or lesion of the immature brain' (Bax 1964). This definition remained unchanged for 40 years when a task force was formed in 2004 to reformulate the definition for both research and clinical purposes. The new and currently accepted definition is as follows:

> Cerebral palsy is a group of disorders of the development of movement and posture, causing activity limitation, that are attributed to non-progressive disturbances that occurred in the developing fetal or infant brain.

> The motor disorders of CP are often accompanied by disturbances of sensation, perception, cognition, communication, and behavior; by epilepsy, and by secondary musculoskeletal problems. (Rosenbaum, Paneth et al. 2007)

This definition is an expansion over prior versions to include a minimal severity clause (e.g. causing activity limitation) and a second sentence that acknowledges the co-morbid neurologic impairments and complications often associated with the motor deficits.

Diagnosis and evaluation

Making the diagnosis of CP has not changed in several decades. It is a clinical diagnosis based on the early presence of motor delay or differences together with abnormalities of movement, reflexes and muscle tone without evidence of clinical/neurological deterioration and where the clinical picture fits the definition. It is a "phenomenological" (rather than an etiological) diagnosis, akin to DSM-5 diagnoses such as Autism, Intellectual Disability, and ADHD. As such, it is dependent on clinical history and physical examination and requires some skill on the part of the examiner. An important practice parameter was published in 2004 delineating the evidence for diagnostic testing after clinical diagnosis (Ashwal, Russman et al. 2004). Important features are the strong recommendation for a brain MRI to corroborate clinical findings, evaluation looking for associated impairments and secondary conditions, consideration of additional hematologic evaluation in cases of apparent stroke, and genetic evaluation when MRI shows evidence of malformation or phenotypic differences are observed (Fig. 1.1). All children with a clinical diagnosis of CP should obtain a brain MRI, vision and hearing testing, and a developmental assessment. Additional investigations more recently suggest that genetic evaluation should be considered more often as studies have shown 7–15% prevalence of chromosomal deletions or duplication in CP (similar to those now being identified in association with autism).

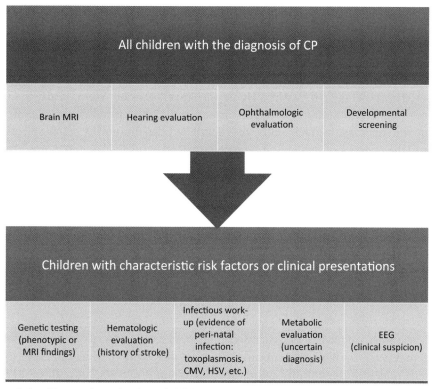

Figure 1.1 Diagnostic evaluation of children with cerebral palsy based on common etiologies, associated conditions and risk factors.

Classification of CP

As the definition of CP has evolved over the years, so have the classification systems applied to the condition. The traditional "anatomic" classification included two main types: pyramidal (spastic) and extra-pyramidal (non-spastic). Pyramidal CP referred to children with the presence of spasticity (velocity-dependent hypertonia, characteristic of involvement of the pyramidal tracts) and was sub-classified by the anatomic distribution of that spasticity on the child. Classically this included hemiplegia (spasticity on one half of the body (left/right) with upper extremity generally more involved), diplegia (spasticity predominantly in the lower extremities, with upper extremities only minimally involved) and quadriplegia (all extremities relatively equally involved). Because children did not always follow a classic distribution of spasticity, non-classic descriptors evolved such as triplegia (diplegia with super-imposed hemiplegia and one relatively un-involved upper extremity) and double hemiplegia (all extremities involved, often asymmetrically, with upper extremities generally more involved than lower extremities). Extra-pyramidal CP (suggesting involvement of parts of the brain outside the pyramidal tracts) was sub-classified by the appearance of the underlying movement disorder: hypotonia, chorea, athetosis, dystonia, and ataxia. Additionally, 'mixed' types involving spasticity and non-spastic movement disorders were also prevalent in this paradigm.

Attempts to study CP within such a framework demonstrated that this scheme is unreliable and overly subjective (e.g. no clear boundary between diplegia and quadriplegia, asymmetry problematic to classify). Hence the Surveillance of Cerebral Palsy in Europe network (SCPE-NET) (Gainsborough, Surman et al. 2008) developed a classification scheme with demonstrated reliability. They simplified classification by describing first and foremost the presence of spasticity. If present, unilateral or bilateral manifestation is noted. Next, the presence of dyskinesia (movement disorder), ataxia or significant hypotonia are identified. If possible, the dyskinesia is described further as chorea, athetosis or dystonia.

The workgroup on the definition and classification of CP sought to improve on the SCPE-NET schema by adding a framework for classification that includes additional elements. This framework shown in Table 1.1 includes four components: (1) motor abnormalities (includes the SCPE scheme noted above plus an assessment of functional severity), (2) anatomic (distribution of motor abnormalities) and radiologic findings, (3) associated impairments, and (4) causation and timing.

The development of reliable tools to assess functional severity has revolutionized the field of cerebral palsy. Such assessment can include various types of functional severity and currently may include mobility, hand function, communication, and eating/drinking. The first such assessment to be developed was the Gross Motor Function Classification

Table 1.1   Proposed framework for classification of cerebral palsy*

Primary Component	Potential Sub-Component	Example
Motor Abnormalities	Motor Typology	Spasticity & dystonia
	Functional Status	GMFCS IV, MACS III
Associated impairments	Neurological comorbidities	Seizures, ID**, CVI***, dysphagia
	Medical/Orthopedic secondary conditions	Contractures at elbows, knees, hips; constipation; malnutrition; drooling
Anatomic & Radiologic Findings	Anatomic distribution of spasticity	Bilateral, asymmetric (R>L)
	Neuroimaging findings/ classification	Malformation: schizencephaly
Causation and Timing	Genetic ("intrinsic") factors	Gene deletion syndrome
	Medical ("extrinsic") factors	Cocaine exposure in utero
	Timing of injury or perturbation	Early second trimester; born at term

*Adapted from (Rosenbaum, Paneth et al. 2007)
**intellectual disability, ***cortical visual impairment

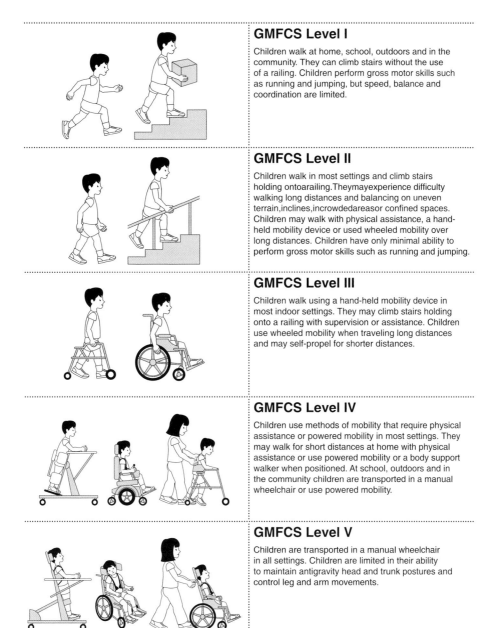

GMFCS Level I

Children walk at home, school, outdoors and in the community. They can climb stairs without the use of a railing. Children perform gross motor skills such as running and jumping, but speed, balance and coordination are limited.

GMFCS Level II

Children walk in most settings and climb stairs holding ontoarailing.Theymayexperience difficulty walking long distances and balancing on uneven terrain,inclines,incrowdedareasor confined spaces. Children may walk with physical assistance, a hand-held mobility device or used wheeled mobility over long distances. Children have only minimal ability to perform gross motor skills such as running and jumping.

GMFCS Level III

Children walk using a hand-held mobility device in most indoor settings. They may climb stairs holding onto a railing with supervision or assistance. Children use wheeled mobility when traveling long distances and may self-propel for shorter distances.

GMFCS Level IV

Children use methods of mobility that require physical assistance or powered mobility in most settings. They may walk for short distances at home with physical assistance or use powered mobility or a body support walker when positioned. At school, outdoors and in the community children are transported in a manual wheelchair or use powered mobility.

GMFCS Level V

Children are transported in a manual wheelchair in all settings. Children are limited in their ability to maintain antigravity head and trunk postures and control leg and arm movements.

Figure 1.2 Gross Motor Function Classification System.
Palisano et al (1997), CanChild: www.canchild.ca; Illustrations Version 2 © Bill Reid, Kate Willoughby, Adrienne Harvey and Kerr Graham, The Royal Children's Hospital Melbourne ERC 151050

System (GMFCS) (Palisano et al. 1997). The GMFCS ranks gross motor (independent mobility) function into five categories of severity, GMFCS IV and V being the more "severe" end of the spectrum (Fig. 1.2). The system has proven to be quite robust in predicting outcomes and associated problems, facilitating communication, clinical work and research. The GMFCS has been embraced by the field and, though relatively straightforward, it may be the single most important advance of the last twenty years.

The anatomic distribution of the motor abnormalities is simply descriptive (e.g. bilateral versus unilateral). Radiologic findings reflect abnormalities seen by neuro-imaging, which can include ultrasound and a computed tomography (CT) scan, but now generally refers to brain MRI. As noted, the practice parameter from the American Academy of Neurology recommends that all children with the diagnosis of cerebral palsy undergo a brain MRI. The age at which the MRI should be obtained has not been standardized; however, studies have led to a harmonized classification system based on MRI findings, the MRICS (MRI Classification System) (Himmelmann et al. 2017). The harmonized system includes five categories: maldevelopments, predominant white matter injury, predominant grey matter injury, miscellaneous, and normal. The system has been shown to be easy to use and reliable with a web-based manual available for training. MRI findings vary with motor abnormalities. In children with bilateral spastic CP, for example, abnormal MRI findings were found in 90%, with 60% predominant white matter injury, 15% predominant grey matter injury, and 10% brain maldevelopments (Krägeloh-Mann and Cans 2009). On the other hand, in children with unilateral spastic CP (hemiplegia), 90% of MRIs were abnormal with 16% maldevelopment (mainly focal cortical dysplasia or unilateral schizencephaly), 36% periventricular white matter injuries or post-hemorrhagic porencephalic lesions, and 31% infarcts of the middle cerebral artery (Krägeloh-Mann and Cans 2009). Studies in children with dyskinetic and ataxic CP have demonstrated abnormal MRI findings in only 68% and 39% respectively (Krägeloh-Mann and Cans 2009); such clinical presentations with normal MRI findings often warrant more extensive genetic and metabolic evaluations, searching for underlying causation. In general MRI is useful as it often reflects pathogenic patterns related to the timing of the disruption of brain development and specific causes.

Epidemiology and causal pathways

The overall prevalence of cerebral palsy has remained fairly constant in recent years, despite increased survival of low birthweight infants. A recent systematic review and meta-analysis of worldwide data determined a pooled prevalence of 2.11 per 1000 live births (Oskoui, Coutinho et al. 2013). Most recently available data from the United States (US) was similar with a prevalence of 1.8 per 1000 live births (Van Naarden Braun, Doernberg et al. 2016). CP prevalence in the US using a different methodology, showed prevalence of 2.9 children per 1000 live 8-year old children in 2010, a rate that was down from 3.5 children per 1000 8-year olds in the same surveillance area in 2006 (Durkin, Benedict et al. 2016). Prevalence varies significantly by birthweight and gestational age with rates as high as 56 per 1000 births below 1000gs and 82 per 1000 births under 28 weeks' gestation (Oskoui et al. 2013).

Table 1.2 Mechanisms leading to cerebral palsy *

Timing	Type of Mechanism	Examples
Pre-natal	Intrauterine pathological processes	Placental vascular disease
		Intrauterine growth retardation
		Infection with fetal inflammatory response
		Congenital/genetic anomalies
Peri-natal	Peri-partum events	Birth asphyxia
		Chorioamnionitis
		Placental abruption
Post-natal	Neonatal complications	Intraventricular hemorrhage
		Sepsis/meningitis
		Periventricular leukomalacia
	Late complications	Hypoxic-ischemic brain injury
		Non-accidental trauma
		Meningitis/encephalitis

*Adapted from Figure 1, (Stavsky, Mor et al. 2017)

The causes of cerebral palsy are numerous as any process that disrupts early brain development can lead to the condition. The timing of disruptive processes spans prenatal, perinatal, and early post-natal time periods. Causes of cerebral palsy are often described by a number of risk factors that combine into causal pathways leading to alterations in early brain development causing the motor impairments of cerebral palsy and the associated neurological impairments. Well recognized risk factors include: congenital malformations, fetal growth restriction, multiple gestations, infections during the fetal and neonatal period, birth asphyxia, preterm delivery, untreated maternal hypothyroidism, perinatal stroke and thrombophilia (Stavsky, Mor et al. 2017). Congenital malformation and specific genetic diagnoses are often associated with a clinical diagnosis of CP. One way to organize pathophysiologic mechanisms leading to cerebral palsy is illustrated in Table 1.2.

The International Classification of Functioning, Disability and Health

The impact of CP can be quite broad in its scope for an affected child, and the above-mentioned definition and classification schemes do not address the full spectrum of that

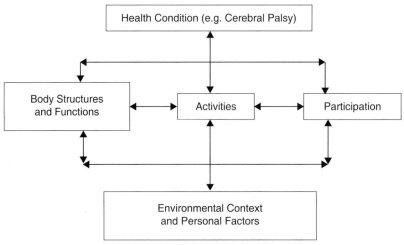

Figure 1.3 International Classification of Functioning, Disability and Health. Reproduced with permission from WHO, 2001.

impact. The primary manifestation of CP is activity limitation secondary to abnormal motor control. However, it is often the associated conditions of altered sensation, perception, cognition, communication, behavior, epilepsy and musculoskeletal complications that most dramatically affect a child's function and quality of life. For children with complex CP there can be additional far-reaching consequences for multiple body systems, each with potential great impact. All of these elements affect a child's ability to engage in activities, participate in their environment and frequently affect family dynamics.

Caring for a child with CP poses unique challenges to the provider. The range of medical complications requiring management can be broad and, additionally, children with complex CP are often dependent on technologies such as gastrostomy tubes, tracheostomies and baclofen pumps. The core healthcare team can be large, including multiple specialty providers, therapists and specially trained educators. Additionally, a variety of community support systems can be involved such as home nursing, equipment and supply vendors, complex insurance mechanisms and specialized educational, therapeutic and recreational programs. The challenge for the medical provider playing a central role in the care for a child with complex CP lies in anticipating commonly encountered conditions and situations, both physiologic and otherwise, and managing them in an organized fashion to promote a child's well-being.

The International Classification of Functioning, Disability and Health (ICF), a classification system put forward by the World Health Organization in 2001, provides a framework for thinking about an individual's overall health and function, and is frequently used in assessing and monitoring children with CP. The ICF reflects health and ability as a dynamic entity and does not focus exclusively on a condition or disease. It looks at physiology, activity, and participation in the context of environmental and personal factors (WHO 2001) (Fig. 1.3). As such, it provides an integrated, holistic perspective on a child's life.

Applying ICF components to general domains of care

The ICF when used formally includes a coding system. However, for the purposes of painting an integrated picture of a child's abilities, function and challenges, the ICF components in and of themselves can provide a functional and clinical framework for considering the child with CP (Glader, Plews-Ogan et al. 2016). There are five components to the ICF.

Body functions and structures

For a child with CP, this component of the ICF model includes the primary brain injury/perturbation causing the motor impairment, plus the range of secondary complications and associated conditions. Fundamentally, the body functions and structures domain is based on organ systems (e.g. neurological, pulmonary, etc.). Thus, it would include a description of the structural brain abnormalities associated with the CP (e.g. schizencephaly, or periventricular leukomalacia) and the functions affected by the brain anomalies (e.g. spasticity or dystonia). It would also include entities such as: neurologic sequelae (i.e. intellectual disability, learning disabilities and seizure disorders); respiratory concerns like a chronic inflammatory lung disease secondary to aspiration and obstructive sleep apnea; gastrointestinal issues such as malnutrition, intestinal dysmotility, gastroesophageal reflux and constipation; and musculoskeletal complications such as joint contractures, hip subluxation, scoliosis, and osteopenia.

Activity

Activity relates to how a child is able to perform a task or action. Fundamentally, this domain relates to task at the level of the whole body or body segments. For the child with CP, this includes volitional movement, coordination, and cognition, all of which combine to allow them to accomplish activities such as standing, walking, wheelchair mobility, communication, feeding, and toileting. Defining how well a child is able to accomplish these tasks has significant ramifications for creating appropriate and effective interventions. This includes strategies for bracing, therapies, choosing equipment, tone management, and potential surgeries.

Participation

A child's participation is reflected in how they are able to be involved in their world. Thus, this domain relates to how a person fulfills their social role in the family, school, and in the larger community. This is intimately dependent upon optimization of underlying medical and developmental concerns as well as the employment of effective strategies such as equipment choice and environmental modification.

Participation spans all aspects of a child's life, from engaging in meals with the family to attending school or a recreational program, or simply going to the movies or a sporting event.

Environment
Many factors beyond a child's innate medical complications, abilities and use of empowering strategies influence their overall functioning. This can include factors such as physical access, transportation, safety concerns and community resources as well as attitudinal and belief systems held by important people and institutions within the child's world.

Personal factors
Intrinsic characteristics of a child play a critical role in their participation, health and general well-being. For example, a child's age, sex, cultural context, spiritual beliefs or practices, and resilience can dramatically impact his or her ability to cope with a chronic condition as well as acute issues as they arise.

Additional considerations (the expanded environment/context)

The five components outlined above reflect those defined in the ICF. Of particular interest to medical providers caring for children with CP are the very specific topics of technology utilization, family dynamics and team management. These could be considered within the traditional environmental component or could be considered independently given the significance of their importance in the care of children with complex CP (Fig. 1.4). In either case, the concept of dynamic interactions between the child with complex CP and all of these elements results in a holistic description of functional life for the child.

Technology
Children with severe CP are often dependent on a variety of technologies to maintain basic bodily function as well as to enhance their activity and participation. These technologies include, for example, gastrostomy and endotracheal tubes, baclofen pumps, vagal nerve stimulators, urinary catheterization and central vascular access. Mobility and communication devices, while not indwelling, enhance physiologic function and are equally important. Patients, families and clinicians alike must be familiar with the risks and benefits of considering these devices, their care and maintenance, as well as their complications.

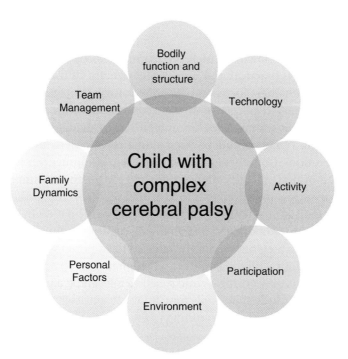

Figure 1.4 Adapted ICF framework for children with complex CP: a dynamic construct.
ICF, International Classification of Functioning Disability and Health

Family dynamics

In the US, children below the age of 18 and those above the age of 18 who have intellectual disability are not independent decision-makers. In other countries, such as the United Kingdom, the age of competence may be defined differently. The management of their health as well as the advocacy for tools and interventions to optimize their function and participation often falls solely on their caregivers. As a result, the strengths and coping of the family as a whole becomes central to a child's health and well-being. The medical provider for a child with CP must be aware of parental mental health concerns, a child's living circumstances, the family's financial situation and more.

Team management

A child with complex CP often has a large multidisciplinary team involved in different aspects of their care. This spans a broad range, from clinicians, to therapists, educators, religious leaders, home care providers, agency representatives and more. Communication between different types of providers thus becomes extremely important, whether around decision-making or delegation of responsibilities. It behoves the central medical provider for a child with severe CP to be cognizant of the extent of the team and to develop a plan with the family and other providers regarding these dynamics.

Putting It all together

The ICF outlines a systematic way of approaching the broad impact of complex CP on a child's life that is practical and useful. The content of this book reflects those components. Many chapters focus on pathophysiology, management and treatment of commonly encountered associated medical conditions for the child with severe CP, laying down a foundation for anticipatory and preventive management. Other chapters focus on optimizing a child's abilities, which ultimately impact participation, through a variety of interventions, from therapeutic to surgical to equipment choices. Navigating decision-making around potential interventions and considering the impact of interventions can be challenging. Improvements to structural problems (e.g. orthopedic surgery) may or may not translate to changes in activity level or participation in the community. The ICF creates a framework that can facilitate discussions around interventions and their impact. Other chapters are specifically targeted to empower providers to steer these important conversations with the families and children they serve. Utilizing the ICF as a general template for monitoring a child's well-being can be a useful strategy. At the end of this book we include Care Tools for Clinical Practice which details approaches to care for the individual with CP according to the ICF components.

Conclusions

Children with complex CP are broadly affected by their diagnosis. They experience impacts on movement and coordination that in turn affect function, participation and self-efficacy. Associated conditions are common, as are secondary complications. Although the child is primarily affected, in fact the entire family system experiences the impact of the diagnosis. As health care providers managing the well-being of children with complex CP, the range of issues for which we are responsible is equally broad. Depth of knowledge about commonly associated conditions and secondary complications is critical, as is developing skills around assessing equipment needs, frequently utilized technologies, family resilience and managing a frequently large health care team. It is our hope that this handbook goes some distance towards illuminating the nuances of caring for children with complex CP and provides a basis for enhanced clinical care.

Key points

- Cerebral Palsy is a complex syndrome of the motor manifestations of brain abnormalities/differences, coupled with associated impairments and secondary conditions.

- Classification of CP includes a description of the findings related to motor abnormality, anatomic distribution of those abnormalities, associated impairments, and causation and timing.

- When the diagnosis of CP has been made the most essential evaluations include brain MRI to try to link anatomic findings to clinical presentation, hearing and ophthalmologic assessments given the known associated risks for impairment, and developmental screening.

- Standardized classification systems which define functional aspects of CP, such as the Gross Motor Function Classification System, have evolved which allow for a common language in studying and talking about children with CP.

- The International Classification of Functioning, Disability and Health (ICF) presents a useful framework for considering the broad impact of CP on a child's life and can provide useful structure for the clinician responsible for managing and monitoring a myriad of factors.

References

Ashwal S, Russman BS, Blasco PA, et al. (2004) Practice parameter: diagnostic assessment of the child with cerebral palsy: report of the Quality Standards Subcommittee of the American Academy of Neurology and the Practice Committee of the Child Neurology Society. *Neurology* **62**: 851–863.

Bax MCO (1964) Terminology and classification of cerebral palsy. *Dev Med Child Neurol* **6**: 295–307.

Durkin MS, Benedict RE, Christensen D, et al. (2016) Prevalence of cerebral palsy among 8-year-old children in 2010 and preliminary evidence of trends in its relationship to low birthweight. *Paediatr Perinat Epidemiol* **30**: 496–510.

Gainsborough M, Surman G, Maestri G, et al. (2008) Validity and reliability of the guidelines of the Surveillance of Cerebral Palsy in Europe for the classification of cerebral palsy. *Dev Med Child Neurol* **50**: 828–831.

Glader L, Plews-Ogan J, Agrawal R (2016) Children with medical complexity: creating a framework for care based on the International Classification of Functioning, Disability and Health. *Dev Med Child Neurol* **58**: 1116–1123.

Himmelmann K, Horber V, de la Cruz J, et al. (2017) MRI classification system (MRICS) for children with cerebral palsy: development, reliability, and recommendations. *Dev Med Child Neurol* **59**: 57–64.

Krägeloh-Mann I, Cans C (2009) Cerebral palsy update. *Brain Dev* **31**: 537–44.

Morris C (2009) Definition and classification of cerebral palsy: a historical perspective. *Dev Med Child Neurol Suppl* **49**(s109): 3–7.

Oskoui M, Coutinho F, Dykeman J, et al. (2013) An update on the prevalence of cerebral palsy: a systematic review and meta-analysis. *Dev Med Child Neurol* **55**: 509–519.

Palisano R, Rosenbaum P, Walter S, et al. (1997) Development and reliability of a system to classify gross motor function in children with cerebral palsy. *Dev Med Child Neurol* **39**: 214–223.

Palisano et al. (1997), CanChild: www.canchild.ca; Illustrations Version 2 c Bill Reid, Kate Willoughby, Adrioenne Harvey and Kerr Graham, The Royal Children's Hospital Melbourne ERC 151050.

Rosenbaum P, Paneth N, Leviton A, et al. (2007) A report: the definition and classification of cerebral palsy April 2006. *Dev Med Child Neurol* Supplement **109**: 8–14.

Stavsky M, Mor O, Mastrolia SA, et al. (2017) Cerebral palsy-trends in epidemiology and recent development in prenatal mechanisms of disease, treatment, and prevention. *Front Pediatr* **5**: 21.

Van Naarden Braun, K, Doernberg N, Schieve L, et al. (2016) Birth prevalence of cerebral palsy: a population-based study. *Pediatrics* **137**. doi: 10.1542/peds.2015-2872. Epub 2015 Dec 9.

WHO (2001) *International Classification of Functioning, Disability and Health*. Geneva: World Health Organization.

Chapter 2

Functional assessment and goals of management

Jilda N. Vargus-Adams and Andrea L. Paulson

Overview of function as a key piece of care planning

Cerebral palsy (CP) is a far-reaching diagnosis and represents an extremely heterogeneous group of clinical presentations (Bax et al. 2005). Efforts to describe CP often center on the creation of sub-types or classifications, the most impactful of which typically address function. Function can be understood largely as a reflection of all domains of the International Classification of Functioning, Disability, and Health (ICF 2001) including body structures and function, activity, and participation (see Chapter 1 for a detailed description of the ICF). Not only does a clear description of function help clinicians, researchers, community organizations, and families better understand CP, it also helps these stakeholders anticipate needs and create effective care plans for each individual child.

Deficits in any realm of function increase the risk of complications or comorbidities; for example, concerns at the ICF level of body structures and function, such as hip subluxation, bone fragility (osteopenia and osteoporosis), scoliosis, constipation, and skin breakdown, are all associated with reduced functional mobility. Functional mobility, largely an ICF activity level construct, may be strongly associated with participation, especially in settings where environmental adaptations are not standard. Facets of adult life, independent living and employment are also correlated with functional status and current functional level can help to predict future function. The Gross Motor Function Measure (GMFM); (Palisano et al. 2000), a clinical and research tool designed to evaluate change in the gross motor function in children with CP, assesses gross motor function during activities like lying, rolling, running and jumping. Rosenbaum et al. (2002) plotted the GMFM scores for children with CP over time and created distinct motor growth curves to describe typical gross motor development stratified by Gross Motor Function Classification System (GMFCS) level (see Chapter 1), which has become the criterion standard for describing functional abilities in children with CP.

Using these motor development curves, we can anticipate future gross motor functional abilities with families and individuals with CP, which can be important when discussing goals for care. In addition to gross motor function (mobility) other key arenas of function to consider are feeding, cognition, communication, and fine motor function.

Using validated ways to describe current function and to understand likely patterns of development helps providers to predict future function and inform the care that each individual receives. It also provides care providers, individuals, and families with a framework for the discussion of future needs and concerns. Care teams can consider each patient's current status exploring issues across the ICF spectrum, evaluating connections, and planning for the future. One way to accomplish this is to create and use evidence-based care pathways or algorithms. Individuals and families can use the care pathway to think and plan ahead with regard to care and needs and to focus discussions with their care providers. Moreover, care pathways help providers to adhere to best practices and to have a clear expectation of progress over time.

Assessment

Essential pieces of the history and physical examination reflect an individual's current function. Some of these important areas to consider include describing general functional status, understanding cognition and communication, understanding gross motor function and mobility, and understanding fine motor function and self-care (including feeding). Providers should be sure to inquire about age of attainment of typical developmental milestones, but should also assess development and the current level of function more broadly for individuals with CP.

Functional classification variables permit efficient description of a person's general abilities. In CP, several classification systems have been established in key functional domains. The construct of each is similar, with five strata of function with Level I demonstrating the fewest impairments and Level V reflecting greater limitations. The Gross Motor Function Classification System (GMFCS) (described in Chapter 1) addresses mobility and gross motor skill. The Manual Abilities Classification System (MACS) (Eliasson et al. 2006) describes how a child over 4 years old handles objects in important daily activities (see Box 2.1).

MACS I	Handles objects easily and successfully
MACS II	Handles most objects but with somewhat reduced quality and/or speed
MACS III	Handles objects with difficulty; needs help to prepare and/or modify activities
MACS IV	Handles a limited selection of easily managed objects in adapted situations
MACS V	Does not handle objects and has severely limited ability to perform even simple actions

The Communication Function Classification System (CFCS) (Hidecker et al. 2011) establishes how consistently and effectively an individual can communicate with others (see Box 2.2).

CFCS I	Effective sender and receiver with unfamiliar and familiar partners
CFCS II	Effective, but slower-paced sender and/or receiver with unfamiliar and familiar partners
CFCS III	Effective sender and effective receiver with familiar partners
CFCS IV	Inconsistent sender and/or receiver with familiar partners
CFCS V	Seldom effective sender and receiver with familiar partners

Communication (see also Chapter 10) includes all methods of sharing information (National jJoint Committee for theCommunicative Needs of Persons with Severe Disabilities, 1992). Although verbal communication is often thought of first, individuals can use nonverbal cues like facial grimacing or groaning to signal discomfort, eye contact or facial expressions for choice selection, sign language, written language or an augmentative and alternative communication (AAC) device. Although language development is a reflection of cognitive status, in young children or those with intellectual disability, oromotor impairment, or other concerns, verbal communication may not develop typically. Families should be asked about communication behavior including how they understand a child's state of mind (facial expressions, gestures, specific sounds), how the child interacts with toys or technology, whether the child can make choices or follow instructions, and what purposeful things the child can do. These investigations may be supplemented with formal, standardized assessments. Communication is a broad construct that encompasses the ICF domains of body structures and function (e.g. oromotor ability), activity (speaking), and participation (ordering lunch in the community). As a child grows and develops, providers should continue to explore if and how each child obtains a means of effective communication to make choices, ask questions, and participate in and manipulate their environment.

Gross motor function is the realm of mobility and encompasses everything from walking with or without adaptive equipment to crawling or scooting, to using a gait trainer, walker, or wheelchair. An individual's preferred method of mobility may be different in the home when compared to school or in the community. When assessing mobility for individuals with CP who are not ambulatory, it is important to consider head control and trunk control, sitting ability, and transfer needs, as well as bed mobility. Again, the ICF can be applied across all domains from muscle strength to standing ability to riding the school bus.

Fine motor function is essential for self-care activities and activities of daily living. Self-care activities include feeding, continence and toileting, dressing, bathing and the manipulation of technology. Specific examination and history components may include grip strength, grasp and release ability, and fine motor manipulation. Like gross motor

Table 2.1 Common patient/parent reported outcome tools

Tool	Application	Domains Addressed	Reference
Pediatric Evaluation of Disability Inventory – computer-adaptive test (PEDI-CAT)	Parent or clinician reported functional outcome measure useful in clinical research as well as practice	Daily activities, mobility, social/cognitive function and responsibility	Haley et al. 2005
Pediatric Outcomes Data Collection Instrument (PODCI)	Parent report to assess changes following pediatric orthopedic interventions for a broad range of diagnoses	Function and quality of life through seven sub-constructs: upper extremity function, transfers and mobility, physical function and sports, comfort (lack of pain), happiness, satisfaction, and expectations	Daltroy et al. 1998 Allen et al. 2008
The Caregiver Priorities and Child Health Index of Life with Disabilities (CPCHILD)	Caregivers' perceptions, sensitive to change even when the individual has severe disability	Health status, comfort, well-being, and ease of care	Narayanan et al. 2006
Cerebral Palsy Quality of Life Questionnaire (CP QOL)	Parent report measure of quality of life for children with CP	Quality of life	Waters et al. 2006
Measure of Processes of Care (MPOC)	Parent reported, family-centered measure of perceptions of the healthcare that a child receives	Enabling and partnership, providing general information, providing specific information about the child, coordinated and comprehensive care, and respectful and supportive care	Dyke et al. 2006

function, fine motor function is salient across the ICF, moving from body function to activity to participation. Families or patients may report alternative strategies or use of assistive devices that compensate for impairments or activity limitations and facilitate the accomplishment of self-care goals.

Specific assessment tools have been developed to better describe function. These assessment tools are either patient reports or therapist/clinician-administered measures and have clinical applicability. Five common patient/parent reported outcome tools are included in Table 2.1: the Pediatric Evaluation of Disability Inventory – computer-adaptive test (PEDI-CAT), the Pediatric Outcomes Data Collection Instrument (PODCI), the Caregiver Priorities and Child Health Index of Life with Disabilities (CP-CHILD), the Cerebral Palsy Quality of Life Questionnaire (CP QOL), and the Measure of Processes of Care (MPOC). Each of these measures assesses items across the ICF spectrum, but they focus on activity and participation as well as quality of life, a construct that is outside the ICF. Four common therapist or clinician administered measures include the GMFM, the Cortical Visual Impairment (CVI) Range, the Canadian Occupational Performance Measure (COPM) and the Goal Attainment Scale (GAS) (see Table 2.2)

Table 2.2   Therapist or clinician administered measures of function

Tool	Application	Domains Addressed	References
Gross Motor Function Measure (GMFM)	Therapist or clinician administered tool to evaluate change in gross motor function in children with cerebral palsy	Assesses the ability to perform certain actions like rolling, walking, running and jumping, focusing on activity level items	Ko and Kim, 2013
Cortical Visual Impairment (CVI) Range (CVI Range)	Functional vision assessment, completed by a trained therapist	Determines, on a scale of 1-10, the child's functional visual capacity reflecting the ICF domain of body functions	Newcomb, 2009
Canadian Occupational Performance Measure (COPM)	Used to detect self-perceived changes in occupational performance over time, completed by a trained therapist	Patient-specific and can encompass virtually any functional domain of import to the patient and thus may reflect the entire spectrum of the ICF	Law et al. 1998
Goal Attainment Scale (GAS)	Used as a technique to evaluate the functional goal attainment of children receiving pediatric therapy services, administered by a therapist or clinician	Each patient has their own outcome measure; however, it undergoes standardized scoring to allow statistical analysis on a five point scale from -2 to +2. Similar to COPM above, patient specific.	Steenbeek et al. 2007

Medical testing can aid understanding of functional status in specific conditions, particularly in the ICF domain of body structures and function. Where there is concern about hip subluxation or scoliosis, X-rays can be performed. Where there is concern about osteoporosis or osteopenia, tests that assess bone health (calcium and vitamin D levels, DXA scans) can be performed (see Chapter 4 on Orthopedic Management and Chapter 6 on Osteoporosis). When cognition and thinking need to be further evaluated, neuropsychological testing can be performed.

Because individuals with CP are dynamic and ever-changing, providers should be vigilant about reassessing functional status over time. Some aspects of function are known to decline with time in some populations, such as mobility skills (Bottos et al. 2001), whereas others may be fairly static.

The Role of interdisciplinary teams with families

Interdisciplinary teams facilitate a rich model of care for families of children with cerebral palsy (King et al. 2004). Key components of successful team care delivery include skilled management of information, collaborative decision-making, and effective communication within and outside of the team. However, not all children have access to an interdisciplinary team. Such a team may be quite effective in a more virtual model of delivery, with providers seeing patients on different days and, often, in different locales. The challenges in this common scenario lie in pooling information effectively to promote collaborative team management.

When many providers with wide-ranging backgrounds and expertise are included on a team, the breadth of pertinent information can be significant. Pre-visit planning helps to optimize the efficiency of information accrual and to reduce the burden on families to answer lots of questions. This process can include chart review, contact with families by paper or electronic survey or telephone, and/or solicitation of information from other providers. Teams may also choose to define specific tasks or responsibilities amongst team members, often dividing work by discipline and setting clear expectations for how assessments, decision-making, and communication will proceed.

Collaborative decision making is a hallmark of a high performing interdisciplinary team. Various models may be employed and can be effective, depending on the needs and preferences of the practice setting and team members. Key components include utilizing the expertise and knowledge of all team members, which includes patients and families, exploring priorities, considering concerns across the entire ICF, and presenting options (Stille et al. 2013). With involvement of the whole team, a prioritized and feasible plan of care can be created. Models of care such as pathways, algorithms, or care maps can be instrumental in guiding this process.

Teams need to be explicit about what they do and be clear in communicating with primary providers. These primary providers, both physicians and therapists, should be informed about the plan of care and have an open line of communication with the interdisciplinary team members. Frequently, an interdisciplinary care team serves as a panel of consultant specialists who work together to provide advice regarding treatment plans but do not provide the bulk of a child's therapy or medical treatment directly. However the team's role may be defined, all other providers should also understand it and there should be flexibility to adapt and to accommodate family preferences, geography, alterations in resources, or any other need.

Therapeutic decision making

As teams and families work together they must focus on ensuring that standards of care are met and on setting goals with the patient and family.

Goal setting is an iterative and ongoing process. Patient and family preferences form the foundation for goals. Questioning, listening, and conversation can facilitate an understanding of patient and family desires (Costa et al. 2017). When meaningful goals are established, patients and families demonstrate greater adherence to treatment plans and experience better outcomes. Providers may want to utilize standardized outcome measures including the GAS or the COPM as quantifiable mechanisms to define and measure progress toward goals.

Conversations addressing goal setting may take considerable time and information sharing. Providers and families will want to address important points of information, including prognosis and anticipated changes in functional capacity. As part of the interchange, team members should aid families in setting realistic goals but allowing for 'stretch' goals when appropriate. Additional visits may be needed to fully elucidate patient and family goals and the process may be facilitated by training team members in techniques and encouraging families to break down big goals into smaller goals that can be approached step by step.

Some aspects of care address health maintenance and are fairly consistent from patient to patient. Children with functional deficits have specific needs that should be incorporated into decision making, including greater attention to nutrition and preventive services. Many children with mobility impairment require health surveillance because of increased risk of complications such as hip dislocations or osteoporotic fractures. These needs should be met either in the setting of medical home or in a specialty practice; either way, primary care providers must be partners in the process (Stille et al. 2013).

Comfort and ease of care are primary drivers of therapeutic decision making for many children with significant functional deficits. Providers should be vigilant in their efforts to assess the presence of pain or discomfort and to understand its severity and causes. Many medical issues, outside of straightforward functional limitation, may impede comfort or ease of care. These concerns include spasticity and other movement disorders, gastroesophageal reflux, gastric motility issues, menstruation, contractures, and others. Patients may benefit from interventions aimed at these medical concerns (see relevant Chapters). Provision of equipment and environmental modifications may be very impactful in improving the burden of care for families (see Chapter 5 for a discussion on Equipment).

Quality of life is often the most important outcome for patients and families. Quality of life is not accurately defined as function as reflected in the ICF. Rather, exactly what constitutes quality of life may vary from person to person and generally reflects an overall sense of contentment with one's life. Child factors that contribute to quality of life include sleep, level of alertness, behavior, and psychiatric concerns. Family life plays a role in terms of relationships with family members, stressors on family time or finances, and parent stress. Participation in the community with school, recreation, and peer activities is another component of quality of life. Understanding the barriers that patients and families face in these realms will allow providers to partner with them, establish achievable goals, and implement a plan of care that can further those goals (Costa et al. 2017).

Care map

Care maps are a mechanism to aggregate recommendations for surveillance, care, and treatments for a particular diagnosis or clinical group. Frequently, a care map will be constructed to demonstrate treatment guidelines, prevention strategies, or other standards of care in an easy to interpret format. For individuals with CP, many care pathways or algorithms have been developed addressing issues from bone health to drooling. Care maps can seek to reference and combine pertinent evidence-based pathways into a single source to guide care. Functional status can be a key component of care map differentiation.

One example of a care map is shown in Fig. 2.1. The care map was developed for an interdisciplinary CP specialty clinic through a consensus process with team clinicians. Although some of the content reflects published research, much of it is based on typical practice and expert opinion. The three sections include medical care, therapy and equipment, and support and resources. The care map is used by the team to ensure that important components of care and planning are addressed and it is used by families as an overview of care and a way to start thinking about future needs. A vertical line is drawn on the map to correspond with the child's age and then notes can be made about concerns, needs, options, or plans along each row. Some of the sections merely reference more detailed care, such as the 'bone health' item which connects to additional documentation in the form of a care pathway that recommends particular populations to have lab monitoring as well frequency of testing and standard dosing for identified deficiencies. Other sections are fairly comprehensive, such as the list of spasticity management options or areas to assess for equipment needs. Regardless, the care map serves as a starting place and an initial checklist for clinic visits and planning.

An example of how the care map might be used in the context of an interdisciplinary clinic visit follows.

Case study

Jayden, a 4-year-old boy in GMFCS level IV MACS level III, CFCS level II with bilateral spastic-dystonic CP related to preterm birth, is a new patient in the CP clinic. When he arrives with his parents they are given a copy of the care map with a vertical line drawn at 4 years old and they are told about how the care map is used. During their visit a team member will write on the care map with recommendations and clarifications for the family. The team will use the care map to guide the topics they address. This would include talking with the family about all the arenas that the vertical line transects: For example, after confirming his placement in GMFCS level IV, the physical therapist in clinic would look at the parent-provided responses about Jayden's use of a stander since she is aware of the recommendations for 2 hours daily in weight bearing. After seeing that this is part of Jayden's school program, notation would be made to "continue with 2 hours in stander every day." The occupational therapist would explore if Jayden has the right sort of supported seating for toileting at home and at preschool. The physician would confirm that Jayden's constipation is well controlled with diet and that he is starting to be successful with continence training intermittently. Any recommendations would be written or circled on the care map. If Jayden's weight gain is poor the dietitian would work with the family and create a plan for increased caloric intake. Together, the physician and therapists would examine and observe Jayden and consider input from his primary therapy team as they recommend botulinum toxin injections for some lower extremity muscles. They might also recommend specific therapy such as a strengthening program and introduce the idea of transitioning into a model of episodic physical therapy over the next year or so. Finding that Jayden's braces are becoming too small, a prescription for new orthoses would be produced and noted on the care map. The social worker would ask about Jayden's developmental preschool and the plans to transition to kindergarten next fall. Perhaps the care map would remind a team member to double check on something like an overdue surveillance hip X-ray or a referral to a recreational aquatics program. Jayden's family might look at the care map again and ask about timing for a neuropsychological evaluation in the next year. At the end of the visit a team nurse would review the care map and all the notes with the family before giving it to them to take home.

The care map serves to enable better communication, comprehensive care, and targeted age- and function-specific recommendations. These concepts, pursued in the setting of an engaged treatment team, family, and patient set the stage for success. In the setting where a physical interdisciplinary team is not available, a central provider, often a child's pediatrician, can utilize a care map to ensure that appropriate referrals and follow-ups are occurring. Please see Chapter 23 for additional tools that may facilitate a decentralized team approach with the primary care provider at its center.

Conclusion

Understanding function is critical to optimal care for children with CP and their families. Providers can use standard assessments to develop a rich description of function for each patient and to guide recommendations and interventions. Function encompasses all of the ICF domains, from body structures to activity to participation. As care teams learn about each patient's functional status as well as that patient's and family's goals, they can utilize additional resources, including care maps and algorithms, to refine the care each patient receives. Understanding function enables care teams to know more about each patient's CP and to plan for their current and future needs.

Key points

- For children with complex CP, a clear understanding of functional status informs effective selection and delivery of care and also aids in anticipating future needs.

- The GMFCS predicts functional abilities and guides goals of care.

- Children with complex CP benefit from assessment of functional domains including communication, mobility and self-care. Specific assessment tools are available for these domains.

- Functional status needs to be assessed broadly and repeatedly as children with complex CP may experience fluctuations in functioning over time or between domains.

- CP care pathways guide providers to best practices and to reasonable expectation of change over time.

- Care for children with complex CP may be most effectively delivered via interdisciplinary collaboration allowing joint therapeutic decision making.

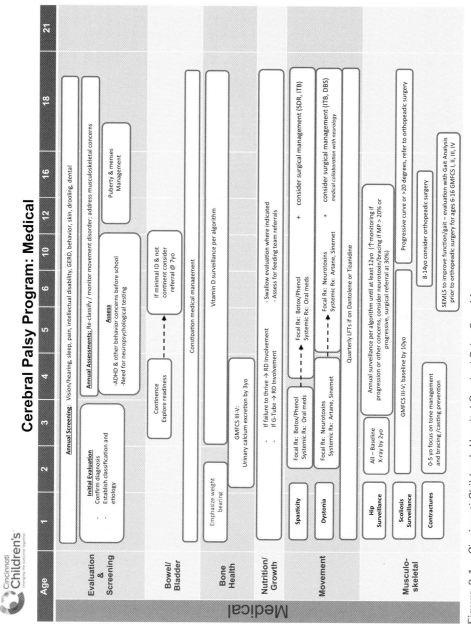

Figure 2.1 Cincinnati Children's Hospital Cerebral Palsy Care Map
Reproduced with permission from Cincinnati Children's Hospital.

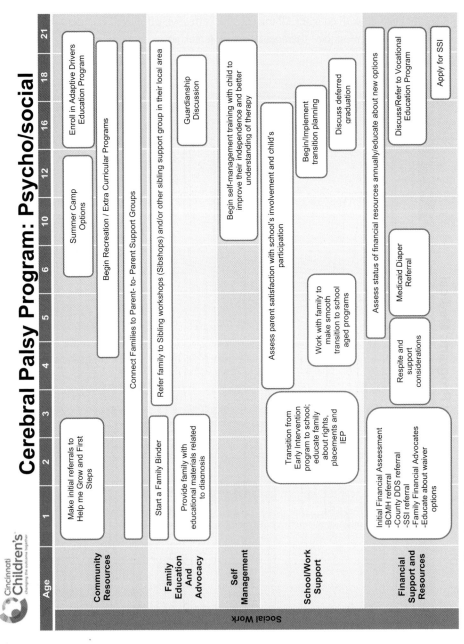

Figure 2.1 (Continued)

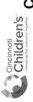

Cerebral Palsy Program: Therapy, Technology and Communication

Age	1	2	3	4	5	6	10	12	16	18	21

THERAPY

GMFCS I–III
- OT/PT/SP evaluation and plan of care development; Early intervention Programs
- Progression of gross and fine motor strengthening, ADLs, mobility, gait training, endurance
- Therapy model may include episodic and/or intensive scheduling bursts (may be related to SEMLS or SDR surgeries), aquatics, or group therapy programs
- Consultative Management
- Annual OT/PT/SLP Re-evaluation and Progression of Therapy Plan of Care
- Closer to 21 years, transition to adult outpatient therapy

GMFCS IV–V
- Early mobility and positioning; Vision evaluation; Aquatics
- Progression of gross and fine motor strengthening, transfer training, bed mobility, gait training for aerobic capacity

TECHNOLOGY & EQUIPMENT

GMFCS I–III
- AT evaluation and plan of care development for power mobility, feeding, bathing, floor sitting, early standing, toileting, car seat, adapted bed, bracing/orthoses
- Annual AT evaluation, Integration of technology and equipment needs to support school performance; adaptive equipment for mobility, feeding, floor sitting, positioning, standing, toileting, hygiene, bracing/orthoses
- Technology Support for reading and writing

GMFCS IV–V
- Investigate loaner options and adapted commercial products
- AAC / Communication Evaluation; Introduce AT in the home; Early Power Mobility
- Annual Re-Evaluation of Seating and Positioning; Home Modifications Evaluation and continued assessment
- Maintain yearly connection to Technology Center for equipment; Explore community technology/communication groups
- Assessment for assistive driving equipment

COMMUNITY

GMFCS I–III
- Explore Community Wellness options
- Explore community wellness options
- Assessment for assistive driving equipment
- Explore Community Transportation Options
- Community Wellness Vocational Evaluation

GMFCS IV–V
- Begin recreational and/or adaptive sports (individual and team); Home Exercise equipment or adapted bikes

Figure 2.1 (Continued)

References

Allen DD, Gorton GE, Oeffinger DJ, et al. (2008) Analysis of the Pediatric Outcomes Data Collection Instrument in ambulatory children with cerebral palsy using confirmatory factor analysis and item response theory methods. *J Pediatr Orthop* **28**: 192–8.

Bax M, Goldstein M, Rosenbaum P, et al. (2005) Proposed definition and classification of cerebral palsy. *Dev Med Child Neurol* **47**: 571–6.

Bottos M, Feliciangeli A, Sciuto L, et al. (2001) Functional status of adults with cerebral palsy and implications for treatment of children. *Dev Med Child Neurol* **43**: 516–28.

Chen KL, Wang HY, Tseng MH, et al. (2013) The Cerebral Palsy Quality of Life for Children (CP QOL-Child): evidence of construct validity. *Res Dev Disabil* **34**: 994–1000.

Costa UM, Brauchle G, Kennedy-Behr A (2017) Collaborative goal setting with and for children as part of therapeutic intervention. *Disabil Rehab* **39**: 1589–600.

Dyke P, Buttigieg P, Blackmore AM, Ghose A, et al. (2006) Use of the measure of process of care for families (MPOC-56) and service providers (MPOC-SP) to evaluate family-centred services in a paediatric disability setting. *Child Care Health Dev* **32**: 167–76.

Eliasson AC, Krumlinde-Sundholm L, Rösblad B, Beckung E, Arner M, Öhrvall AM, et al. (2006) **48**: 549–54.

Haley SM, Raczek AE, Coster WJ, et al. (2005) Assessing mobility in children using a computer adaptive testing version of the pediatric evaluation of disability inventory. *Arch Phys Med Rehabil* **86**: 932–9.

Hidecker MJC, Paneth N, Rosenbaum PL, et al. (2011) Developing and validating the Communication Function Classification System (CFCS) for individuals with cerebral palsy. *Dev Med Child Neurol* **53**(8): 704–10.

ICF (2001) International Classification of Functioning, Disability and Health [Online]. World Health Organization. Available at: http: //www.who.int/icf.

King S, Teplicky R, King G, Rosenbaum P (2004) Family-centered service for children with cerebral palsy and their families: a review of the literature. *Semin Pediatr Neurol* **11**: 78–86.

Ko J, Kim M (2013) Reliability and responsiveness of the Gross Motor Function Measure-88 in children with cerebral palsy. *Phys Ther* **93**: 393–400.

Law MC, Baptiste S, Carswell A, et al. (1998) *Canadian Occupational Performance Measure*. Ottawa: Canadian Association of Occupational Therapists.

Narayanan UG, Fehlings D, Weir S, et al. (2006) Initial development and validation of the Caregiver Priorities and Child Health Index of Life with Disabilities (CP-CHILD). *Dev Med Child Neurol* **48**: 804–12.

National Joint Committee for the Communicative Needs of Persons with Severe Disabilities (1992) Guidelines for meeting the communication needs of persons with severe disabilities. *ASHA* **7**: Suppl 1–8.

Newcomb S (2009) *Reliability of the CVI Range: A Functional Vision Assessment for Children with Cortical Visual Impairment*. ProQuest. University of Maryland.

Palisano RJ, Hanna SE, Rosenbaum PL, et al. (2000) Validation of a model of gross motor function for children with cerebral palsy. *Phys Ther* **80**: 974–85.

Rosenbaum PL, Walter SD, Hanna SE, et al. (2002) Prognosis for gross motor function in cerebral palsy: creation of motor development curves. *JAMA* **288**: 1357–63.

Steenbeek D, Ketelaar M, Galama K, Gorter JW, et al. (2007) Goal attainment scaling in paediatric rehabilitation: a critical review of the literature. *Dev Med Child Neurol* **49**: 550–6.

Stille CJ, Fischer SHLA, Pelle N, et al. (2013) Parent partnerships in communication and decision making about subspecialty referrals for children with special needs. *Academic Pediatrics* **13**: 122–32.

Waters E, Davis E, Boyd R, et al. (2006) *Cerebral Palsy Quality of Life Questionnaire for Children (CP QOL-Child) Manual*. Melbourne: Deakin University.

Chapter 3

Hypertonia

Darcy Fehlings, Cecilia Lee,
Amber Makino and Anne Kawamura

Definitions and overview

Hypertonia is defined as an abnormally increased resistance to passive stretch of the muscle across a joint. The two main forms of hypertonia in individuals with cerebral palsy (CP) are spasticity and dystonia. Spasticity is the presence of increasing tone with increasing speed of muscle stretch (Sanger et al. 2003). Dystonia is a movement disorder in which involuntary sustained or intermittent muscle contractions cause twisting and repetitive movements, abnormal postures or both. Hypertonia can be generalized, involving many muscles in the body, or focal. This chapter will provide a practical overview of pharmacological and neurosurgical approaches to hypertonia management in CP including oral medications, botulinum toxin and chemodenervation, intrathecal baclofen pumps and selective dorsal rhizotomy. The roles of rehabilitation interventions such as splinting and orthopedic surgery are outside of the scope of this chapter.

Impact on function and activities

Hypertonia, like poor motor control or weakness, can negatively impact motor function, comfort and care. If a muscle group has a high level of hypertonia it can contribute to difficulties moving the joint through the available range, which can limit motor function. Hypertonia is a common cause of pain, which can be focal such as muscle spasms, or more generalized. Stretching a hypertonic muscle or 'getting stuck' in dystonic postures can be uncomfortable. Generalized hypertonia can decrease seating tolerance and cause frequent night awakenings requiring repositioning. Significant hypertonia can make caregiving tasks such as dressing, bathing, and lifting, challenging. In contrast, some individuals with hypertonia utilize their tone for function (e.g. tone through the quadriceps can help to prevent excessive knee flexion during standing/transferring activities, particularly in individuals functioning at a Gross Motor Function Classification system (GMFC, see Chapter 1) level of IV). Assessment and management of hypertonia needs to be undertaken on an individual basis.

Overview of hypertonia management strategies

A careful baseline assessment of the individual with CP is required to assess the impact of hypertonia on motor function, comfort and care. Fig. 3.1 is a flow diagram of an overall management approach to pharmacological and neurosurgical options. A history is critical to elucidating information to shape a management plan. The physical examination should include a neurological examination to determine if spasticity, dystonia or mixed tone is present. A tool called the Hypertonia Assessment Tool (HAT) can be used for this purpose (Jethwa et al. 2010). The examination should quantify the severity of the hypertonia with established tools such as the modified Ashworth scale, the Australian Spasticity Assessment Scale (ASAS), the modified Tardieu scale for spasticity or the Barry Albright Dystonia or Burke Fahn Marsden scales for dystonia. An assessment of overall health with a focus on musculoskeletal status and nutrition should be completed. In addition to a baseline assessment, ongoing follow-up and periodic evaluation are required as the impact of hypertonia evolves over time. Paradoxically, hypertonia treatment occasionally results in diminished function. An assessment of the response to hypertonia intervention should be integrated into future treatment plans.

Before embarking on any management strategy for hypertonia, it is important to identify the goals of treatment with the child and their family. When a management plan is implemented, individualized goals, utilizing a tool such as the Canadian Occupational Performance Measure (COPM), should be established and the response to the intervention monitored. As a general guideline, rehabilitation strategies such as splinting and positioning should routinely be implemented. For focal hypertonia goals that require additional intervention, chemodenervation strategies can be utilized. For generalized hypertonia goals, oral medications are often considered a first line approach with the introduction of more invasive treatments, such as intrathecal baclofen, selective dorsal rhizotomy or deep brain stimulation, being reserved for individuals with severe generalized hypertonia associated with pain or severe challenges with care giving. It is also important to note that there may be *focal* hypertonia reduction goals for an individual with generalized hypertonia (e.g. reducing adductor tone for ease of diapering/groin care). Here, focal chemodenervation can play a role, often in combination with other treatment options. Two websites that outline guidelines and care pathways for hypertonia management in CP are the following:

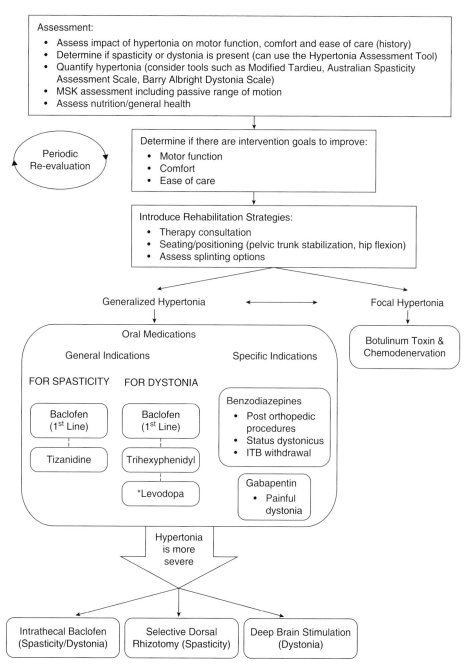

Figure 3.1 Flow diagram for hypertonia management in individuals with cerebral palsy (GMFCS levels IV & V).

*Substantial improvement with a trial of levodopa suggests DOPA-responsive dystonia (DRD). Due to concerns regarding limited effectiveness in secondary dystonia, some clinicians restrict use of levodopa to a trial to rule out DRD.

- https://pathways.nice.org.uk/pathways/spasticity-in-children-and-young-people (National Institute for Health and Care Excellence 2017)

- https://www.aacpdm.org/publications/care-pathways/dystonia (American Academy for Cerebral Palsy and Developmental Medicine 2016)

Oral pharmacotherapy for hypertonia management in severe cerebral palsy

There are a variety of oral pharmacotherapy options to treat hypertonia in children and youth with CP functioning at GMFCS levels IV and V. Oral pharmacotherapy is the preferred first-line choice for the treatment of generalized spasticity and dystonia that is symptomatic. While medications are non-invasive treatments that can be easily administered, the evidence to support oral medications in general is weak, leading to practice variation, and their side effects are often systemic. Due to the chronic nature of hypertonia, use of oral medications should be limited to those with specific indications. Common indications in this population include chronic pain, sleep disturbance, challenges with caregiving and hygiene, and discomfort with seating. The decision to treat with oral medications should include a careful assessment of the individual's symptoms and medical comorbidities in order to balance the potential benefits with the side effects of medication use. For example, an individual with appendicular spasticity may have axial weakness that becomes more pronounced with spasticity treatment resulting in untoward side effects such as poor head control and a compromised airway. In general, one medication is maximized before a second medication is started. Table 3.1 shows the practical aspects of medication usage including suggested dosages, formulations, and common side effects. A helpful website to support clinical drug information is the following:

- http://www.wolterskluwercdi.com/lexicomp-online/ (Lexicomp Online)

Baclofen (spasticity and dystonia)
Baclofen is a gamma-aminobutyric acid (GABA) agonist that binds at GABA-B receptors on pre- and post-synaptic neurons in the spinal cord and brain, resulting in the inhibition of mono- and polysynaptic spinal reflexes. The American Academy of Neurology (AAN) systematically reviewed evidence for pharmacotherapy for spasticity management in CP, and found only three studies of limited quality that addressed the effect of baclofen in this population (Delgado et al. 2010). This review found insufficient evidence to support or refute the use of oral baclofen to treat spasticity or to improve motor function. Despite limited evidence for the effectivness of baclofen, it is commonly used for hypertonia that causes pain or discomfort, interferes with caregiving, or disrupts sleep patterns because of its relatively safe side effect profile and ease of administraton. Oral baclofen is widely used in clinical practice as a first-line treatment in those with generalized spasticity, dystonia, or both.

Tizanidine (spasticity)
Tizanidine is an alpha-2 adrenergic agonist that enhances noradrenergic presynaptic inhibition at the level of the brain and spinal cord. It was found to be possibly effective in the treatment of spasticity based on one small placebo-controlled study, which found an improvement in spasticity in 10 children over 6-months' duration (Delgado et al. 2010). Due to the paucity of studies in children, there is little information available to inform the use of this medication, but it may be considered as a second-line treatment option for spasticity.

Benzodiazepines (spasticity and dystonia)
Benzodiazepines result in GABA-A mediated inhibition in the brain. Two studies that met AAN criteria found an improvement in spasticity management with the use of diazepam, resulting in their recommendation that diazepam is probably effective for short-term treatment of spasticity in CP (Delgado et al. 2010). Benzodiazepines can be very effective at decreasing dystonic spasms, such as those seen in periods of dystonic storms, or reducing muscle spasms in the short-term in individuals with CP after orthopedic surgery. Although there are concerns around cognitive side effects (e.g. drowsiness) and dependence on benzodiazepines, which limit their potential for long-term use in individuals with CP, they may be considered as an option to treat generalized tone that is difficult to manage. Care should be taken to avoid respiratory depression.

Dantrolene (spasticity)
Dantrolene is a hydantoin derivative that inhibits the release of calcium at the sarcoplasmic reticulum in skeletal muscle. Previous studies have shown conflicting data regarding its effect on reducing spasticity (Delgado et al. 2010). In the AAN practice parameter on pharmacological treatment of spasticity in children it was noted by the expert panel to rarely be used (Delgado et al. 2010). Adverse effects associated with dantrolene include diffuse weakness and hepatotoxicity and should be considered prior to the initiation of this medication.

Trihexyphenidyl (dystonia)
Trihexyphenidyl is an anticholinergic agent that aims to treat dystonia by re-establishing balance between dopaminergic and cholinergic innervation, though the precise mechanism is unknown. The overall level of evidence is limited. One randomized, double-blinded, placebo-controlled crossover trial found no significant improvement in dystonia (Rice and Waugh 2009). An open-label study with 23 participants revealed improved upper arm function, with a delay in the effect of the medication of 15 weeks (Sanger et al. 2007). Despite limited evidence regarding its effects on dystonia, trihexyphenidyl continues to be considered for individuals to reduce severe generalized dystonia associated with symptoms such as pain or caregiving challenges. It has also

Table 3.1 Summary of oral pharmacotherapy in hypertonia management in cerebral palsy

Medication (potential mechanism of action)	Hypertonia sub-type	Suggested dosing	Formulation[a]	Selected adverse effects	Comments
Baclofen (GABA agonist)	Spasticity (first-line), dystonia (first-line)	Starting dose: 2.5–5 mg/day (Lexicomp Online) Slow titration to maximum 2 mg/kg/day or 80 mg total dose (>2 years) divided TID or QID (He et al. 2014)	Tablet: 10 mg, 20 mg Compounded form available	Sedation, urinary retention (high dose), constipation, weakness, orthostatic hypotension	Withdrawal symptoms if abrupt discontinuation (seizures, increased spasticity, hallucinations, confusion, hyperthermia)
Tizanidine (alpha-2 adrenergic agonist)	Spasticity (second-line)	0.05 mg/kg/day div BID-QID (Delgado et al. 2010) Maximum adult dose: 36 mg/day; Pediatric maximum dose unknown (Lexicomp Online) Author's note: Adolescents – starting dose 2 mg TID	Tablet: 2 mg, 4 mg Capsule (US only): 2 mg, 4 mg, 6 mg	Not well studied in children; enuresis, aggression, hypotension, sedation, dry mouth, weakness, hepatotoxicity	Monitor liver function tests and blood pressure
Diazepam (binds to GABA-A receptors)	Spasticity or dystonia (specific indications)	Dose should be individualized and titrated to effect Weight-based dosing: 0.01–0.3 mg/kg/day divided BID –QID (Lexicomp Online) Fixed Dosing: Child ≥5 years and adolescents – starting dose: 1.25 mg TID, may titrate to 5 mg QID (Lexicomp Online)	Tablet: 2 mg, 5 mg, 10 mg	Sedation, cognition and memory impairment, respiratory suppression, and paradoxical reactions	Withdrawal symptoms if abrupt discontinuation (irritability, tremor, agitation, seizures)

Drug	Indication	Dosing	Formulations[a]	Side effects	Comments
Dantrolene (Hydantoin derivative)	Spasticity (rarely used in children with hypertonia)	Starting dose: 0.5 mg/kg/dose BID Maximum dose: 12 mg/kg/day or 400 mg/day divided TID or QID (Lexicomp Online)	Tablet: 25 mg, 100 mg	Weakness, drowsiness, irritability, vomiting, diarrhea, hepatotoxicity	Monitor liver function tests
Trihexyphenidyl (anticholinergic)	Dystonia (second-line)	Starting dose: 0.1–0.2 mg/kg/day divided TID for the first week (Lexicomp Online, Rice and Waugh 2009) Dose range: 0.05–2.6 mg/kg/day divided TID (Rice and Waugh 2009)	Tablet: 2 mg, 5 mg Elixir: 0.4 mg/mL	Constipation, urinary retention, agitation, xerostomia, blurred vision and photosensitivity	Improves drooling Use with caution in individuals with increased intraocular pressure
Carbidopa/ Levodopa (dopaminergic)	Dystonia (second-line)	Starting dose (levodopa): 1 mg/kg/day (Mink 2003) Maintenance dose: 4–5 mg/kg/day (levodopa) in divided doses Maximum dosage usually does not exceed 10 mg/kg/day or 600 mg/day (Mink 2003)	Tablet (25/100): Carbidopa 25 mg, Levodopa 100 mg Compounded form available	Somnolence, nausea, dyskinesia, headache, mood disturbance	A trial of Levodopa is recommended if dopamine responsive dystonia is suspected. Genetic evaluation is recommended if a response to medication is seen
Gabapentin (GABA analogue)	Dystonia (associated with pain)	Starting dose: 2–3 mg/kg/dose (author suggestion) (up to 300 mg/dose) once daily; Work up to 5 mg/kg/dose TID; further titration to effect (Lexicomp Online) Mean reported dose: 18.1 mg/kg/dose TID (Liow et al. 2016) Maximum dose: 3,600 mg/day (Lexicomp Online)	Capsule: 100 mg, 300 mg, 400 mg Tablet: 600 mg, 800 mg	Sedation	Higher dose required for dystonia compared to pain relief alone

aFormulations available in the United States and Canada unless otherwise specified
BID, twice daily; TID, three times daily; QID, four times daily

been found to decrease excessive drooling, which may warrant a reduction or cessation of anticholinergic agents, such as glycopyrrolate, for those already receiving treatment for sialorrhea.

Levodopa (dystonia)

Levodopa increases dopamine transmission in the basal ganglia. Although levodopa is an effective treatment for primary dystonia, few studies have examined its effectiveness in treating dystonia in the context of CP. While cases studies have shown some benefit, a randomized, double-blinded, placebo-controlled crossover study with nine participants with CP and upper arm dystonia found no improvement in dystonia compared to placebo (Pozin et al. 2014). In the clinical setting, levodopa may be used in some individuals with dystonia specifically to rule out at DOPA-responsive dystonia.

Gabapentin (dystonia)

Gabapentin is a GABA analogue that interacts with alpha subunits of voltage-gated calcium channels and overall inhibits the synthesis of glutaminergic excitatory synapses. Currently, only one 4-year retrospective study has explored the effect of gabapentin on severe childhood dystonia, in which 25 of 69 individuals were diagnosed with CP (Liow et al. 2016). While the results were not differentiated based on the etiology of dystonia, improvements overall were seen in the areas of sleep amount and quality, mood, pain, tone, and seating tolerance. A higher mean dose was required for management of dystonia versus for pain relief alone. Gabapentin can play a role in dystonia management, especially if pain is a significant factor.

Intrathecal baclofen

It has been nearly 25 years since Albright and colleagues published their findings on the first series of paediatric patients with CP receiving continuous intrathecal baclofen (ITB) therapy with implanted pumps (Albright et al. 1993). Since then, ITB therapy has become widely acknowledged as clinically effective for treating intractable spasticity and dystonia in individuals with CP.

ITB is delivered by a surgically implanted and externally programmable pump positioned in the abdomen containing a refillable drug reservoir connected to a catheter that enters the intrathecal space. When baclofen is taken orally there is limited crossing of the blood-brain barrier. Baclofen administered into the intrathecal space has direct access to GABA-B receptors distributed in the superficial dorsal layers of the spinal cord. Low doses produce high concentration in the cerebrospinal fluid (CSF) resulting in a therapeutic effect with virtually undetectable plasma levels. For dystonia, the site of action may be at the cortical level from retrograde flow of the CSF where baclofen inhibits stimulation of the premotor and supplementary motor cortex.

Evidence

Current evidence for the effectiveness of ITB in the treatment of spasticity and dystonia in CP is limited. Evidence is constrained by a shortage of controlled and randomized studies, small sample sizes and a lack of long-term follow-up and focus on important outcome measures such as participation, and patient and caregiver quality of life. A 2015 Cochrane Review found some evidence from randomized control trials suggesting that trial doses of ITB are effective for reducing spasticity in children in the short-term but found that long-term outcomes of ITB are uncertain and the validity of the current evidence is affected by methodological issues (Hasnat and Rice 2015). One randomized control trial demonstrated that ITB reduces pain, increases ease of care and improves multiple domains of health-related quality of life for children with severe CP and their caregivers (Hoving et al. 2009). For dystonia in individuals with CP, high-level evidence for ITB is not yet available. Cohort studies suggest ITB leads to improvements in tone, comfort and ease of care in children with severe dystonic CP (Albright et al. 2001).

Patient selection

Placement of an ITB pump is an invasive procedure that can be associated with significant complications, therefore, careful selection of candidates is vital to achieving optimal outcomes. Ideally, evaluation should be a multidisciplinary assessment involving the individual and their caregivers, as well as the surgeon, and the medical and therapy team with expertise in general hypertonia and ITB. There is no absolute age or weight requirement but patients need sufficient body size to accommodate the pump. Amongst individuals with CP, candidates for ITB will have generalized moderate to severe spasticity and/or dystonia symptoms that are poorly controlled despite maximal therapy with, or limited tolerance of, less invasive modalities. Their hypertonia is either causing significant discomfort or impeding care. Realistic treatment goals should be established before implantation. Risks related to surgery, infection, pump and catheter malfunction as well as potential for overdose and withdrawal need to be outlined. Individuals and caregivers must be motivated and prepared for a long-term commitment and able to adhere to the requirements of treatment, including frequent appointments for pump refills every 1 to 6 months, and subsequent surgical procedures for pump replacement due to battery life and possibly repairing or repositioning catheters. Accessibility to the specialized medical care required is an important consideration.

Therapeutic trial

Traditionally, a trial dose of ITB is administered to assess the candidate's response before pump placement, although due to limitations, some centers have abandoned trials and proceed directly to implantation. Trials are commonly administered as a bolus dose by lumbar puncture. The typical starting bolus is 50mcg and may need to be repeated at higher doses to see an effect, especially for dystonia. Alternatively, intrathecal catheters can be inserted and can be kept in place for repeat doses or continuous infusion via an external pump, but may carry a higher risk of complications. Trials need to be done in a setting where adverse effects can be managed. Although a response can be seen a few hours after a bolus dose for spasticity, effects on dystonia typically take longer, up to several days and trial effects do not reliably predict long-term outcomes.

Implantation

Medical status should be stable before pump implantation. The pump is placed subcutaneously or subfascially in the abdominal wall under general anaesthesia. Recommendations vary for placement of the catheter tip which is traditionally placed in the middle to upper thoracic region. Cervical placement has been recommended for increased efficacy or when treating dystonia (Dan et al. 2010), although supporting evidence is lacking.

Titration and Maintenance

After implantation, ITB is initiated as a simple continuous infusion with the traditional starting daily dose of twice the effective bolus trial dose. The dose can be increased by 5–15% daily for in-patients post-operatively and every 1 to 2 weeks when seen as an outpatient. Oral hypertonia medications may be weaned in parallel. The dose is titrated individually and based on therapeutic response that meets the individual's goals, thus the effective dose varies widely with average doses being reported in the range of 400–500 mcg per day (Boster et al. 2016), with higher doses typically required for dystonia. After the daily dose has been optimized, fine-tuning by programming variable rates during different times of the day can optimize comfort or care for each individual. Establishing optimal dosing and programming may take time – up to 6 months. Periodic reservoir refills are performed percutaneously with a needle using sterile technique in an outpatient setting with frequency depending on pump reservoir size and dosing.

Complications and troubleshooting

It is estimated that about 30% of pediatric patients receiving ITB will experience a major complication (Dan et al. 2010). Pump and catheter infections occur in about 10% of children with CP, half during the first few months after implantation (Bayhan et al. 2016). Catheter-related complications (e.g. disconnection, obstruction, migrations, breakage) are also common but have decreased with modern catheter design.

Individuals on ITB who present with increased hypertonia must be evaluated carefully for the underlying cause of increased tone. Noxious stimuli including pain, constipation and infection may trigger increased tone. Rebound hypertonia due to withdrawal from pump or catheter related malfunction must also be considered. Evaluation should include a focused history and physical examination, judicious use of laboratory and radiologic testing, and pump assessment (Saulino et al. 2016). Pump interrogation should occur to check dosing parameters. Unexpected "extra" residual volume in the reservoir suggests a blockage in the catheter or a problem with the pump. The presence of a pump alarm occurs with low battery or reservoir volume. Rising serial creatine kinase levels is suggestive of withdrawal. Plain X-ray of the abdomen, and lateral lumbar and thoracic spine series to check catheter continuity and look for disconnection or migration should be performed. Dye studies of the catheter under fluoroscopy can be performed to look for a blockage or leak if the initial workup is unrevealing.

Acute baclofen withdrawal symptoms can present within a few hours to days with variable intensity. Symptoms include rebound hypertonia, itching without rash, fever, altered mental status, hemodynamic instability, seizures, rhabdomyolysis and multisystem organ failure. The most effective treatment is prompt restoration of ITB therapy. If this is not possible, benzodiazepines along with supportive measures are first-line treatment of acute withdrawal. Overdoses are not usually a result of pump error but of human error in programming or refill procedures. Respiratory depression progressing to coma may result. Treatment involves turning off the pump temporarily and supporting respiration until the drug has been metabolized.

Caution should be used with ITB in individuals with nocturnal hypoventilation and overnight oximetry or a sleep study may be informative. Current data suggest that ITB does not affect the natural history of scoliosis in CP and does not seem to aggravate or induce seizure activity. In relation to life expectancy, the best available evidence does not show increased mortality from ITB use (Dan et al. 2010).

Selective dorsal rhizotomy

Lumbosacral selective dorsal rhizotomy (SDR) is a neurosurgical procedure where some dorsal nerve rootlets are permanently severed. This leads to a permanent decrease in spasticity in the lower limbs. Importantly it does not reduce dystonia. The main selection criteria for SDRs includes children who are ambulatory with bilateral spastic CP, (spastic diplegic sub-type). However, SDR has also been used for children who are non-ambulatory with significant lower extremity spasticity impacting on ease of care and comfort. The majority of evidence for SDR involves children who are ambulatory; however there are select studies that have evaluated SDR's impact on children who have spasticity who are non-ambulatory (Health Quality Ontario 2017). There is some evidence for non-ambulatory children with spasticity improving mobility skills such as crawling and sitting. Improvements have also been identified in functional independence and self-care.

Reviewing practical considerations for SDR in non-ambulatory children with bilateral spastic CP (i.e.-spastic diplegic or quadriplegic sub-types), it is important to highlight that as more research/evidence is produced for this sub-group, SDR's position in the overall management of hypertonia is likely to evolve. There is significant variability in how different centres integrate SDR into their treatment recommendations. The evidence does support consideration of SDR in children who are functioning at a GMFCS level of IV, whose goals are for improved sitting balance or crawling mobility. However, if the main goal of the SDR is to enhance standing mobility it is important to highlight that eliminating spasticity can adversely affect physical function, particularly when the child uses hypertonia to assist with transfers and standing. Similarly, care must be taken in considering SDR in individuals with significant dystonia (relative contraindication) as the procedure will reduce the spasticity but not affect the dystonia.SDR can also be considered for spasticity reduction where the main goals are to improve comfort. Here it is important to note that dystonia is not reduced post- SDR and a careful assessment of the relative contribution of spasticity and dystonia to the individual's hypertonia needs to be undertaken. In general, SDR procedures are safe with minimal peri-operative complications. Long-term bladder dysfunction and sensory disturbances are also uncommon. Decision-making regarding SDR is best accomplished with multi-specialty evaluation.

Chemodenervation agents: botulinum toxin type A, phenol and ethanol

Chemodenervation agents such as botulinum toxin A (BTA), phenol and ethanol are used to treat focal hypertonia in individuals with CP in GMFCS levels IV and V. These agents are effective in reducing pain, decreasing muscle spasms and promoting ease of caregiving. In this section, we will review the mechanism of action, indications and practical aspects when using these agents to treat hypertonia in severe CP.

Botulinum toxin type A (BTA)
Mechanism of action
Botulinum toxin type A (BTA) has clear advantages for treating hypertonia in individuals with CP. It is an effective medication for reducing focal hypertonia because of its predictable effects on the muscle. Botulinum toxin reduces hypertonia by acting at the neuromuscular junction. The toxin is a protease that cleaves vesicle fusion proteins at the neuromuscular junction and prevents release of acetylcholine inducing muscle weakness and blocking the spinal reflex contributing to spasticity. Botulinum toxin is produced by the bacterium, *Clostridium botulinum*. There are seven serotypes, two of which have been approved for use by the United States (US) Food and Drug Administration (FDA): (BTA) & botulinum toxin type B (BTB). BTA is manufactured as 'Botox' (Allergan Inc., Irvine, CA, US), 'Dysport' (Ipsen Ltd., Slough, United Kingdom), and 'Xeomin' (Merz North America). BTB is manufactured as 'MyoBloc' (US) and 'Neurobloc' (Europe).

For the purposes of this chapter, we will focus on the use of BTA due to its wide availability and reduced risk for side effects (Brandenburg, et al. 2013). It is important to note that different formulations of BTA (e.g. Botox and Dysport) have different dosing equivalents, therefore, caution must be exercised to ensure that the correct dosing is being used for each medication to prevent serious side effects.

Indications and evidence for use

There is good evidence to support the use of BTA to reduce localized spasticity and improve function in children with CP (Delgado et al. 2010). Two international consensus papers have reported that there is level A evidence for tone reduction in lower extremities, functional gait improvements and attainment of individualized goals for upper extremities. In children and youth with CP, functioning at GMFCS levels IV and V, BTA can be used to achieve goals such as improved ease of transferring with medial hamstring injections or targeted hand use (e.g. use of a switch for communication).

Importantly, BTA has been used in this group of individuals with CP for management of pain, ease of care (e.g. dressing, hygiene) and positioning (e.g. seating). One in four children with CP is identified as having chronic pain that limits activities and participation (Penner et al. 2013). This chronic pain may be caused by muscle spasms related to dystonia or stretch of spastic muscles. Prolonged muscle spasms due to dystonia, such as those seen in dystonic storms, can be painful which can trigger increased muscle spasms. BTA can be effective at reducing dystonia in these cases thereby breaking the cycle of muscle spasms and pain that is disruptive to daily functioning and sleep patterns. Hypertonia in the adductors may also make caregiving, such as dressing and perineal hygiene, difficult. Copeland et al. (2014) demonstrated through a double-blinded, randomized, sham-controlled trial that BTA can reduce pain and improve ease of care for non-ambulatory children with CP.

Children and youth with CP in GMFCS levels IV and V are at high risk of hip subluxation and dislocation. While ambulatory status and weight bearing play important roles in the growth and development of the proximal femur, hip subluxation and dislocation is a complex process that may in part be due to spastic adductor muscles. There is some evidence that while repeated BTA injections combined with SWASH (sitting, walking and standing hip orthoses) may at least prolong the need for preventative surgery (i.e. adductor releases), they may not prolong or prevent the need for reconstructive surgery (Willoughby et al. 2012). Variability in indications for surgery across centers and individual patient differences has made studying the role of BTA in the management of hip subluxation and dislocation challenging. Many centers continue to use BTA in the management of tight adductor and hip flexor muscles in non-ambulatory children with CP, particularly if there is pain associated with the hip subluxation or caregiving has become an issue.

Safety concerns
In 2008, the US FDA increased label warnings for commercially available BTA products. Nine deaths had been reported in children with CP after intramuscular injections with BTA resulting in a black box warning being issued, warning of the spread of BTA beyond the injection site. BTA can enter the blood stream and weaken distal muscles involved in swallowing and breathing resulting in dysphagia, aspiration, pneumonia and death. Children with CP in GMFCS levels IV and V have higher rates of comorbidities, such as feeding and respiratory difficulties, active gastroesophageal reflux, and gastrostomy feeding. Therefore, clinicians administering BTA must weigh the benefits and potential side effects of this medication carefully when offering this treatment to children and their families. Monitoring individuals after BTA administration for signs and symptoms of distal spread such as drooling, dysphonia, dysphagia, aspiration, respiratory difficulties and muscle weakness is important.

Despite this risk, a recent randomized, double-blinded, sham-controlled trial in children with CP (GMFCS levels IV and V) showed no statistically significant differences between BTA and control groups in the rate of moderate and serious adverse events (Edwards et al. 2015). Moreover, there was no added risk of having a second set of BTA injections after a 6 month period. While BTA continues to carry a boxed warning regarding distal spread of medication causing weakness of distal muscles, it remains an important medication for treatment of hypertonia in this population when used with care and individuals are informed of potential side effects.

Practical aspects
BTA acts quickly with an onset of action of 1–3 days. It peaks in 7–14 days and has a total duration of action of 3–6 months. While this duration of action often necessitates repeated injections of BTA into targeted muscle groups every 3–6 months, it can also be viewed as an advantage, as any side effect such as unintended muscle weakening, is reversible in the same time frame. Repeat injections are not recommended at intervals shorter than 3 months due to the potential formation of antibodies that can reduce the effectiveness of the medication.

Clinicians may use techniques to identify target muscles appropriately, particularly those in the upper extremity where the muscles are smaller and close together. Ultrasound visualization of muscles is used commonly in children as it is noninvasive and painless; however, electromyography (EMG) and electrical stimulation are additional methods used for the same purpose. Procedures to minimize pain associated with injection should be used and may include pain medications and local anesthetics (e.g. ice, EMLA, Ametop), distraction techniques (e.g. music therapy) or general anesthesia.

Phenol and ethanol
Phenol causes protein denaturation and reversible Wallerian degeneration of axons. It produces a focal reduction in spasticity that lasts up to 12 months following an injection.

Injections with phenol have largely been replaced by or used in conjunction with BTA. One of the main uses of phenol is to allow for an increased number of muscle groups that can be injected in a single session without exceeding the dosage limitations for either BTA or phenol. In addition, phenol provides an immediate onset of action, a longer duration of effect compared to BTA, and is lower in cost.

Administration of phenol requires considerable skill on the part of the injector. It is injected directly adjacent to a motor nerve (perineural), either where it enters the muscle (motor nerve block) or at a branching of the nerve within the muscle (motor point block). The nerve or motor point must be localized by electric stimulation and since this is poorly tolerated by children, phenol injections require general anesthesia. Most studies examining the effectiveness of phenol have been conducted in adults with few studies having been completed in children.

Phenol is felt to be a relatively safe medication. There may be local discomfort at the site of the injection site, perhaps related to the acidity of the phenol and its tendency not to diffuse well resulting in a local tissue inflammatory response. The obturator nerve (for adductor hypertonia) and musculocutaneous nerve (for shoulder and elbow flexor tone) are most often targeted as they are motor nerves that do not have a sensory component, thereby reducing the risk of dysesthesias. Overall, the risk of dysesthesias is low with a recent retrospective review reporting an incidence of 0.4% (Kolaski et al. 2008). Cardiac arrhythmias have been reported intraoperatively with halothane inhalation anesthesia and intramuscular phenol. Arrhythmias may be less common when using a total intravenous anesthesia regimen and perineural technique. Overall, the risk of cardiac dysrhythmia is felt to be low.

Ethanol has a similar mechanism of action to phenol and is administered using similar techniques. It possesses a shorter duration of action but diffuses through the muscle better than phenol. Dysesthesias are possible with ethanol but are rare.

Summary

In summary, this chapter has provided an overview of hypertonia management strategies for individuals with CP who are non-ambulatory. The majority of these individuals will have significant hypertonia and benefit from hypertonia reduction strategies over the lifespan. Such strategies should be combined with rehabilitation where feasible. The importance of setting targeted goals with individuals and families and monitoring progress towards the goals has been highlighted as well as the need for periodic re-evaluation. Determining whether spasticity, dystonia or both are present has also been stressed as there are differential treatments for each hypertonia sub-type. Intervention approaches for generalized versus focal hypertonia have been presented with more invasive hypertonia reduction strategies reserved for individuals where hypertonia is significantly impacting on their comfort and quality of life.

Key Points

- An effective hypertonia management plan starts with a baseline assessment of motor function, comfort and care leading to individualized goal setting. Ongoing management requires monitoring of progress towards goals and reassessment over time.

- Treatments of hypertonia are tone specific. Determining whether spasticity, dystonia or both are present by physical exam is essential.

- Rehabilitation strategies, such as splinting and seating, should be considered as part of any hypertonia management plan.

- For generalized hypertonia requiring intervention, oral medications are considered first-line treatment, though supporting evidence guiding medication use in individuals with CP is weak leading to variations in practice. Oral baclofen is often given as the initial medication for spasticity, dystonia or mixed tonal patterns.

- Intrathecal baclofen pump therapy (spasticity and dystonia) and deep brain stimulation (dystonia only) can be considered for individuals with generalized hypertonia who are poorly controlled despite therapy with, or limited tolerance of, less invasive modalities.

- Selective dorsal rhizotomy (SDR) permanently decreases spasticity in the lower limbs. The role of SDR in non-ambulatory individuals with CP is not well established and requires additional research.

- Chemodenervation strategies are effective and can be utilized for focal spasticity and dystonia. Botulinum toxin A is the most widely used agent.

Useful websites

https://pathways.nice.org.uk/pathways/spasticity-in-children-and-young-people (National Institute for Health and Care Excellence 2017)

https://www.aacpdm.org/publications/care-pathways/dystonia (American Academy for Cerebral Palsy and Developmental Medicine 2016)

References

Lexicomp Online.

Albright AL, Barron WB, Fasick MP, Polinko P, Janosky J (1993) Continuous intrathecal baclofen infusion for spasticity of cerebral origin. *JAMA* **270**: 2475–2477. doi: 10.1001/jama.1993.03510200081036

Albright AL, Barry MJ, Shafton DH, Ferson SS (2001) Intrathecal baclofen for generalized dystonia. *Dev Med Child Neurol* **43**: 652–657. doi: 10.1111/j.1469-8749.2001.tb00137.x

American Academy for Cerebral Palsy and Developmental Medicine (2016) *Care pathways: dystonia* [Online]. Available: https://www.aacpdm.org/publications/care-pathways/dystonia [Accessed 05 April 2017].

Bayhan IA, Sees JP, Nishnianidze T, Rogers KJ, Miller F (2016) Infection as a complication of intrathecal baclofen treatment in children with cerebral palsy. *J Pediatr Orthop* **36**: 305–309. doi: 10.1097/BPO.0000000000000443

Boster AL, Adair RL, Gooch JL, et al. (2016) Best practices in intrathecal baclofen therapy: dosing and long-term management. *Neuromodulation* 19: 623–631. doi: 10.1111/ner.12388

Brandenburg JE, Krach LE, Gormley ME, Jr. (2013) Use of rimabotulinum toxin for focal hypertonicity management in children with cerebral palsy with nonresponse to onabotulinum toxin. *Am J Phys Med Rehabil* **92**: 898–904. doi: 10.1097/PHM.0b013e31829231fa

Copeland L, Edwards P, Thorley M, et al. (2014) Botulinum toxin A for nonambulatory children with cerebral palsy: a double blind randomized controlled trial. *J Pediatr* **165**: 140–146 e4. doi: 10.1016/j.jpeds.2014.01.050

Dan B, Motta F, Vles JS, et al. (2010) Consensus on the appropriate use of intrathecal baclofen (ITB) therapy in paediatric spasticity. *Eur J Paediatr Neurol* **14**: 19–28. doi: 10.1016/j.ejpn.2009.05.002

Delgado MR, Hirtz D, Aisen M, et al. (2010) Practice parameter: pharmacologic treatment of spasticity in children and adolescents with cerebral palsy (an evidence-based review): report of the Quality Standards Subcommittee of the American Academy of Neurology and the Practice Committee of the Child Neurology Society. *Neurology* **74**: 336–343. doi: 10.1212/WNL.0b013e3181cbcd2f

Edwards P, Sakzewski L, Copeland L, et al. (2015) Safety of Botulinum Toxin Type A for Children With Nonambulatory Cerebral Palsy. *Pediatrics* **136**: 895–904. doi: 10.1542/peds.2015-0749

Hasnat MJ, Rice JE (2015) Intrathecal baclofen for treating spasticity in children with cerebral palsy. *Cochrane Database Syst Rev*, CD004552. doi: 10.1002/14651858.CD004552.pub2

He Y, Brunstrom-Hernandez JE, Thio LL, et al. (2014) Population pharmacokinetics of oral baclofen in pediatric patients with cerebral palsy. *J Pediatr* **164**: 1181–1188. doi: 10.1016/j.jpeds.2014.01.029

Health Quality Ontario (2017) Lumbosacral dorsal rhizotomy for spastic cerebral palsy: a health technology assessment [Online]. Available: http://www.hqontario.ca/Portals/0/Documents/evidence/reports/hta-dorsal-rhizotomy-04-07-2017-en.pdf [Accessed 26 April 2017].

Hoving MA, Van Raak EP, Spincemaille GH, et al. (2009) Efficacy of intrathecal baclofen therapy in children with intractable spastic cerebral palsy: a randomised controlled trial. *Eur J Paediatr Neurol* **13**: 240–246. doi: 10.1016/j.ejpn.2008.04.013

Jethwa A, Mink J, Macarthur C, Knights S, Fehlings T, Fehlings D (2010) Development of the Hypertonia Assessment Tool (HAT): a discriminative tool for hypertonia in children. *Dev Med Child Neurol* **52**: e83–e87. doi: 10.1111/j.1469-8749.2009.03483.x

Kolaski K, Ajizian SJ, Passmore L, Pasutharnchat N, Koman LA, Smith BP (2008) Safety profile of multilevel chemical denervation procedures using phenol or botulinum toxin or both in a pediatric population. *Am J Phys Med Rehabil* **87**: 556–566. doi: 10.1097/PHM.0b013e31817c115b

Liow NY, Gimeno H, Lumsden DE, et al. (2016) Gabapentin can significantly improve dystonia severity and quality of life in children. *Eur J Paediatr Neurol* **20**: 100–107. doi: 10.1016/j.ejpn.2015.09.007

Mink JW (2003) Dopa-responsive dystonia in children. *Curr Treat Options Neurol* **5**: 279–282. doi: 10.1007/s11940-003-0033-9

National Institute for Health and Care Excellence (2017) *Spasticity in children and young people overview* [Online]. Available: https://pathways.nice.org.uk/pathways/spasticity-in-children-and-young-people [Accessed 05 April 2017].

Penner M, Xie WY, Binepal N, Switzer L, Fehlings D (2013) Characteristics of pain in children and youth with cerebral palsy. *Pediatrics* **132**: e407–e413. doi: 10.1542/peds.2013-0224

Pozin I, Bdolah-Abram T, Ben-Pazi H (2014) Levodopa does not improve function in individuals with dystonic cerebral palsy. *J Child Neurol* **29**: 534–537. doi: 10.1177/0883073812473645

Rice J, Waugh MC (2009) Pilot study on trihexyphenidyl in the treatment of dystonia in children with cerebral palsy. *J Child Neurol* **24**: 176–182. doi: 10.1177/0883073808322668

Sanger TD, Bastian A, Brunstrom J, et al. (2007) Prospective open-label clinical trial of trihexyphenidyl in children with secondary dystonia due to cerebral palsy. *J Child Neurol* **22**: 530–537. doi: 10.1177/0883073807302601

Sanger TD, Delgado MR, Gaebler-Spira D, Hallett M, Mink JW, Task Force on Childhood Motor Disorders (2003) Classification and definition of disorders causing hypertonia in childhood. *Pediatrics* **111**: e89–e97. doi: 10.1542/peds.111.1.e89

Saulino M, Anderson DJ, Doble J, et al. (2016) Best practices for intrathecal baclofen therapy: troubleshooting. *Neuromodulation* **19**: 632–641. doi: 10.1111/ner.12467

Willoughby K, Ang SG, Thomason P, Graham HK (2012) The impact of botulinum toxin A and abduction bracing on long-term hip development in children with cerebral palsy. *Dev Med Child Neurol* **54**: 743–747. doi: 10.1111/j.1469-8749.2012.04340.x

Chapter 4

Musculoskeletal and orthopedic management

Mark J. Romness and
Victor Anciano

Orthopedic management of children with severe cerebral palsy (CP) strives to be consistent with the functional goals of management defined in previous chapters. While children with complex CP will do limited if any ambulation, management is important to maintain function for activities of daily living that help with quality of life, comfort and care. Loss of even simple functional abilities (e.g. comfortable sitting) can significantly impair quality of life and increase the need for additional assistance. On the contrary, sometimes simple additions or assistive devices can significantly help with functional abilities, and maintaining or supplementing what function the patient has is important throughout their life.

Orthopedic management generally consists of treatments to prevent and correct contractures, maintain hip reduction and manage scoliosis. Unfortunately, fractures are common in this population and they require unique management and treatment techniques compared to able-bodied patients. Collaboration between all the patient's providers and orthopedists is of utmost importance. Many children with complex CP are seen on a more frequent and regular basis by teachers, therapists and primary medical providers who represent the first-line of evaluation and referral, than by orthopedists. The ability to recognize early signs of developing orthopedic complications allows for early management and prevention of more severe problems. Standardized orthopedic exams allow monitoring of changes over time that may not be obvious to those who see the child more frequently.

Joint care

Factors that lead to joint problems in children with severe CP include asymmetric or unbalanced muscle tone across the joints, decreased active and passive use and decreased external forces on the joints. Based on these factors, the natural history is for joint contractures to develop and progress if joint mobility is not monitored and addressed prophylactically.

Muscle function tends to be more impaired in muscles that are considered 'two joint muscles' (Gage 1993). These are muscles that cross two different joints and may have different effects at the joints they cross. Because of their more complex function they are felt to be more susceptible to the loss of cortical control and increased spasticity. In the upper extremity this includes the long head of the biceps and many of the forearm muscles for both flexion and extension of the wrist and hand. In the lower extremities the primary two joint muscles are the psoas at the hip, the hamstrings, the rectus femoris, the gastrocnemius and most of the ankle and toe muscles. Increased spasticity in these muscles helps explain why contractures occur, as well as why treatments are focused primarily on these muscle groups.

As discussed in Chapter 3, tone management remains the primary method to control the spasticity, yet asymmetric tone across the joints often continues. Regular therapy including positioning, transfers and specific joint range of motion are important activities that need to be incorporated into the patients' daily routines. This can include formal therapy and caregiver-directed activities. Formal therapy with an occupational or physical therapist is beneficial for the use of specialized equipment that the therapist has access to and for their expertise with specific treatment modalities. While formal therapy has not been shown to prevent contractures, regular activity is still beneficial for maintaining daily function. Even standing with the use of standing devices has been shown to positively affect bone mineral density, hip stability, hip, knee and ankle range of motion and spasticity (Paleg et al. 2013).

The use of bracing (orthoses) may help prevent contractures but the primary use of bracing is for function in daily activities. In general, bracing is used during the day for functional reasons but can be beneficial in non-functional times, such as during sleep, to hold a joint in a stretched position.

When joint stability and range of motion cannot be maintained by non-operative measures, surgical intervention is warranted to prevent progressive fixed contractures which interfere with daily activities and become more difficult to treat as their severity increases. Smaller contractures can often be improved with soft tissue procedures to release the spasticity on one side of the joint or to balance the muscle forces across the joint. More extensive procedures are required once contractures become severe including incision of the joint capsules for more extensive release, osteotomy to redirect the joint surfaces or joint fusions (arthrodesis) to prevent any motion through the joint. Deciding which procedure is best for each patient requires careful and thorough evaluation of the patient including current physical condition and abilities, functional goals and family support.

An important aspect of joint care in children with severe CP is hip surveillance. The risk of hip displacement in children with CP is related to their level of function with 0% in children with Gross Motor Function Classification System (GMFCS) level I to a more concerning 90% in children with GMFCS level V (Hägglund et al. 2005). Based on the high incidence of hip subluxation, hip screening programs have been developed and validated as preventing the need for more extensive surgery or hip dislocation. The primary study in Sweden showed a decrease in hip dislocation from 8% in a historical comparison group to 0.5% in a surveillance group over a 7-year period (Hägglund et al. 2005). This was compared to a group in Norway over the same period that did not have a reduction in dislocations.

Signs and symptoms of hip problems can be non-specific, but when presenting in conjunction in patients with severe CP suspicion should arise for hip displacement. Physicians should ask about pain arising from the hip, deterioration in sitting or standing capacity, and/or increasing difficulty with perineal care or hygiene. On the physical exam, special attention should be paid to apparent leg length discrepancies, deterioration in hip abduction (adduction contractures) or other motion at the hip, and increasing muscle tone in the affected hip.

Per screening protocol, children in GMFCS level II should have an anteroposterior pelvis X-ray at age 2 and 6 years. Children in a GMFCS levels of III–V should undergo radiographic examination at the time of diagnosis. After the initial X-ray, patients should have radiographic monitoring at least yearly until 8 years of age. If there is mild radiographic abnormality in children in GMFCS levels IV–V, radiographs should be carried out every 6 months (Hägglund et al. 2007). Children in GMFCS level I do not need screening X-rays unless there is concern based on examination, such as asymmetric motion or tone.

The key radiographic indicator of hip dysplasia used for hip surveillance is the migration percentage. This is a measurement of the portion of the femoral head that is not covered by the pelvic socket or acetabulum on a standard anteroposterior pelvis radiograph (Fig. 4.1). Since it does not measure actual migration, it is also referred to as the percent uncovered or Reimers' Index in some publications.

If the migration percentage is more than 33% or concerning signs and symptoms are present, these patients may require more regular radiographic examinations. General guidelines recommend referral to an orthopedist if there is hip migration greater than 33% (Mugglestone et al. 2012). Patients with hip displacement showing a migration percentage of 40% or more may require hip containment surgery (Ramstad et al. 2017).

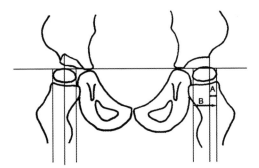

Figure 4.1 Calculation of migration percentage.
Migration percentage is the portion of the femoral head that is not covered by the acetabular roof on a standard anteroposterior pelvis X-ray with the legs in neutral position. The measurement is also referred to as the percent uncovered or Reimers' Index. MP = A/B x 100.

The American Academy for Cerebral Palsy and Developmental Medicine has developed a Care Pathway for Hip Surveillance (available at https://www.aacpdm.org/publications/care-pathways/hip-surveillance.) An application for mobile devices has been developed by Shriners Hospitals for Children called HipScreen that is available at no charge. These resources have similar guidelines for hip monitoring and are extremely helpful in the clinical setting and for learning the monitoring standards.

Soft tissue surgery

The term soft tissue surgery is used to describe surgical procedures on muscles, tendons and joints that do not include osteotomy or cutting of the bones. These procedures are perceived to be 'less involved' by families and caretakers as they often require less extensive restrictions or rehabilitation following the procedure. Generalized goals for soft tissue procedures are release of soft tissue contractures, balancing forces across a joint and improving functional motion if possible.

The most common procedures for the upper extremity are release of contractures about the shoulder, elbow, wrist and fingers. These releases usually are of the two joint muscles in the upper extremity such as the biceps and forearm muscles. Wrist fusion, while not purely soft tissue surgery, requires minimal rehabilitation and is a common procedure for this population. The fusion stabilizes the wrist in a neutral position and can allow the patient better use of the arm as a helper and better use of the fingers for motor activities, as the stabilized wrist allows better finger function (Fig. 4.2). Patients that may benefit from this surgery include skeletally mature patients with severe fixed wrist deformity and poor motor control. Fusion outcome studies have shown significant improvement in standardized disability assessment scores when comparing preoperative and postoperative values. Satisfaction scores were also shown to be improved.

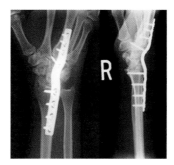

Figure 4.2 Anteroposterior and lateral X-rays of a wrist following fusion with a dorsal plating technique.
The fusion procedure usually includes resection of some of the carpal bones to allow better positioning and less tension on the finger flexor tendons.

a.   b.   c.

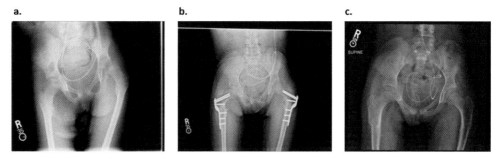

Figure 4.3 Proximal femoral osteotomy
a. Preoperative radiographs of a 6-year-old patient with cerebral palsy demonstrating left femoral head subluxation and bilateral poor acetabular coverage of the femoral heads. b. Postoperative radiographs of same patient 5 months after performing bilateral proximal femoral osteotomies and soft tissue releases with improved femoral head position in acetabulum. c. Radiographs of same patient after hardware removal and two years following original operation, demonstrating maintained reduction and femoral head coverage.

In the lower extremities, release of contractures is very common for the hips and knees. Surgery for the ankles and feet are directed at obtaining a plantigrade foot that tolerates bracing if necessary. Tendon transfers have a less predictable outcome in the non-ambulatory patient, but may be considered in the less involved and less disabled patients.

Osteotomy

Generalized goals for osteotomies are to redirect and maintain joint reduction and to improve joint position and motion for daily function. The most common osteotomy in this population of children with complex CP is a proximal femoral osteotomy for hip reduction. Hip dislocation is common and proportional to the severity of involvement as noted earlier. The osteotomy redirects the femoral head into the center of the acetabulum to improve joint stability and encourage acetabular development (Fig. 4.3).

Remodeling or improved development of the acetabulum often occurs in the younger patients with just correction of the femoral head position but older patients may require additional osteotomy in the pelvis to improve hip stability. The femoral osteotomy also allows correction of excessive femoral anteversion which is common in this population and causes internal positioning of the legs.

Osteotomies about the knee are primarily to correct flexion contractures which do not improve adequately with soft tissue release. Likewise, foot osteotomies are used to correct contractures that interfere with foot positioning and bracing. Arthrodeses or fusions are commonly used in the foot for recurrent or severe contractures, but this is usually reserved until after growth of the foot bones has completed.

Scoliosis

The development of scoliosis in children with severe CP has been shown to cause both physiologic and functional impairment for the patient (Park et al. 2006, Kwon and Lee 2015). Since the incidence of developing scoliosis is proportional to the severity based on the GMFCS levels (Fig. 4.4), most children with severe CP will develop some degree of scoliosis. While there is no established surveillance program similar to the hip, all patients with severe CP should have spinal examination as part of their routine scheduled evaluations.

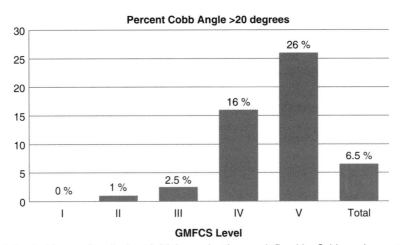

Figure 4.4 Incidence of scoliosis at initial examination, as defined by Cobb angle greater than 20 degrees, increases with increased severity of involvement based on GMFCS Level. There is also increased incidence with age of the patient. (Persson-Bunke et al., 2012)

In an epidemiological total population study, scoliosis was diagnosed in most children with CP after 8 years of age. Curvature noted on exam in children under age 8 is usually positional and related to poor trunk control. Children with CP and a GMFC level of IV or V had approximately a 50% risk of developing moderate to severe scoliosis by the time they were 18 years old. This is compared to children in GMFCS levels of I or II who had almost no risk of developing scoliosis (Persson-Bunke et al. 2012).

Radiographic evaluation with anteroposterior and lateral thoraco-lumbar spine views should be done if there is clinical evidence of scoliosis – especially if there is no flexibility to passive correction nor correction in the supine position. Sitting views are preferred by surgeons, but supine views are adequate for screening purposes. Radiographic measurement of the Cobb angle is used as the primary indicator of severity. This is measured on the anteroposterior view based on the angle between the vertebral bodies with the most tilt as diagramed in Fig. 4.5.

A Cobb angle over 10 degrees is required for the diagnosis of scoliosis and progression is considered significant with increase of more than 10 degrees in this population of patients. Risk factors for curve progression include: spinal curve of 40 degrees before age 15, having total body involvement (GMFCS level V), being bedridden, with thoracolumbar curves. Patients with these risk factors should be evaluated by a spine surgeon (Saito et al. 1998).

Treatment considerations include the patient's age, definition and extent of the curve, the generalized health condition of the patient and life expectancy. Treatment options

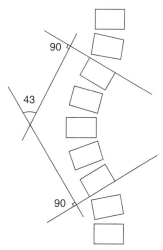

Figure 4.5 Calculation of Cobb Angle.
Maximum tilt is measured at 43 degrees in this diagram. Curves measuring less than 10 degrees do not meet the criteria for a diagnosis of scoliosis (Cobb Angle, no date).

are generally the three 'O's of observation, orthosis or operation. Smaller curves in younger patients are often only positional in that the degree of curvature is related to the positioning of the patient when the radiograph is taken. These curves may not be present in the supine position but are more noticeable in sitting when the patient cannot support the trunk against gravity. Clinically there is passive flexibility of the spine and radiographically these curves do not demonstrate rotation of the vertebral bodies. The smaller curves can usually be controlled with proper positioning including modifications to the patient's seating devices.

As the patients age, the curves progress and become more rigid. Softer or less rigid bracing may help with positioning for activities of daily living, but more rigid bracing is required to affect the scoliosis. Bracing has been shown to delay but not prevent progression of the curve in patients with neuromuscular associated scoliosis (Halawi et al. 2015, Roberts and Tsirikos 2016). Various types of braces have been developed to address the different types of curves while accommodating medical devices that these complex patients have, such as tracheostomies and feeding tubes. More rigid bracing has been shown to affect the chest anatomy and this negative effect needs to be considered when utilizing bracing for these medically challenging patients.

Surgery for scoliosis in this population of patients with complex CP has evolved over the last few decades to include more extensive preoperative evaluation, intra-operative spinal cord monitoring, stronger instrumentation and multi-specialty postoperative management. Surgery has been shown to be effective for deformity correction with positive trends in caregiver and quality of life outcomes, but minimal change in function (Toovey et al. 2017).

Bracing

The use of bracing is a common and important aspect of daily care for individuals with severe CP. The general goal of bracing is to improve function without impairment of other activities. Even a small gain in function can make a dramatic difference in the daily activities of this patient population. A common example for children with severe CP is the ability to bear bodyweight through their lower extremities. If they are able to bear at least some of the weight themselves they often can be transferred with one person assisting, whereas if they cannot tolerate any weight they require a two person assist or a mechanical lift. Bracing of the ankle and foot can often provide the stability needed to allow single assist transfers.

The primary brace utilized in the upper extremity is to stabilize the wrist. This prevents wrist drop, which interferes with use of the hand as a helper, and also interferes with the function of the fingers as they have lost their stable base. The other type of bracing used in the upper extremities is to prevent contractures with either static or dynamic braces. Static braces hold the joint in a specific position which is usually the position of maximum stretch. Dynamic braces provide a force to counteract the contracture while allowing some motion but are often too weak to counteract the spasticity or too complex for the patient and family to tolerate or use properly.

The most commonly used lower extremity brace is an ankle foot orthosis (AFO). As its name implies, an AFO primarily controls the ankle and foot position; however, it can also have an influence on the leg including stabilization of the knee and can help with overall leg position and body stability.

There are many different styles or types of AFOs and each has positive and negative attributes that need to be considered when ordering. A proper order requires knowledge of the patient's physical condition and abilities and the goals of the brace. There are also multiple modifications that can be made to the AFOs for problems such as excessive pronation, hallux valgus and skin issues that need to be considered (Fig. 4.6).

Other braces commonly used in the lower extremity include hip abduction braces and knee extension braces. As in the upper extremity, bracing can be for functional purposes or to prevent contractures. Functional bracing at the hip is utilized to prevent scissoring in both the sitting and upright positions. Fixed abduction hip bracing may help prevent adduction contractures but has not been shown to prevent hip dislocation (Hägglund et al. 2007, Miller et al. 2017). Functional bracing across the knee is not commonly utilized as the braces tend to be bulky with limited benefit above that which can be obtained by using AFOs. More commonly, bracing across the knee is aimed at preventing knee flexion contractures.

Despite the benefits of bracing, it does increase the burden of care for this patient population. Therefore, bracing goals need to be specific and reevaluated on a regular basis. With each new order or renewal order these questions have to be asked: What are the

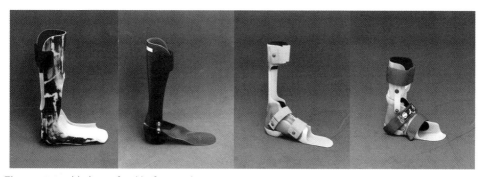

Figure 4.6   Variety of ankle foot orthoses.
Modifications can be made to allow for different functionality. The variety exists due to the different goals of bracing and the variability of foot problems in children with cerebral palsy.

goals of the brace? Is this the best brace for the goal? Does the patient need and benefit from the brace? Can the patient tolerate the brace?

Fracture care

Unfortunately, the incidence of fracture in the child with severe CP is higher than the less severely affected child and is often a warning that the child is not adequately nourished. Fracture risk is related to osteopenia (see Chapter 6) from decreased activity and metabolic issues such as general malnutrition, insufficient mineral intake, and vitamin D deficiency. Because of their decreased bone mass and non-ambulatory status, fracture treatment in non-ambulatory children varies from that for fractures in ambulatory children. Consideration of the bone quality and fracture location help determine best treatment option, but in general fixation should be with load sharing implants and post-procedure immobilization should be as minimal as possible. Medically fragile children may be better treated with non-operative means if similar long-term goals can be maintained, but often surgery allows faster recovery with less pain for the patient and less burden for the care team during healing.

Pre-surgical preparation

Comprehensive pre-surgical planning benefits the patient, the family and the providers. This begins with well-defined indications and goals for the procedure. As presented earlier in this chapter, the indications for hip and spine surgery are fairly well defined, but indications for some of the other procedures such, as soft tissue releases, are not as well defined. The family needs to be involved with the decision for surgery with understanding of why the surgery is being recommended and how the surgery will help the patient and caregivers, both short and long term.

Medical optimization for children with severe CP is primarily focused on general nutritional status, seizure control/medications, pulmonary risks, urinary retention or infections, and gastrointestinal issues such as feeding tubes and constipation, which are common comorbidities in this population. Preoperative assessment of nutritional status found that patients with serum albumin levels less than 3.5 g/dl and total lymphocyte count less than 1 500 cells per mm^3 had an increased rate of infection, longer intubation, and longer hospitalization (Jevsevar and Karlin 1993). Less frequent are dental and skin issues that need to be addressed, but any active infection in these areas should be resolved before surgery as this increases the risk of surgical site infection, which can be a severe and difficult problem to treat, especially if implants were left in vivo for the procedure.

Planning for the surgical procedure includes scheduling and availability of appropriate equipment and implants as well as any casting or bracing that will be utilized following the procedure. Bracing that will be utilized immediately after surgery should be ordered early enough to be ready for use when needed. Advanced preparation of discharge medication and equipment is key to a smooth transition from the hospital. This includes confirmation of who will be available and able to assist the patient after discharge. Arrangements for either home or facility based therapy should be considered and arranged preoperatively as needed. Finally, clear expectations of the recovery pathway and time frame help all participants plan their schedules.

Post-surgical care

Post-surgical complication rates in patients with CP are increased compared to the average population due to underlying comorbidities. Severe cases of CP are associated with decreased pulmonary function, inadequate nutritional status, decreased mobility, and cognitive impairment.

Complications following surgical procedures in patients with cerebral palsy are variable and dependent on the kind of surgery. Patients undergoing spine surgery have high risk of postoperative complications, with incidence reported between 17–68% (Cloake 2016). In a 2013 meta-analysis of complications following surgery for neuromuscular scoliosis, pulmonary complications were found to be most common (22.7%), followed by implant complications (12.5%) and infections (10.9%) (Sharma et al. 2013). While post-operative illness and increase over baseline constipation are common in children with complex CP undergoing major surgery, true gastrointestinal complications are rare. However, preoperative poor nutritional status has been associated with increased rate of digestive complications in spinal surgery performed on patients with CP (Pesenti et al. 2016).

Other surgeries carry less risk. For example, wrist fusions have over 90% successful union rates (Van Heest and Strothman 2009). Patients who undergo proximal femoral osteotomy surgery have a risk of developing avascular necrosis of the femoral head that ranges significantly across studies but with an average rate of 7.5% (Hesketh et al. 2016). Additionally, patients in GMFCS levels IV and V have increased risk of hardware-related complications and implant related fractures (Chung et al. 2017).

Primary providers should be suspicious of acute changes in physical exam in patients with severe CP in the postoperative period. Unstable vital signs, changes in passive joint motion, or sudden onset of pain at the surgical site should trigger more in-depth evaluation such as a chest X-ray and basic inflammatory serology. Recognizing postoperative complications and addressing them as soon as possible is important in preventing poorer outcomes.

The time needed to return to regular daily activities is based on what procedure was performed and what restrictions are needed, but in general patients can return to their preoperative activities such as school and therapy once narcotic medications are no longer needed for pain control and the patient can tolerate the activities planned. Bracing may resume once the patient is comfortable with use and serves to maintain range of motion and/or protect from harmful movements that may jeopardize the recent surgery.

Conclusion

Patients with CP who experience severe functional impairments have higher risks of developing musculoskeletal problems. These musculoskeletal issues can affect soft tissues, joints and bones. Contractures are the most common problem encountered in this population due to the high degree of spasticity and low level of functional abilities. Hip displacement and scoliosis have a strong association with the spasticity found in patients with CP which helps explain the correlation to GMFC level. Non-operative modalities exist to help many early aspects of musculoskeletal problems, so primary providers should be familiar with first-line treatments of bracing and physical therapy. Progression of musculoskeletal impairment may benefit from orthopedic surgery, so it is important to be familiar with common parameters to trigger orthopedic consultation.

Key points

- Children with severe CP are at high risk for developing joint contractures, hip dysplasia and scoliosis – all of which can have significant impairment in their activities of daily living and quality of life.

- Regular monitoring of joint range and simple treatments such as positioning, passive range of motion or orthoses can prevent more severe deformity requiring more extensive treatments.

- Hip screening protocols have been established and for patients with GMFC levels IV–V, an anteroposterior pelvis X-ray should be taken at time of diagnosis and then every 6 months until 7 years old. From 7 to 16 years of age, annual X-rays are recommended.

- The development and severity of scoliosis is proportional to the GMFC level with 50% risk of moderate to severe curves in CP patients GMFC levels IV–V.

- Orthoses for scoliosis may help with daily activities and positioning but have not been shown to prevent progression in neuromuscular scoliosis.

- Ankle foot orthoses (AFOs) are regularly used even in non-ambulatory children with CP to prevent contractures and help with positioning or transfers.

- Fractures are common even with minimal injury in non-ambulatory patients due to osteopenia, decreased activity and metabolic issues.

References

Applied Biomechanics Guelph' Applied Biomechanics Orthotics and Bracing. Available at: https:// appliedbiomechanics.com/services-guelph/orthopedic-bracing/bracing-for-children/.

Chung MK, Kwon SS, Ho BC, et al. (2018) Incidence and risk factors of hardware-related complications after proximal femoral osteotomy in children and adolescents. *J Pediatr Orthop B* **27**: 264–270.

Cobb Angle (no date) CLEAR Scoliosis Institute. Available at: https://www.clear-institute.org/ learning-about-scoliosis/cobb-angle/.

Gage JR (1993) Gait analysis. An essential tool in the treatment of cerebral palsy. *Clin Orthop Relat Res* **288**: 126–134.

Hägglund G, Lauge-Pedersen H, Wagner P (2007) Characteristics of children with hip displacement in cerebral palsy. *BMC Musculoskelet Disord* **8**: 101.

Halawi MJ, Lark RK, Fitch RD (2015) Neuromuscular scoliosis: current concepts. *Orthopedics* **38**: e452–e456.

Hesketh K, Leveille L, Mulpuri K (2016) The Frequency of AVN Following Reconstructive Hip Surgery in Children With Cerebral Palsy: A Systematic Review. *J Pediatr Orthop* **36**: e17–e24.

Jevsevar DS, Karlin LI (1993) The relationship between preoperative nutritional status and complications after an operation for scoliosis in patients who have cerebral palsy. *J Bone Joint Surg Am* **75**: 880–884.

Kwon YH, Lee HY (2015) Differences in respiratory pressure and pulmonary function among children with spastic diplegic and hemiplegic cerebral palsy in comparison with normal controls. *J Phys Ther Sci* **27**: 401–403.

Miller SD, Juricic M, Hesketh K, et al. (2017) Prevention of hip displacement in children with cerebral palsy: a systematic review. *Dev Med Child Neurol* **59**: 1130–1138.

Mugglestone MA, Eunson P, Murphy MS, et al. (2012) Spasticity in children and young people with non-progressive brain disorders: summary of NICE guidance. *BMJ* **345**: e4845.

Paleg GS, Smith BA, Glickman LB (2013) Systematic review and evidence-based clinical recommendations for dosing of pediatric supported standing programs. *Pediatr Phys Ther* **25**: 232–247.

Park ES, Park JH, Rha DW, Park CI, Park CW (2006) Comparison of the ratio of upper to lower chest wall in children with spastic quadriplegic cerebral palsy and normally developed children. *Yonsei Med J* **47**: 237–242.

Persson-Bunke M, Hägglund G, Lauge-Pedersen H, Wagner P, Westbom L (2012) Scoliosis in a total population of children with cerebral palsy. *Spine (Phila Pa 1976)* **37**: E708–E713.

Pesenti S, Blondel B, Peltier E, et al. (2016) Experience in perioperative management of patients undergoing posterior spine fusion for neuromuscular scoliosis. *Biomed Res Int* **2016**: 3053056.

Ramstad K, Jahnsen RB, Terjesen T (2017) Severe hip displacement reduces health-related quality of life in children with cerebral palsy. *Acta Orthop* **88**: 205–210.

Roberts SB, Tsirikos AI (2016) Factors influencing the evaluation and management of neuromuscular scoliosis: A review of the literature. *J Back Musculoskelet Rehabil* **29**: 613–623.

Saito N, Ebara S, Ohotsuka K, Kumeta H, Takaoka K, et al. (1998) Natural history of scoliosis in spastic cerebral palsy. *Lancet* **351**: 1687–1692.

Sharma S, Wu C, Andersen T, Wang Y, Hansen ES, Bünger CE, et al. (2013) Prevalence of complications in neuromuscular scoliosis surgery: a literature meta-analysis from the past 15 years. *Eur Spine J* **22**(6): 1230–1249.

Terjesen T (2012) The natural history of hip development in cerebral palsy. *Dev Med Child Neurol* **54**: 951–957.

Toovey R, Harvey A, Johnson M, Baker L, Williams K (2017) Outcomes after scoliosis surgery for children with cerebral palsy: a systematic review. *Dev Med Child Neurol* **59**: 690–698. doi: 10.1111/dmcn.13412.

Van Heest AE, Strothman D (2009) Wrist arthrodesis in cerebral palsy. *J Hand Surg Am* **34**: 1216–1224.

Chapter 5

Seating, mobility, and equipment needs

Christopher D. Lunsford and Jonathan Greenwood

Introduction

For children with cerebral palsy who are classified as Gross Motor Function Classification System (GMFCS) levels III through V, durable medical equipment (DME) often has a significant positive effect on function, seating and mobility. Moreover, these children have a very high usage of equipment throughout their lifespan compared to those with less complex motor challenges. The equipment reviewed in this chapter is by no means an exhaustive list, but rather a starting point for patient and provider alike. Identifying this need can be a complex process that is best conducted by an interdisciplinary team including the child and family. This process can look very different depending on geographic restrictions, regional laws, medical/community resources, and family preferences. However, wherever possible it is best to follow a model as adapted from equipment delivery resources from the Rehabilitation Engineering and Assistive Technology Society of North America (RESNA) (Box 5.1) (Arledge et al. 2011, Meehl et al. 2012).

General principles
Referral and intake
Some communities will have access to a medical equipment clinic where the referral and intake process will be established. Referral and intake can take many forms. First, primary care providers, therapists, or families themselves may make a referral. The

Box 5.1: Equipment evaluation and delivery

Step 1 Referral and intake process
Step 2 Team assembly and client arrival
Step 3 Client assessment
Step 4 Equipment trial and decision
Step 5 Funding/resource review
Step 6 Delivery, fitting, education and follow-up

Adapted from equipment delivery resources from the Rehabilitation Engineering and Assistive Technology Society of North America (RESNA).

intake process often includes asking some basic questions of the referrer and family to clarify the appropriateness of the referral and begin to identify goals. The family should be introduced to the basic structure of the whole process and timeline in order to be informed on what to expect. Setting expectations and goals early helps to improve satisfaction and outcomes.

Team assembly and client arrival

An interdisciplinary team can be advantageous, but it is not always possible. In addition to the child and family, this team could include a developmental pediatrician, physiatrist, orthotist, rehabilitation engineer, vendor representative as well as occupational, physical, and speech language therapists. Clearly, not all families will have access to facilities that can assemble such a team; the most basic team can be a therapist and an equipment provider. The roles of the client/caregiver, therapist/medical provider and vendor are equally important so that the collaborative effort can foster decision making to meet the needs of the end-user. Some facilities are also able to have representatives from multiple vendors participate in the process to expose the client to a wider variety of options.

Client assessment

Perhaps the most important step is assessment of the client. Assessment includes evaluating the range of motion, strength, tone, and body habitus as needed. Review may also include pertinent medical history and assessment of physical, sensory, cognitive, and functional aspects to the clinical presentation. Most importantly, the team must understand the goals of the client and family. One way to do this is to utilize the International Classification of Functioning, Disability, and Health (ICF) as a tool in approaching the equipment evaluation (World Health Organization 2007). The ICF organizes the concepts of function and disability by factors related to body function, family/social function, and societal function (see Chapter 1). This dynamic understanding of a patient and their real-life circumstances helps the team more reliably act in the patient's best interest. Using the ICF, current mobility status and activities of daily living (ADLs) should be reviewed. Parts of the assessment process may actually need to occur during the screening and intake so the team and vendors can make sure to have appropriate devices available during the session.

Device availability

Based on the assessment of the client and his goals, the team can begin to conceptually narrow down the list of devices that might be useful. Deciding what equipment will be needed depends both on the specific goals as well as potential barriers to avoid. The team should ask the family if they have seen or heard of equipment that they would think would fit the goals. Pros and cons should be reviewed by all members of the team to identify a short list of devices to trial. To increase the chances that the device can be funded, the team should also strive to choose the least costly device that achieves all stated goals.

Equipment trial and decision

Trialing equipment during the session can be logistically difficult, but it should be pursued where possible. This trial can offer the chance to gauge expected fit, further define medical need, comfort, tolerance, and functional use. Lack of an appropriate trial can contribute to delivery complication and device abandonment. Given insurance reimbursement protocols, equipment often must be used for as long as 5 years, further highlighting the need for appropriate trials. In-home trials can be better than office/clinic trials. Regardless of location, the team should strive to mimic the day to day use of the device. The final decision should be the result of the assessment, discussion of devices, trial, and review. While the ultimate decision should rest with the family, often the family will look to the team to help make this decision. The ordering process as well as funding review sometimes takes several weeks to months, so the family often returns to clinic for final device delivery.

Funding/resource review

Funding should ideally flow from the demonstrated medical necessity of the ordered device. However, the process is rarely this straightforward. The client and family may have their own resources, but often third-party payers are utilized (e.g. medical insurance, state-based resources). The justification for any DME should include why similar equipment will not meet the goals of the client. If other less expensive options are not addressed in the assessment, then this is likely to be flagged by an insurance provider for likely denial. Remember to highlight the medical necessity and not solely convenience as many third-party payers will not recognize convenience as sufficient justification. If the selected device is unlikely to be funded, the team should return to the decision-making process to arrive at an option that is more likely to be funded or decide as a team that the device selected will likely need to be appealed if denied. The client and family should be educated on the remaining options and next steps.

The client and team should explore community resources including charities. Some organizations offer trade-in and borrowing programs, but the available choices may be more limited in this case. When children no longer need their DME either due to growth or improved function, some organizations will take donations of the soon to be abandoned equipment. These organizations typically recycle/repair/reuse the equipment to make it available to children/families with fewer funding resources. Such donation organizations/pathways may include early intervention therapy programs, school districts therapy offices, or peer to peer social networks. Whether donating or receiving donated equipment, the team must ensure the equipment is functioning properly and not in disrepair.

Delivery, fitting, education, and follow-up
The team should plan to have the client and family return once the device is prepared for delivery. The delivery date may be several weeks or months after the trial and device ordering process was initiated. Occasionally, adjustments are needed based on client growth or other factors that have changed since the original assessment. Education and review of device function and maintenance are important during delivery. Additionally, the team should explain how the family can get more information after they leave clinic on function, maintenance or repairs. Both secondary fitting and device education are crucial to maximize the end-user experience. Ideally, the client should return again several weeks after device delivery to review the original goals and ensure that no further education or modifications are needed.

Equipment

In planning for the lifetime needs of patients with cerebral palsy, it can be difficult to determine the most appropriate device at the most appropriate time. The best starting place for this is to assess according to the motor function and age of the patient. The DME Blueprints system shown in Table 5.1 is a conceptualization of common equipment needs for individuals with cerebral palsy indexed by GMFCS level and age. With age, comes a general estimate of the size of the patient and expected cognitive function; however, these will vary from patient to patient which the team must recognize. The Blueprints can help families and providers prepare for the sheer volume of equipment that might be needed over time as well as help the team anticipate needs. Many of these devices will be reviewed more specifically, but this chart is not exhaustive. The Blueprints are meant to be used as a starting place for the team and family.

Table 5.1 DME Blueprints system showing common equipment needs for individuals with cerebral palsy indexed by GMFCS level and age.

Age		GMFCS III	GMFCS IV	GMFCS V
At birth				Medical stroller
1 year	Early intervention	Medical stroller vs manual wheelchair Posture control walker Feeder seat	Medical stroller vs Tilt-in-space wheelchair Stander	Stander
2 years		Power wheelchair trial	Gait trainer Tub seat / Shower chair	Gait trainer Tub seat / Shower chair
3 years	Pre-school		Power wheelchair trial	Tilt-in-space Wheelchair
4 years				Hospital bed system
5 years	Elementary school	Hospital bed system Tub seat / Shower chair	Hospital bed system	
6 years		Manual wheelchair Posture control walker	Tilt-in-space Wheelchair Stander	Stander
7 years		Power wheelchair	Gait trainer Tub seat / Shower chair	Gait trainer Tub seat / Shower chair
8 years				Tilt-in-space wheelchair
9 years			Power wheelchair trial	
10 years		Tub seat / Shower chair		
11 years		Manual wheelchair Posture control walker	Tilt-in-space wheelchair Stander	Power wheelchair trial

Table 5.1 (Continued)

12 years	Middle school	Power wheelchair	Gait trainer Tub Seat / Shower chair	Stander Lift system
13 years				Tilt-in-space wheelchair Shower chair
14 years			Lift System	Hospital bed system
15 years	High school	Hospital bed system Tub seat / Shower chair	Hospital bed system	
16 years		Manual wheelchair Posture control walker	Tilt-in-space wheelchair Stander	
17 years		Power wheelchair	Tub seat / Shower chair	
18 years				Tilt-in-space wheelchair Shower transfer system
19+ years	Secondary education / Adulthood	Replacement of older DME	Replacement of older DME	Replacement of older DME

Copyright Jonathan Greenwood. Used with permission.

Seating

Due to the nature of complex cerebral palsy, many children spend a majority of their day in a seated position and the ideal seating system may need to be customized for the child with cerebral palsy. This is in part to accommodate the spasticity and/or low truncal tone that may be present as well as to ensure that asymmetric forces on the trunk and pelvis do not lead to pain and impaired skin integrity. Seating systems may or may not also be used for transportation and mobility. With regards to seating in wheelchairs, please refer to the Wheelchair section. Both wheeled and stationary seating must be closely reviewed.

Positioning and activity chairs

Pediatric clients may present with unique positioning needs throughout their day. Positioning and activity chairs may provide minimal to moderate postural support (see Figs. 5.1 and 5.2). These devices are often used in the classroom, especially when the primary mobility based seating system is not adequate for the needed function such as feeding or floor time with other children. Maintaining the principles of seating, positioning, and alignment are essential when selecting positioning and activity chairs.

Car seats, car beds, and transportation restraints

As children grow too large for commercial car seats and booster seats, the team should prepare to transition them to medical car seats or adaptive transportation systems. Medical car seats typically provide additional support such as lateral trunk and head supports and accommodate higher user weights than commercial car seats (Fig. 5.3). Medical car beds allow for safe transport of users who are unable to maintain a seated position and provide padding and strapping for support and added safety in supine, prone, and side-lying positions. Transportation restraints such as belts and vests may provide a safety component to transportation, but do not provide postural support. Special considerations for use of medical car seats include the need for proper installation in accordance with manufacturer guidelines and the avoidance of post-market alterations due to crash testing regulations.

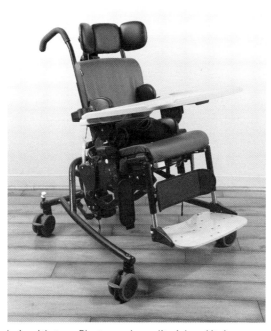

Figure 5.1 Activity chair with tray. Photograph credit: Adam Litvin

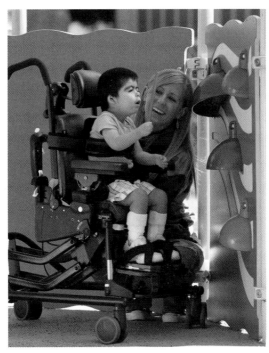

Figure 5.2   Child in activity chair. Photo © 2015 by Rifton Equipment. Used with permission.

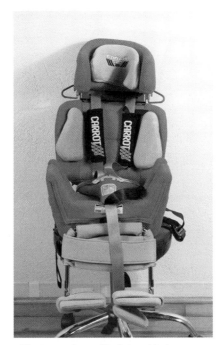

Figure 5.3   Medical car seat. Photograph credit: Adam Litvin.

Standing and upright activities

Pediatric clients with complex cerebral palsy and classified as GMFC levels IV and V will often be candidates for standing in devices. Standers are positional devices intended to place a child in the best possible upright standing position for prolonged weight bearing. Standing programs mitigate the impact of primary and secondary co-morbidities of immobility. For example, standing regimens have been shown to improve bone mineral density, hip stability, range of motion of the lower extremities, and spasticity measurements (Paleg et al. 2013). Stander variations include static upright standers, prone standers, supine standers and dynamic/mobile standers (Figs. 5.4–5.8). Standers can have unique features to meet the positional and functional needs of the child and family as well as functional features to add to daily enrichment goals. For example, sit-to-stand standers can provide for easy transition from one position to the other during the course of a school day (Fig. 5.9). These sit-to-stand devices are a functional hybrid between activity chairs and standers.

Gait trainers

Gait trainers should be considered for the child classified as GMFCS level IV, but may not always be helpful and should be reviewed on a case by case basis. For younger children who have not reached their functional potential, these devices are used to train

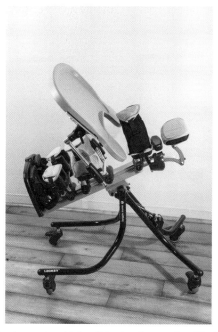

Figure 5.4 Supine stander in supine. Note: this stander can be tilted to a fully upright position. Photograph credit: Adam Litvin.

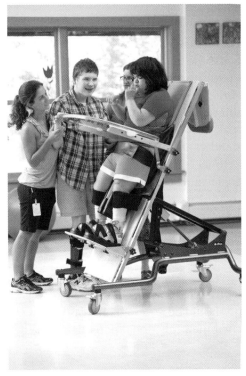

Figure 5.5   Child in supine stander. Photo © 2015 by Rifton Equipment. Used with permission.

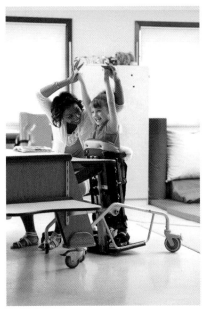

Figure 5.6   Child in prone stander. Photo © 2015 by Rifton Equipment. Used with permission.

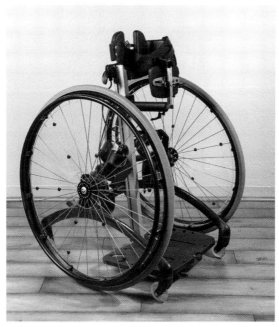

Figure 5.7 Mobile stander. Photograph credit: Adam Litvin.

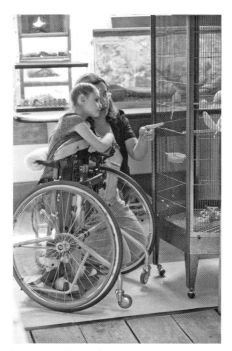

Figure 5.8 Child in mobile stander. Photo © 2015 by Rifton Equipment. Used with permission.

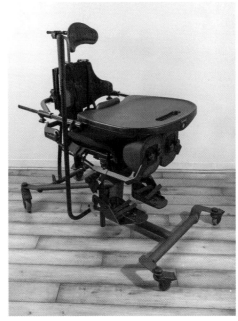

Figure 5.9 Sit-to-stand stander in seated position. Note the similarity to an activity chair. Photograph credit: Adam Litvin.

gait and some users move on to using a walker or other ambulatory devices. However, for most GMFCS level IV patients, gait trainers can be a long-term option for exercise and independent mobility. Gait trainers can provide variable amount of truncal and weight support as well as prevent leg adduction that can be a major obstacle to walking (Figs. 5.10–5.11). The front wheels of the gait trainer can be locked in one direction or allowed to swivel; locking them provides more stability when ambulating in one direction at the cost of increased difficulty with turns. Additional variations and supports vary by type of gait trainer.

Walkers

As a class, walkers provide children who have higher baseline postural control the ability to maintain upright and midline positioning with minimal balance as stability is achieved through upper limb contact with the device. Unlike gait trainers, walkers provide no weight-bearing or truncal support. Some gait trainers can be 'converted' to walkers, because the supports can be removed. Children who will benefit from walkers must be able to hold onto the device through the upper limbs or else they may fall through the device. However, this can be achieved without significant hand function through the use of platforms allowing for device control and support at the forearm, upper arm and/or shoulder girdle. For children, walkers are most often posterior or rear-facing and the child walks by pulling or rolling the device forward with her.

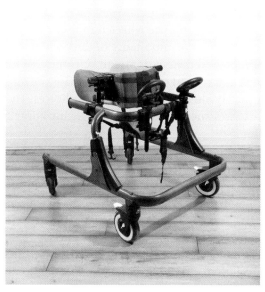

Figure 5.10   Gait trainer. Photograph credit: Adam Litvin.

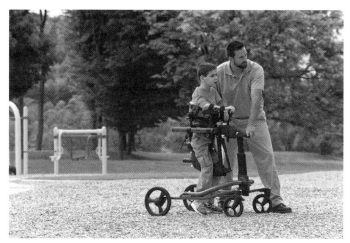

Figure 5.11   Child in gait trainer. Photo © 2015 by Rifton Equipment. Used with permission.

Anterior or forward-facing walkers can be considered, but often require additional push-ing force and postural control, which puts the child at risk of walking with a stooped posture or losing her center of gravity anteriorly and falling. Another option for a walker is a fold-down seat to be used at rest only; while not very supportive, it can be helpful if endurance is an issue.

Wheeled mobility

The equipment evaluation and delivery pathway (Box 5.1) is of utmost importance when assessing for the most appropriate wheeled mobility device. Specific to the process of obtaining wheelchairs is the importance of three variables: the wheelchair user, the wheelchair technology, and the environment or context of the user (Batavia et al. 2001). The environment and context of the user is perhaps the most difficult to capture at times and can completely alter the range of viable choices. The ICF framework can again be helpful in this assessment (World Health Organization 2007).

Adaptive strollers

Younger children and their caregivers may desire more commercial looking positioning devices such as adaptive strollers (Fig. 5.12). These devices are not true wheelchairs. Adaptive or medical strollers provide minimal to moderate dependent positioning, but require caregiver-dependent propulsion. These devices typically allow for a single system approach to positioning, where a manufacturer produces components unique to a single stroller type; these accessory components can be mounted on to the stroller and removed as needed. Medical strollers are designed to also provide more convenience and portability due to folding features, which some families need due to vehicle size restrictions.

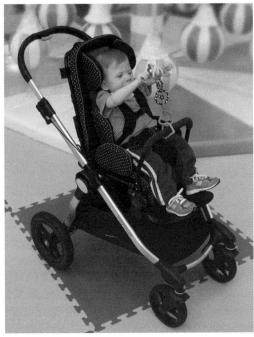

Figure 5.12   Zippie Voyage Medical Stroller © Sunrise Medical.

Wheelchairs

What truly separates adaptive strollers from wheelchairs is the amount of available postural support and the option for independent mobility. Families may struggle with the transition from a stroller to a wheelchair due to image concerns or worry of how the child will react to this change, as well as size concerns as the wheelchair may not be as portable. Due to this, the family may want to delay this transition or avoid it all together. However, usually the size of the child and/or the need to begin working on independent mobility require that the team and family work together to achieve this transition. Usually the obstacles and concerns of the family can be addressed with resource support and counseling. Any associated stigma that the wheelchair may have is often lessened by early conversation and education. Despite the wide range of wheelchair types most wheelchairs include the following components:

- base frame type and style (i.e. ultralight weight manual wheelchair, tilt-in-space manual wheelchair, power wheelchair);

- seating components (i.e. seat cushion, back cushion, lateral supports, headrest, additional positional supports);

- wheel type;

- accessories for additional medical supplies and other needs.

i. Base frame When assessing the needs of a wheelchair user and choosing a base, the team should consider several factors, including the level of cognitive function, environmental safety awareness and decision-making capabilities of the user. Environmental safety awareness and decision-making capabilities of the user relate directly to the expected functional independence. Visual, auditory and other sensory considerations should be closely evaluated; however, less than perfect skills in these areas do not preclude the ability to be independent. Do not assume all clients who have near full motor function of their upper extremities need a manual wheelchair frame as they may benefit from power-assisted mobility due to easy fatigability with self-propulsion. An example of a manual wheelchair is seen in Figure 5.13. In the same fashion, not all functionally dependent users will need powered mobility. Powered mobility does help maintain independence with mobility if that is a goal, but for the patient classified as GMFCS level V who does not have the fine motor skills or cognitive abilities required to operate a powered device then a non-powered option may be best for the family. An example of a powered wheelchair is seen in Figure 5.14.

The needs of the user versus cost and portability will be the most important considerations. Power wheelchairs can have many power drive options including mid wheel, rear wheel, or front wheel drive function, and can be driven by the user or the care giver depending on the setup. Advanced electronics options are available for switch drive access and

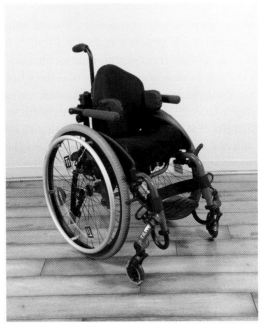

Figure 5.13   Manual wheelchair. Photograph credit: Adam Litvin.

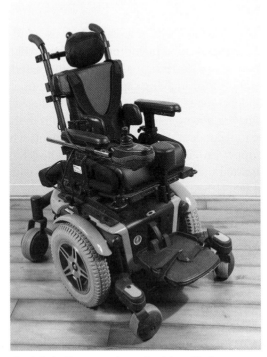

Figure 5.14   Power wheelchair. Photograph credit: Adam Litvin.

environmental controls for user access to ensure independent mobility. With powered mobility, changes to the sensitivity on the joystick as well as lowering maximum device speed can make an unsafe user into an independent user. However, all of these devices are bulky and difficult to transfer without a specialized vehicle.

Another option built into a base is tilt-in-space, which can help with gravity assisted re-positioning and skin pressure relief related to seating. Additionally, assessing for the need for seat recline and sit-to-stand options are important (Dicianno et al. 2015). Tilt-in-space, recline, and sit-to-stand options do not require a powered base, but often are considered with powered chairs.

ii. Wheelchair seating The primary seating system for many children with motorically complex cerebral palsy is the seat in the wheelchair. A primary seating system needs to be dynamic enough to provide good postural support and functional positioning for the widest range of daily activities while respecting anatomical and neuromuscular needs of the user. Special considerations for seating include pressure distribution needs, positional support and accommodating growth. For children with severe scoliosis, a custom molded seating system may be able to provide comfortable positional support. If a child wears a spinal orthosis for positioning and not slowing curve progression, then the custom molded seating can sometimes replace the need for the spinal orthosis. Dynamic spring loaded reclining can be very helpful to the child with dystonic posturing so that the chair can accommodate this posturing. Otherwise the child will have postural reactions that move them out of good positioning in the seat. Seating options may be customized to the user and often updated or changed while keeping the wheelchair base frame the same.

iii. Wheel type Wheel type is important to consider with respect to the expected level of independence by the user as well as terrain in which the chair will be used. The location and type of wheels are important. For manual wheelchair users, increasing camber or stability of the wheel base can be important as well as having wheels with different levels of shock absorption. Also, the wheels must be forward enough to reach for propulsion. For power wheelchairs, the wheels are usually smaller in diameter but more sturdy to accommodate the weight of the device.

iv. Accessories This chapter is not able to cover many of the potentially helpful wheelchair accessories for users and care providers. However, some of the most helpful accessories are removable trays to provide a place for eating, learning, play and communication. These are also useful on activity chairs and standers. Additional accessories might include postural and positional supports, pommels, holders for oxygen tanks, feeding pumps, suction machines, ventilators or other medical supplies, depending on the child's needs. Accessories should be manufacturer approved and reviewed for safety by the clinical team whenever possible. For example, electronics accessories should be integrated into powered chairs by the manufacturer whenever possible to prevent malfunction leading to significant battery drain or failure.

Other assistive and adaptive technology
While seating, standing and mobility are important for the child with motorically complex cerebral palsy, assistive and adaptive technology can also help improve other areas of daily life including but not limited to bathing, sleeping, transfers, recreational sports, head control, communication, hand function, ergonomics, or visual/sensory enrichment. Devices that augment these areas can range from 'low-tech,' such as a foam handle for a spoon, to 'high-tech,' such as proprietary communication hardware. Recreational sports devices, including adaptive sports equipment, are popular but can be difficult to fund with third-party payers. One example of adaptive sports equipment is an adaptive tricycle or trike (Fig. 5.15). The remainder of this section highlights transfer systems, medical beds, and bathroom equipment.

Transfer systems
Transfer systems can be vital to the safety patient and care provider by preventing falls and caregiver lifting injuries. Transfer systems include lifts and ceiling track systems. The most basic transfer system is a manual hydraulic lift (Fig. 5.16). Proper training on lift use is essential. The lift sling is the fabric portion that holds the user and is important to trial as body habitus and musculoskeletal deformities can preclude safe use of the lift. Electronic lifts are also available, but are less often funded by third-party payers. Ceiling track systems work similarly in that a sling holds the patient but the lift mechanism is installed into the ceiling component of the track system. While this is also difficult to fund, it has the benefit of taking up less floor space than a lift for the trade-off of less flexibility in where to take the patient.

Medical beds
Specialized bedding may be recommended to promote a safe sleep environment for children with various conditions where commercially available bedding does not meet their medical needs. These beds may be in the form of manual or electric hospital beds, medical cribs and full/partial enclosure beds. Specialized bedding may provide various adaptations such as head of bed elevation for respiratory or digestive conditions which require the head of the bed to be elevated during the night; foot of bed elevation for lower extremity positioning at night; high–low elevation of the bed surface to provide improved functional transfers or improved safety of transfers; specialized mattresses to provide adequate pressure relief to protect skin during sleep; or full/partial enclosures to provide safety to the child exhibiting extraneous involuntary movements or volitional self-injurious movements during the night. Specialized beds come in many forms; however, it is essential to ensure that the bed is able to target the specific safety, medical and functional needs of the child.

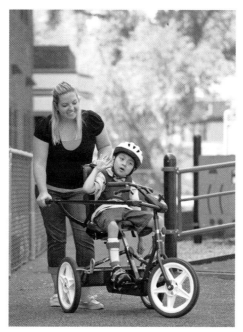

Figure 5.15   Child in adaptive tricycle. Photo © 2015 by Rifton Equipment. Used with permission.

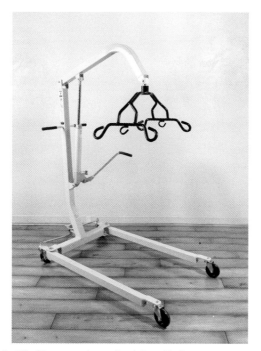

Figure 5.16   Hydraulic lift. Photograph credit: Adam Litvin.

Bathroom equipment

Bathing and toileting are two daily activities that can pose specific challenges for the child with motorically complex cerebral palsy. Whether a child is independent or dependent for the activities, proper equipment can be very helpful. The goal of the equipment is to promote good positioning and ergonomics as well as prevent injury from lifting or falls. Examples of toileting systems are seen in Figures 5.17 and 5.18. A bath or shower chair can vary in how much postural support is offered and examples are seen in Figures 5.19 and 5.20. Also, a bath lift for a tub can be very helpful for a user due to the low height of most tubs (Fig. 5.21).

Conclusion

Medical equipment prescription and delivery is a chance for the family and clinical team to connect on what is important for the child and how to optimize daily function. Devices can be offered, but they only really become important and helpful when the team and family agree on a certain recommendation. This highlights why family and patient participation in the development of goals, selection of equipment, and training with equipment cannot be understated. Periodic reassessment of equipment

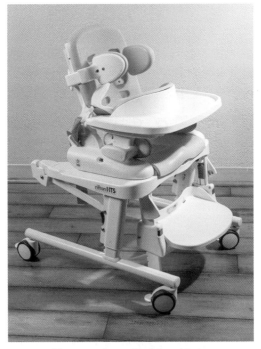

Figure 5.17   Toileting system. Photograph credit: Adam Litvin.

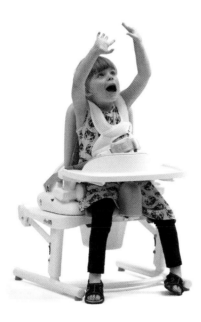

Figure 5.18 Child in toileting system. Photo © 2015 by Rifton Equipment. Used with permission.

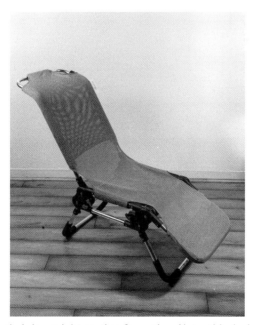

Figure 5.19 Shower chair in upright seating formation. Note: this device can be adjusted to be fully flat to allow the child to be in supine positioning. Photograph credit: Adam Litvin.

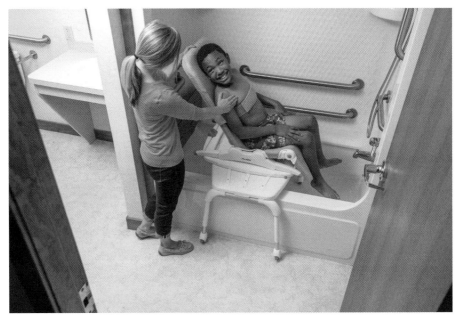

Figure 5.20 Child in seated shower chair. Photo © 2015 by Rifton Equipment. Used with permission.

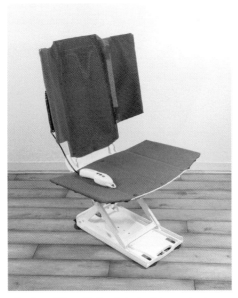

Figure 5.21 Tub lift in raised position. Note: this device can be lowered all the way to the ground electronically to allow for bathing in a tub. Photograph credit: Adam Litvin.

appropriateness and fit where applicable should be pursued. In particular a re-evaluation is needed after major surgeries that can impact positioning, such as spinal fusion, bilateral osteotomies, and baclofen pump placement. When following these guidelines, the positive impact of equipment and devices on the lives of children with complex cerebral palsy can be enormous.

Summary points

- Anyone on a child's healthcare team can identify the need for an equipment evaluation. While it is ideal to have an interdisciplinary team for the evaluation, this is not always possible and should not prevent attempts to obtain equipment.

- Client assessment (Box 5.1: Step 3) is likely the most important component of the equipment evaluation and delivery process, because understanding a child's functional status in the context of her (and her family's) goals is crucial.

- Equipment trials should be pursued prior to purchase, if at all possible.

- Equipment must be monitored for maintenance, adjustments, and timely replacement due to growth, surgical interventions, and other factors which may change over time.

- Clinicians can use the DME Blueprints (Table 5.1) to prescribe equipment based on age and motoric function and predict future needs over the lifespan of a child.

Acknowledgments

Special thanks to Adam Litvin, RN, BSN for photography expertise. Special thanks to Andrew Lewandowski, RTS/ATP and National Seating and Mobility for access to equipment for photography.

Resources

For up to date guidelines and recommendations on many types of equipment.

Websites
http://www.resna.org/at-standards
https://www.disability.gov/resource/disability-govs-guide-assistive-technology/
http://www.seatingandmobility.ca/Education.aspx

Book
Ann-Christian Eliasson, Patricia Burtner, editors (2008) Improving Hand Function in Children with Cerebral Palsy. Theory, Evidence and Intervention. Mac Keith Press. ISBN: 9781898683537.

Conferences

http://www.seatingsymposium.com/

https://www.atia.org/conference/

References

Arledge S, Armstrong W, Babinec M, Dicianno BE, Di Giovine C, Dyson-Hudson T et al. (2011) *RESNA Wheelchair Service Provision Guide*. Rehabilitation Engineering & Assistive Technology Society of North America. https://www.resna.org/sites/default/files/legacy/resources /position-papers/RESNAWheelchairServiceProvisionGuide.pdf.

Batavia M, Batavia AI, Friedman R (2001) Changing chairs: anticipating problems in prescribing wheelchairs. *Disabil Rehabil* **23**(12): 539–548.

Dicianno BE, Lieberman J, Schmeler MR, Souza AE, Cooper R, Lange M et al. (2015) Rehabilitation Engineering and Assistive Technology Society of North America's position on the application of tilt, recline, and elevating leg rests for wheelchairs literature update. *Assistive Technology* **27**(3): 193–198.

Meehl S, D iGiovine C, Berner T (2012) Seating and mobility service delivery process. RESNA Annual Conference, June 28–July 3.

Paleg GS, Smith BA, Glickman LB (2013) Systematic review and evidence-based clinical recommendations for dosing of pediatric supported standing programs. *Pediatric Physical Therapy* **25**(3): 232–247.

World Health Organization (2007) *International Classification of Functioning, Disability, and Health: Children & Youth Version: ICF-CY*. World Health Organization. http://www.who.int /classifications/icf/en/.

Chapter 6

Osteoporosis and fractures

Steven J. Bachrach and Heidi H. Kecskemethy

Introduction

Children with severe cerebral palsy (CP) are at increased risk for under-mineralized bones that fracture with minimal trauma. Evaluating bone health in children and young adults with CP can be challenging and requires consideration of many of the following factors for clinical decision-making:

- the patient's nutritional status including type and modality of feeding, nutrient intake, and serum level of specific nutrients

- assessment of medications and their potential effect on bone

- amount and type of weight bearing

- medical history including co-morbidities and fracture history

- stage in puberty

- bone mineral density (BMD) results.

All or a combination of these factors affect a patient's overall picture of bone health. Familiarity with the tools available to assess bone health is important for practitioners. The American Academy for Cerebral Palsy and Developmental Medicine has published a Care Pathway (available at https://www.aaCPdm.org/publications/care-pathways) based on current evidence that outlines the care of the child with osteoporosis and offers practical tools. In this chapter we describe how bone is accrued throughout childhood, aspects that influence the accrual, bone density assessment and interpretation of results, and treatment options for low bone density/fractures. Questions around who should be treated pharmacologically, for how long, and with what drug are discussed. We provide recommendations on methods to maximize bone health in children with CP.

Bone acquisition and normal growth

Bones typically grow quickly throughout childhood and adolescence, achieving approximately 90% of adult, or peak bone mass, by the third decade of life (Bonjour et al. 1991, Heaney et al. 2000). Bones grow through a process of conversion of chondrocytes in cartilage to mineralized bone in the end plates of long bones (endochondral ossification), and through intramembranous ossification of the flat bones. Modeling and remodeling of bone occurs through osteoblasts and osteoclasts and is determined by forces on the bone, by genetics, and by other factors including hormonal status, sex, and diet. Bones adapt based on need, changing internal architecture and shape, described by Wolff's Law.

In childhood, modeling and remodeling results in increasing bone size and accrual of bone mineral content and density over time. Remodeling is required for repair and maintenance, and through remodeling, calcium and phosphorus are liberated from bone to be used for body functions. This modeling and remodeling occur continuously throughout life. Children typically accrue new bone at a greater rate than is lost through remodeling. During adult years, bone mass is usually maintained, and by the fifth decade of life, the rate of remodeling exceeds the rate of deposition resulting in bone loss in later adulthood. If the attainment of peak bone mass is compromised, there is greater risk for fracture and osteoporosis later in life (Melton et al. 1989, Hui et al. 1990).

The mineral portion of bone, hydroxyapatite, serves as a repository of calcium, phosphorus, and magnesium. These nutrients are needed for homeostasis and for body functions. The chief nutrients of concern for bone health are calcium, vitamin D, and phosphorus. Calcium is the foremost mineral in hydroxyapatite, and dietary intake of calcium is frequently insufficient. Vitamin D is essential for bone mineral accretion and intestinal absorption of dietary calcium. Insufficient phosphorus negatively affects mineralization, yet too much phosphorus decreases the circulating levels of the active form of vitamin D. There are other nutrients of concern for bone health, but a varied diet typically provides adequate intake of these nutrients. Nutrient status and amount of weight bearing, as well as bone development and the amount of bone mineral accrued during childhood, are all important contributors to the overall picture of bone health in children with complex or severe CP.

Why this population is at risk

Children with complex CP are at high risk for compromised bone health due to limited or lack of weight bearing, compromised nutritional status, use of medications that compromise bone metabolism, and lack of sun exposure and/or low serum levels of vitamin D (Apkon and Kecskemethy 2008, Szalay and Cheema 2011, Henderson et al. Henderson 2002a, 2004). Medical and disease conditions can also change metabolism and normal bone accrual, negatively impact overall nutritional status and bone health, and increase risk for fracture. The site and mechanism of fracture differs between typically developing children and children with severe CP. The most common site of fracture in typical children is the forearm and occurs due to a fall or trauma (Cooper et al. 2004). Fractures in children with severe CP occur with little or no trauma and most frequently occur in the lower extremities. Once a child with CP has sustained a fragility fracture, they are at even higher risk of sustaining additional fractures (Goulding et al. 2005, Stevenson et al. 2006).

Weight bearing

The effects of no weight bearing or immobilization from casting are well-documented: bone loss occurs resulting in decreased bone mineral density and weaker bones that are more susceptible to fracture (Giangregorio and McCartney 2006, Ceroni et al. 2012). Low BMD of the lower extremities, the most common site to fracture in non-ambulatory children with CP, has been well-described. Compromised lower extremity BMD and history of fracture has been described in children with other non-ambulatory conditions including Duchenne muscular dystrophy (DMD), and spina bifida (Harcke et al. 2006, Haas et al. 2012). In children with CP, a combination of atypical muscle tone combined with lack of weight bearing likely contributes to differences in bone growth and development. Lack of load-bearing results in reduced periosteal expansion. In tibiae of children with CP who are unable to stand or load the bones of their lower extremities, structural differences have been noted: the bones that develop are smaller and thinner (Binkley et al. 2005). Non- and minimally ambulatory children with CP have lower tibial cross-sectional area and cortical bone area than children with CP who can walk (Wren et al. 2011). In addition to the structural differences, the rate of bone accrual is lower in children with severe CP compared to typically developing, weight bearing children.

Nutrition and nutritional status

Nutrition in children with severe CP may be compromised by many factors, including reflexes associated with CP. For instance, a tonic bite reflex and tongue thrust can compromise the amount of food a child can ingest. These children may also have swallowing difficulties, putting them at risk for aspiration, and limiting the amount and the consistency of what they can safely eat. Other issues that can cause limited intake include dental caries and/or gum disease, severe gastro-esophageal reflux and constipation, all of which are more common in this population. Studies have shown that children with severe CP who are oral feeders take longer to feed at each meal, and they receive only a small percentage of what has been offered to them (Gisel and Patrick 1988). Feeding difficulties and their associated nutritional sequelae result in poor growth and nutritional status. Compromised nutritional status, whether from inadequate intake, intolerance to feeds or volume, fatigue, or the inability to digest and absorb nutrients, is a major risk factor for compromised bone health.

Medications
Certain medications are reported to negatively impact bone density by blocking or changing the absorption or metabolism of nutrients or by altering metabolic processes of the body. The medications that can affect bone and/or increase risk for fracture include chronic use of steroids, proton pump inhibitors, some anticonvulsants (particularly phenobarbital and phenytoin), antidepressants, and depot medroxyprogesterone acetate (Kecskemethy and Harcke 2014). It is prudent to consider if an alternative is available to the medication that may negatively affect bone. When the benefits outweigh the risks, beginning or continuing the medication while monitoring bone density may be best for the patient.

Assessment and interpretation of bone density

The most readily available and widely used modality for assessing BMD is dual energy X-ray absorptiometry (DXA). Other imaging modalities, including quantitative ultrasound (Jekovec-Vrhovsek M et al. 2005), quantitative computed tomography (Binkley, Wren) and magnetic resonance imaging (Modlesky et al. 2008), have been used to assess and describe bone in children with CP. The use of these other modalities is limited to research purposes; they have limited clinical utility. DXA is used for clinical assessment of BMD.

Assessment
The recommended body sites to measure by DXA in children are the total body and lumbar spine, and in children with neuromuscular involvement such as complex CP, the lateral distal femur is a suggested alternative (Crabtree et al. 2014). The lateral distal femur (LDF) DXA was developed specifically for children with CP and other neuromuscular conditions because the standard body sites to measure are frequently unobtainable due to excessive movement and positioning limitations and/or from the presence of non-removable hardware (Harcke et al. 1998, Henderson 2002b&c) (Fig. 6.1) Contractures and high muscle tone create positioning challenges, and artifacts from indwelling metal (rods, clips, screws, baclofen pump) or tubes (shunt, feeding tubes or buttons) affect bone density results. The LDF DXA provides information about bone density for the most clinically relevant site – that which is most apt to fracture (Fig. 6.2). The LDF scan is a non-standard scan and is not resident on any bone densitometer machine. Acquisition and analysis protocols have been standardized but training is required to ensure correct use of the LDF DXA technique. LDF DXA normative values are available for Hologic machines only (Zemel et al. 2009).

The decision to order a DXA for a child with complex CP should be individualized. Some suggest getting a DXA on every child with complex CP by approximately age 10,

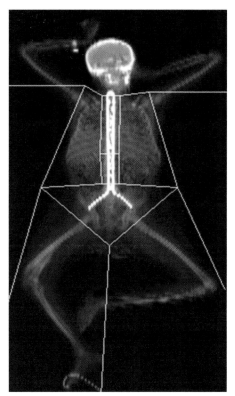

Figure 6.1 Contractures, skeletal deformities, and indwelling metallic artifacts are commonly encountered when measuring bone mineral density by dual energy X-ray absorptiometry in children with severe cerebral palsy. Note artifacts and positioning limitations that affect results: spinal fusion rod, pulse oximeter lead on right toe, and ID band on right wrist.

as most children will have low bone density by that age. However, others think this is not necessary if it will not change treatment. Certainly, any child who has had a non-traumatic fracture, especially if treatment with bisphosphonates is being considered, should have a DXA done. Other children where a DXA should be considered include those where plain X-rays are read as osteopenic by the radiologist, those who will be undergoing major bone surgery where the surgeon is concerned that poor bone quality may negatively impact the surgical outcome, or any child where the results will help manage care and treatment. In most of these situations, a referral to a specialist who manages low bone density in children should be considered. If the DXA is being done as a baseline to document the status of the bone density and to educate the family on the importance of preventive measures (see Prevention below), the primary care provider (PCP) may feel comfortable ordering the study and interpreting it for the parents. If the DXA study is being obtained at an adult imaging center, the PCP should inquire about availability of pediatric software.

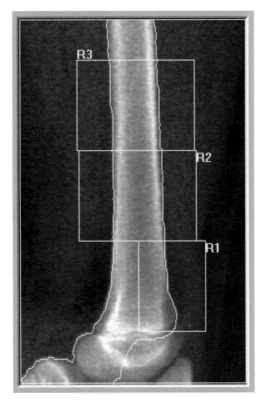

Figure 6.2 The lateral distal femur dual energy X-ray absorptiometry analysis produces information for three regions of interest which reflects differing proportions of trabecular and cortical bone. Region 1 (metaphysis) contains primarily trabecular bone; Region 2 (metadiaphyseal) contains a mixture of trabecular and cortical bone; and Region 3 (diaphyseal) contains primarily cortical bone.

Reproducibility in DXA is very important for accuracy of results. Measuring the growing skeleton poses unique challenges for bone assessment due to growing bones, and this is magnified in children with CP because of skeletal changes over time due to contractures or worsening scoliosis, and the addition of indwelling artifacts (rods, pumps) and fractures. Sometimes sedation is used for acquisition of DXA; however, the clinician should evaluate the value of the information versus the risk of sedation for the patient. It is especially challenging to obtain a technically valid total body DXA as the scan takes from 3–6 minutes to acquire, depending on the scanner, scan modality used, and size of the patient. Lumbar spine DXA acquisition is much quicker, at less than a minute, but artifacts can be common at this body site due to movement, metal scoliosis rods, feeding tubes and buttons, shunt tubing, and/or baclofen pumps. The LDF DXA is acquired in a comfortable side-lying position and it is generally well-tolerated with a scan time of less than 2 minutes. It can almost always be obtained without sedation if the technologist is familiar with both the technique and how to work with children with CP. The ordering physician should have a conversation with the imaging center to determine the center's familiarity with measuring children and scanning techniques used for children with disabilities, before sending a child for a DXA scan. Pediatric software on the bone densitometer is required for correct results. When ordering DXA, it is helpful for the imaging center to know about the patient – the indication for the study, ambulatory status, the presence of metal and other non-removable artifacts, fracture history, medications used (especially bisphosphonate), and Tanner Stage – to guide what body sites should be measured and to aid in the interpretation of results. Unless the imaging center understands the needs of children with disabilities and has the correct pediatric software, the results will likely be difficult or even impossible to interpret.

Interpretation
DXA results are reported as both BMD values (gm/cm^2) and as Z-scores. Z-scores are an indicator of how far the child's BMD value is from the average value for typically developing children of the same age and sex. A Z-score of less than –2.0 is considered 'below normal or low'. It is common for children with severe CP to have low BMD. Evaluating risk factors for low BMD can aid in interpretation of the results. Lack of ambulation is the greatest risk factor for low BMD of the lower extremities. Physical development and pubertal status are also important considerations. Size adjustments to BMD results are recommended, but the type of adjustment depends on the scanner used and body part scanned.

The first scan acquired will serve as the baseline against which all future scans will be compared. Scans acquired on machines from differing manufacturers are not comparable – the machines use different technologies, each have their own set of normative values and they produce different results. Acquisition of as many body sites as is possible at the baseline scan is important because the utility of body sites may decrease over time as hardware is inserted, and bony surgeries or fractures occur. It is important to remember that each patient can serve as their own control over time, even if normative values are not applicable due to technical concerns on the DXA.

For follow-up studies, it is important that the scans be as comparable as possible. It may be impossible to position a child with severe CP in the recommended or optimal position for typical children. Reproducing position from scan to scan is extremely important for serial scans. The effect of bisphosphonates in the growing skeleton is especially apparent in highly trabecular bone regions – at the end of the long bones and in the spine. Normal growth over time is reflected by stable Z-scores. Increasing Z-scores indicate higher than normal bone accrual (increasing BMD), and worsening Z-scores indicate lack of bone accrual. The interval between scans is determined by when meaningful change might occur. The typical time interval for monitoring BMD in children is annually, though this is governed by clinical course, treatment, number and type of risk factors, and age.

Prevention

Nutrition

The main focus on preventing low bone density in this population is assuring the adequate intake of calcium, phosphorus, and vitamin D. There are other micronutrients that are important to bone health, such as zinc and magnesium, which may be deficient with severe malnutrition. The child on a regular diet will meet his phosphorus needs from meat, fish, eggs, and poultry. Calcium is primarily found in dairy products, though there are other good dietary sources of calcium, such as tofu, which can be added into blenderized tube feeds or smoothies (Table 6.1). For the child solely on G-tube feedings, both calcium and phosphorus intake should be evaluated. A quick way to calculate this is to read the label on the container for calcium and phosphorus content and multiply by the number of containers per day the child is getting. The goal is to meet the age-specific dietary reference intake (DRI) for those two minerals (Table 6.2). While the DRI for vitamin D is 600 IU from 1 to 70 years of age, serum levels should be obtained in order to maintain the level of 25-OH-vitamin D in the 'sufficient' range. The Endocrine Society has defined this as a level of 30 ng/mL or higher (Holick et al. 2011), whereas the most recent report from the Institute of Medicine (IOM) defined this as 20 ng/mL or higher, in a healthy population (IOM 2011). Because the non-ambulatory CP population is at high risk for low BMD, we recommend aiming for a level of 30–40 ng/mL. To achieve these levels, many patients will need supplements ranging between 1 000 to 8 000 IU daily, especially those who get little sun exposure (Table 6.3). The IOM report also recommended not exceeding serum levels of 50 ng/mL because of emerging evidence for potential adverse effects, especially at levels above 60 ng/mL. Checking a serum 25-OH-vitamin D level should be done annually beginning around age 3 years, and children with levels below 30 ng/mL should be supplemented with vitamin D.

Weight bearing: standers, gait trainers

As described earlier, lack of stress on the bone from lack of ambulation has a negative effect on BMD and bone morphology (Aguirre et al. 2006). It has been shown that weight-bearing exercise enhances bone mineral accrual in healthy children, particularly during early puberty (Hind and Burrows 2007). Weight bearing in standers and gait trainers is thought to provide several health benefits to children with CP such as improved gastro-intestinal motility, better lung function, increased bone density and improved socialization. However, only a positive effect on bone density and temporary reduction in spasticity has been demonstrated in reports of small numbers of patients in uncontrolled studies (Pin 2007). Well-controlled studies, especially in the non-ambulatory population, are needed (Paleg et al. 2014). On a practical note, positioning children with complex CP in standers can be challenging and few such children tolerate more than an hour a day in a stander. A pediatric physical therapist can best assess which type of stander (prone, supine, sit-to-stand) or gait trainer would be safest and most appropriate.

Table 6.1 Dietary sources of calcium

Dairy products: milk and yogurt	Serving size	Calcium (mg)
Milk, whole, 2%, 1%, skim, lactose-reduced, buttermilk, chocolate	8 oz.	316
Canned, evaporated with added Vitamin A and D	4 oz.	329–371
Milk, dry	¼ cup	377
Yogurt, plain, or flavored	6 oz.	258
Yogurt, fruit bottom	6 oz.	250
Yogurt, Greek, plain	6 oz	187
Yogurt, children's (eg: GoGurt)	1 tube	100
Yogurt smoothie, drinkable	3 oz.	100
Frozen yogurt	8 oz.	174
Ice cream	½ cup	84
Non-dairy beverages	Serving size	Calcium (mg)
Soy Milk, Silk	8 oz.	450
Orange juice (fortified with calcium and vitamin D)	4 oz.	175
Almond Milk, Almond Breeze	8 oz.	450
Soy-based foods	Serving size	Calcium (mg)
Tofu, firm/extra firm, in calcium	½ cup	250
Tofu, silken/regular, in calcium	1 slice	30
Soybeans, cooked	1 cups	260
Soybeans, roasted	1 cup	237
Meats, fish, and poultry products	Serving size	Calcium (mg)
Salmon, pink, canned	3 oz.	51
Sardines, pink, canned with bones	3 oz.	180
Legumes	Serving size	Calcium (mg)
White beans, cooked	1 cup	161
Navy beans	1 cup	126
Pinto beans, chickpeas	1 cup	79
Baked beans	1 cup	80–126

Table 6.1 (Continued)

Other	Serving size	Calcium (mg)
Brown sugar	1 cup	183
Blackstrap molasses	1 tbsp	200
Regular molasses	1 tbsp	41
Egg Custard	½ cup	150
Pancakes, made with milk	3 med.	150
Waffles (eg: Eggo)	1 ea.	132
Puddings, ready-to-eat	4 oz	54
Dairy products: Cheese	**Serving size**	**Calcium (mg)**
Cheese, soft: blue or feta	1 oz (30 g)	150
Cheese, hard: brick, cheddar, Colby, mozzarella, Swiss (includes lower-fat varieties)	1 oz	200–300
Cheese, processed spread	1 oz	130
Cheese, processed slices	1 slice	150
Cheese, grated parmesan	2 tbsp	110
Cheese, ricotta	½ cup	334
Cheese, cottage (1% or 2%)	2 cups	280
Cheese, cottage (nonfat)	2 cups	250
Macaroni and cheese (box mix)	1 cup	160
Fruits	**Serving size**	**Calcium (mg)**
Orange	1 med	60
Figs, dried	1 cup	241
Vegetables (measures for cooked vegetables)	**Serving size**	**Calcium (mg)**
Turnip Greens	½ cup	98.5
Bok choy/Chinese cabbage	½ cup	75
Kale, mustard greens	½ cup	165
Okra, frozen	½ cup	62
Broccoli	½ cup	31
Brussel sprouts	½ cup	28
Rutabaga, mashed	½ cup	21
Seaweed, raw: agar	½ cup	20

Table 6.1 (Continued)

Grain products	Serving size	Calcium (mg)
Oats, instant, enriched	1 pouch	100
Nuts and seeds	**Serving size**	**Calcium (mg)**
Almonds, dry roast	¼ cup	92
Almond butter	2 tbsp	112
Sesame Seeds, toasted kernels	¼ cup	42
Tahini	2 tbsp	130
Hazelnuts, chopped	¼ cup	32

Table 6.2 Dietary reference intake (DRI) for calcium and phosphorus

Age (years)	Calcium (mg)	Phosphorus (mg)
1–3	700	460
4–8	1000	500
9–18	1300	1250
19–50	1000	700
51–70	1000 males/1200 females	700

Table 6.3 Vitamin D intakes recommended for males and females by the Institute of Medicine (IOM) and the Endocrine Practice Guidelines Committee

Age (yr)	IOM recommendations for healthy populations[a]			Endocrine Society recommendations for patients at risk for vitamin D deficiency[b]	
	EAR	RDA	UL	Daily requirement (IU)	UL (IU)
1–3	400 IU (10 µg)	600 IU (15 µg)	2500 IU (63 µg)	600–1000	4000
4–8	400 IU (10 µg)	600 IU (15 µg)	3000 IU (75 µg)	600–1000	4000
9–13	400 IU (10 µg)	600 IU (15 µg)	4000 IU (100 µg)	600–1000	4000
14–18	400 IU (10 µg)	600 IU (15µg)	4000 IU (100 µg)	600–1000	4000
19–70	400 IU (10 µg)	600IU (15 µg)	4000 IU (100 µg)	1500–2000	10000

[a]IOM (2011); [b]Holick (2011)
EAR, estimated average requirement; RDA, Recommended Dietary Allowance; UL, tolerable upper intake level

Table 6.4   Bone Health Assessment Guide for the Primary Care Provider

Evaluate	When	How Often
Growth	Birth	Every well visit
Nutrition		
Feeding modality	Birth	Every well visit
Nutrient intake (in collaboration with dietitian)	2 years	Annually or with change in feeding modality
Medications	Birth	Every well visit
Weight Bearing Activities (in collaboration with PT)	2 years	Every well visit
Serum 25-OH-Vitamin D	3 years of age	Annually

Awareness of medications

As discussed above, certain medications can adversely affect bone density. Clinicians should consider these effects when evaluating drug choices and choose alternatives when possible. For instance, when starting birth control for a young woman with CP, there are many alternatives to depot medroxyprogesterone acetate, which is known to lower bone density even in a healthy, ambulatory population. Specific anti-convulsants, including phenobarbital, phenytoin and valproic acid, can cause decreased vitamin D levels (Kecskemethy and Harcke 2014). While there are many other anticonvuslants available, if a patient's seizures are well-controlled on one or more of these medications, an alternative is to continue their use while monitoring vitamin D levels more frequently and supplementing to maintain an appropriate level. Proton pump inhibitors are another class of medication that can adversely affect bone density, but alternatives are limited. If these drugs are used chronically, then obtaining a baseline DXA may be useful for later comparison.

Table 6.4 summarizes assessment and preventive measures for bone health in children with CP.

Treatments

Nutritional deficiencies and weight bearing

Correcting nutritional deficiencies and maximizing weight bearing have been discussed as preventive measures. However, if a child presents with a fragility fracture and these issues have not been addressed, then they should be addressed promptly. Assess the intake of calcium and phosphorus (consultation with a Registered Dietitian may be helpful), check a 25-OH-vitamin D level, and assess whether the child is able to weight-bear either in a stander or gait trainer. Evaluation with a physical therapist might be helpful.

Vibration

Strain signals, which arise in bone tissue during loading, enhance bone density. The absence of such signals is considered the key factor in the bone fragility of children who are non-ambulatory. Experiments in animals have demonstrated that high frequency (10–90 Hz), extremely low magnitude (<100 microstrain) stimuli are anabolic to trabecular bone (Rubin et al. 2004). Attempts to replicate this effect in children with CP have yielded mixed results (Ward et al. 2004, Wren et al. 2010, Ruck et al. 2010, Duquette et al. 2015, Gusso et al. 2016). Some health benefits have been seen but primarily in children with ambulatory CP. There are limited reports describing the effect of vibration therapy on BMD in the GMFCS IV–V population (who are at the highest risk of low density and fragility fractures); clearly more studies are needed for this population before recommending such therapy with confidence.

Medications

Bisphosphonates are the most commonly used and extensively studied medications to treat osteoporosis. A number of other classes of drugs used in adults are less commonly used in children and some newer drugs are currently being studied.

Bisphosphonates

Bisphosphonates act at the bone tissue level by inhibiting bone resorption. They have been extensively studied for treating osteoporosis in the elderly, and have been approved by the FDA for this purpose. Bisphosphonates have been used for decades to treat children with osteoporosis.

When to treat

Many clinicians treat a child with bisphosphonate when the child has low bone density, the preventive measures noted above have been made, and the child suffers one or more fragility fractures. Other clinicians will opt to treat with bisphosphonates based on low BMD and the presence of other risk factors alone, not waiting for fracture to occur. Subspecialty consultation is advised before beginning treatment with bisphosphonates in a child with complex CP.

Which drug

There are currently several generations of bisphosphonates in use. The two most commonly used bisphosphonates for children with CP are given intravenously, because intravenous infusion assures more complete and uniform drug dosing. Absorption of orally administered bisphosphonates is variable and administration via feeding tube has not been studied.

Pamidronate

In children, the best studied and longest used drug is pamidronate. The most common regimen for pamidronate is to treat with 1 mg/kg/dose (maximum of 60 mg), infused over 4 hours, for 3 consecutive days, every 3–4 months; other doses and schedules have been used. The first 3-day course is often given as half the usual dose (0.5 mg/kg/dose in the most common regimen) so that side effects are minimized. Duration of treatment is variable, and there is little evidence to support any of the different regimens. Suggested treatment regimens include 1 year, 1 year followed by a tapering schedule, treatment until a Z-score of greater than –2.0 is achieved, and treatment until puberty is complete. BMD typically increases during treatment, and then decreases after discontinuation. However, the children remain fracture-free for many years, even though the bone density has returned to its baseline level (Bachrach et al. 2010).

Zoledronate

The other less studied but increasingly commonly used bisphosphonate for children is zoledronate. It is a third generation bisphosphonate, and thus a stronger medication than pamidronate. Zoledronate is much more convenient because it is infused over 30 minutes, once every 6 months. However, it has a higher risk of severe side effects, including at least one case report of shock and admission to the Intensive Care Unit (ICU) (Trivedi et al. 2016). The typical dose for zoledronate is 0.025 mg/kg/dose to 0.05 mg/kg/dose (maximum of 4 mg), with the first dose given as half the usual dose. Lower doses than these are sometimes used for children who are medically fragile or have a tendency toward hypocalcemia. As is the case for pamidronate, the optimal length of treatment for children with CP is unknown.

Oral bisphosphonates, commonly used in adults, are given weekly (alendronate) or monthly (ibandronate), but absorption is very variable, and patients with gastroesophageal reflux are at risk to develop esophagitis. These medications have been used for children in small numbers, but many children with CP have gastroesophageal reflux, and most clinicians have not used the oral medications, at least not until the children are adults.

Side effects

The most common side effects are related to an acute phase reaction, involving fever, chills, bone pain, nausea, and vomiting. These effects are seen in approximately 25% of children given pamidronate, and primarily occur with the initial 3-day course. The incidence is higher in those receiving zoledronate. Some clinicians routinely give acetaminophen or ibuprofen with the first course, while others treat based on the presence of symptoms. These side effects are typically less severe during the second course, and are usually absent by the third course. Hypocalcemia and hypophosphatemia can occur after any of the treatment courses; serum levels need to be monitored, but the drop in levels is usually mild and transient. Testing for 25-OH-vitamin D level should routinely be done before the first course of bisphosphonate is given, with supplementation of vitamin D to get levels above 30 ng/mL, as low levels of vitamin D can predispose to significant hypocalcemia with bisphosphonate treatment. If calcium or phosphorus levels drop significantly, they can be corrected by oral or intravenous supplements, depending on the severity.

In adults, two serious side effects have been described that have not been seen in children. Osteonecrosis of the jaw (ONJ) has been described in a very small percentage of adults who received bisphosphonates. The incidence of ONJ is highest in the oncology patient population (Khan et al. 2015). Known risk factors for ONJ include invasive dental procedures (e.g., tooth extraction, dental implants, boney surgery), cancer diagnosis, concomitant therapy (e.g. chemotherapy, corticosteroids), poor oral hygiene, and comorbid disorders (infection, preexisting dental disease). While it has not been reported in children, it is prudent to have the child evaluated by a dentist prior to starting treatment, looking especially for any teeth that need to be extracted, or any active dental disease. Atypical femur fractures are another side effect described only in adults, leading to clinicians discontinuing the bisphosphonate after 5 years of treatment. The relevance to children is unclear, but may point to a need to limit the length of treatment in children as well.

Other medications

An analogue of PTH (teriparatide) has been used in adults to treat osteoporosis. There is a statistically significant increase in the risk of the development of cancer in patients treated with this medication (compared to placebo), and thus it is not being used in children. Nasal calcitonin is sometimes used in adults and children, but in children has not been shown to improve BMD (Pappa et al. 2011).

A more promising group of medications are the Rank-L inhibitors, one of which, Denosumab, is currently being tested in children with osteogenesis imperfecta. Rank-L activates osteoclast precursors and subsequent osteolysis . Denosumab binds to RANK-L, and prevents osteoclast formation, leading to decreased bone resorption and increased bone mass in osteoporosis. It is given subcutaneously only. Atypical femur fractures and ONJ have been reported in adults receiving Denosumab.

Conclusions

Children with severe CP exhibit many risk factors for compromised bone health. They have smaller, thinner, weaker bones that fracture with minimal trauma. Clinicians should assess for known risk factors and correct where possible: this includes evaluating nutritional intake and status including serum 25-OH-vitamin D level, increasing/encouraging weight bearing, providing adequate nutritional status overall to support growth, avoiding (when possible) medications that have a deleterious effect on bone health, and measuring BMD by DXA, if available. Because the lower extremities are the body site most apt to fracture in non-ambulatory children with CP, the LDF DXA is especially useful. A baseline scan should be performed and BMD monitored every 1–2 years depending on clinical picture. When treating with bisphosphonate, a baseline scan should be obtained, then BMD monitored every 6 months during treatment and annually thereafter. Bisphosphonates are effective at improving or preserving BMD and preventing fractures, but optimal dose, regimen, and duration of treatment have yet to be determined.

Key points

- Children with complex CP who are partially or totally non-ambulatory are at risk for low bone density and fragility fractures.

- Preventive measures can reduce the development of low bone density, and postpone or prevent fractures.

- Preventive measures include optimizing vitamin/mineral intake and correcting deficiencies, standing and/or walking as much as tolerated, and adjusting medications when possible to avoid those that negatively affect bone density.

- DXA is the most readily available, preferred method to measure bone density. A DXA should be obtained on any child who has had a fragility fracture, and in any other child for whom bisphosphonate treatment is being considered.

- Bone assessment in children is challenging and requires specific equipment/software.

- Obtaining DXA measures in children with complex CP is challenging due to positioning concerns, the presence of artifacts (metal, tubes, pumps), and lack of familiarity with handling these children. Children with complex CP should be referred to a center that is experienced with and can accommodate them. For children with fragility fractures, refer to a center that treats children with complex CP. The most common treatment is intravenous bisphosphonate.

References

Aguirre JI, Plotkin LI, Stewart SA, et al (2006) Osteocyte apoptosis is induced by weightlessness in mice and precedes osteoclast recruitment and bone loss. *J Bone Miner Res* **21**: 605–615.

Apkon SD, Kecskemethy HH (2008) Bone health in children with cerebral palsy. *J Pediatr Rehabil Med* **1**: 115–121.

Bachrach SJ, Kecskemethy HH, Harcke HT, Hossain J (2010) Decreased Fracture Incidence after One Year of Pamidronate Treatment in Children with Spastic Quadriplegic Cerebral Palsy. *Developmental Medicine and Child Neurology* **52**: 837–842.

Binkley T, Johnson J, Vogel L, Kecskemethy H, Henderson R, Specker B (2005) Bone measurements by peripheral quantitative computed tomography (pQCT) in children with cerebral palsy. *J Pediatr* **147**: 791–796.

Bonjour JP, Theintz G, Buchs B, Slosman D, Rizzoli R (1991) Critical years and stages of puberty for spinal and femoral bone mass accumulation during adolescence. *J Clin Endocrinol Metab* **73**: 555–563.

Ceroni D, Martin X, Delhumeau C, Rizzoli R, Kaelin A, Farpour-Lambert N (2012) Effects of cast-mediated immobilization on bone mineral mass at various sites in adolescents with lower-extremity fracture. *J Bone Joint Surg Am* **94**: 208–216.

Cooper C, Dennison EM, Leufkens H, Bishop N, van Staa TP (2004) Epidemiology of childhood fractures in Britain: a study using the general practice research database. *J Bone Miner Res* **19**: 1976–1981.

Crabtree NJ, Arabi A, Bachrach LK, et al. (2014) Dual-Energy X-ray Absorptiometry Interpretation and Reporting in Children and Adolescents: The Revised 2013 ISCD Official Pediatric Positions. *J Clin Densitom* **17**: 225–242.

Duquette SA, Guiliano AM, Starmer DJ (2015) Whole body vibration and cerebral palsy: a systematic review. *J Can Chiropr Assoc* **59**: 245–252.

Giangregorio L, McCartney N (2006) Bone loss and muscle atrophy in spinal cord injury: epidemiology, fracture prediction, and rehabilitation strategies. *J Spinal Cord Med* **29**: 489–500.

Gisel EG, Patrick J (1988) Identification of children with cerebral palsy unable to maintain a normal nutritional state. *Lancet* **1**: 283–286.

Goulding A, Jones IE, Williams SM, et al. (2005) First fracture is associated with increased risk of new fractures during growth. *J Pediatr* **146**: 286–288.

Gusso S, Munns CF, Colle P, et al. (2016) Effects of whole-body vibration training on physical function, bone and muscle mass in adolescents and young adults with cerebral palsy. *Sci Rep* **6**: 22518.

Haas RE, Kecskemethy HH, Lopiccolo MA, Hossain J, Dy RT, Bachrach SJ (2012) Lower extremity bone mineral density in children with congenital spinal dysfunction. *Dev Med Child Neurol* **54**: 1133–1137.

Harcke HT, Taylor A, Bachrach S, Miller F, Henderson RC (1998) Lateral femoral scan: an alternative method for assessing bone mineral density in children with cerebral palsy. *Pediatr Radiol* **28**: 241–246.

Harcke HT, Kecskemethy HH, Conklin D, Scavina M, Mackenzie WG, McKay CP (2006) Assessment of bone mineral density in Duchenne's muscular dystrophy (DMD) using the lateral distal femur. *J Clin Neuromusc Dis* **8**: 1–6.

Hartman C, Brik R, Tamir A, Merrick J, Shamir R (2004) Bone quantitative ultrasound and nutritional status in severely handicapped institutionalized children and adolescents. *Clin Nutr* **23**: 89–98.

Heaney RP, Abrams S, Dawson-Hughes B, Looker A, Marcus R, Matkovic V, et al. (2000) Peak bone mass. *Osteoporosis Int* **11**: 985–1009.

Henderson RC, Lark RK, Gurka MJ, et al. (2002a) Bone density and metabolism in children and adolescents with moderate to severe cerebral palsy. *Pediatrics* **110**(Pt 1): e5.

Henderson RC, Lark RK, Kecskemethy HH, Miller F, Harcke HT, Bachrach SJ (2002b) Bisphosphonates to treat osteopenia in children with quadriplegic cerebral palsy: a randomized placebo-controlled clinical trial. *J Pediatr* **141**: 644–651.

Henderson RC, Lark RK, Newman JE, et al. (2002c) Pediatric reference data for dual X-ray absorptiometric measures of normal bone density in the distal femur. *Am J Roentgenol* **178**: 439–443.

Henderson RC, Kairalla J, Abbas A, Stevenson RD (2004) Predicting low bone density in children and young adults with quadriplegic cerebral palsy. *Dev Med Child Neurol* **46**: 416–419.

Henderson RC, Berglund LM, May R, et al. (2010) The relationship between fractures and DXA measures of BMD in the distal femur of children and adolescents with cerebral palsy or muscular dystrophy *J Bone Min Res* **25**: 520–526.

Hind K, Burrows M (2007) Weight-bearing exercise and bone mineral accrual in children and adolescents: a review of controlled trials. *Bone* **40**: 14–27.

Holick MF, Binkley NC, Bischoff-Ferrari HA, et al. (2011) Evaluation, treatment, and prevention of vitamin D deficiency: an Endocrine Society clinical practice guideline. *J Clin Endocrinol Metab* **96**(7): 1911–30. Erratum in: **96**: 3908.

Hui SL, Slemenda CW, Johnston CC Jr (1990) The contribution of bone loss to postmenopausal osteoporosis. *Osteoporos Int* **1**: 30–34.

IOM (Institute of Medicine) (1997) *Dietary reference intakes for calcium, phosphorus, magnesium, vitamin D, and fluoride.* Washington, DC: The National Academies Press.

IOM (2011) *Dietary reference intakes for calcium and vitamin D.* Washington, DC: The National Academies Press.

Jekovec-Vrhovsek M, Kocijancic A, Prezelj J (2005) Quantitative ultrasound of the calcaneus in children and young adults with severe cerebral palsy. *Dev Med Child Neurol* **47**: 696–698.

Kecskemethy HH, Harcke HT (2014) Assessment of bone health in children with disabilities. *J Pediatr Rehabil Med* **7**: 111–124.

Khan AA, Morrison A, Hanley DA, Felsenberg D, et al. (2015) Diagnosis and management of osteonecrosis of the jaw: a systematic review and international consensus. *J Bone Miner Res* **30**: 3–23.

Khoury DJ, Szalay EA (2007) Bone mineral density correlation with fractures in nonambulatory pediatric patients. *J Pediatr Orthop* **27**: 562–566.

Lee JJ, Lyne ED (1990) Pathologic fractures in severely handicapped children and young adults. *J Pediatr Orthop* **10**: 497–500.

Melton LJ, Kan SH, Frye MA, Wahner HW, O'Fallon WM, Riggs BL (1989) Epidemiology of vertebral fractures in women. *Am J Epidemiol* **129**: 1000–1011.

Modlesky CM, Subramanian P, Miller F (2008) Underdeveloped trabecular bone microarchitecture is detected in children with cerebral palsy using high-resolution magnetic resonance imaging. *Osteoporos Int* **19**: 169–176.

Paleg GS, Smith BA, Glickman LB (2013) Systematic review and evidence-based clinical recommendations for dosing of pediatric supported standing programs. *Pediatr Phys Ther* **25**: 232–247.

Pappa HM, Saslowsky TM, Filip-Dhima R, et al. (2011) Efficacy and harms of nasal calcitonin in improving bone density in young patients with inflammatory bowel disease: a randomized, placebo-controlled, double-blind trial. *Am J Gastroenterol* **106**: 1527–1543.

Pin TW (2007) Effectiveness of Static Weight-Bearing Exercises in Children with Cerebral Palsy. *Pediatr Phys Ther* **19**: 62–73.

Presedo A, Dabney KW, Miller F (2007) Fractures in patients with cerebral palsy. *J Pediatr Orthop* **27**: 147–153.

Rubin C, Recker R, Cullen D, Ryaby J, McCabe J, Mcleod K (2004) Prevention of postmenopausal bone loss by a low-magnitude, high-frequency mechanical stimuli: a clinical trial assessing compliance, efficacy, and safety. *J Bone Miner Res* **19**: 343–351.

Ruck J, Chabot G, Rauch F (2010) Vibration treatment in cerebral palsy: A randomized controlled pilot study. *J Musculoskelet Neuronal Interact* **10**: 77–83.

Stevenson RD, Conaway M, Barrington JW, Cuthill SL, Worley G, Henderson RC (2006) Fracture rate in children with cerebral palsy. *Pediatr Rehabil* **9**: 396–403.

Szalay EA, Cheema A (2011) Children with spina bifida are at risk for low bone density. *Clin Orthop Relat Res* **469**(5): 1253–1257.

Trivedi S, Al-Nofal A, Kumar S, Tripathi S, Kahoud RJ, Tebben PJ (2016) Severe non-infective systemic inflammatory response syndrome, shock, and end-organ dysfunction after zoledronic acid administration in a child. *Osteoporos Int* **27**: 2379–2382.

Ward K, Alsop C, Caulton J, Rubin C, Adams J, Mughal Z (2004) Low magnitude mechanical loading is osteogenic in children with disabling conditions. *J Bone Miner Res* **19**: 360–947.

Wren TA, Lee DC, Hara R, Rethlefsen SA, Kay RM, Dorey FJ, Gilsanz V (2010) Effect of high-frequency, low-magnitude vibration on bone and muscle in children with cerebral palsy. *J Pediatr Orthop* **30**: 732–738.

Wren TA, Lee DC, Kay RM, Dorey FJ, Gilsanz V (2011) Bone density and size in ambulatory children with cerebral palsy. *Dev Med Child Neurol* **53**: 137–141.

Zemel BS, Stallings VA, Leonard MB, et al. (2009) Revised pediatric reference data for the lateral distal femur measured by Hologic Discovery/Delphi dual energy x-ray absorptiometry. *J Clin Densitometry* **12**: 207–218.

Chapter 7

Feeding and nutrition

Mary C. Bickley, Eva Delaney and Valentina Intagliata

Introduction

Feeding disorder from oral-motor impairment is one of the comorbid impairments in children with cerebral palsy (CP). Prevalence varies among studies, but one estimate is that as many as 90% of preschool children with CP have oral-motor dysfunction (Reilly et al. 1996). Some studies report that even children with mild CP show evidence of oral-motor dysfunction impacting functional feeding skills (Gisel et al. 2000).

Children with CP have a spectrum of feeding abilities. Some children with oral-motor impairment are prohibitively unsafe to eat orally due to the risk of aspiration. Others cannot handle solids, but may be able to eat safely and grow adequately on purees or specific food/liquid consistencies. Many children with severe CP are inefficient eaters. These children may be able to chew and swallow safely, but may take excessive time to eat, and fatigue easily doing so.

In the most severe cases of feeding disorder, children require placement of a feeding tube to maintain adequate nutrition and/or to ensure safe feeding. Other children may be able to learn strategies to help them with certain problematic textures of food. Often, the stress of the feeding disorder can have a profound impact on the family dynamics around mealtimes and the child's feeding behaviors.

In this chapter, we provide an overview of feeding, nutrition and growth in children with complex CP including oral motor dysfunction, feeding assessment and interventions, evaluation of nutrition and physical growth. Other issues related to feeding and nutrition are covered in Chapter 8 (dysphagia, constipation, gastroesophageal reflux, gastrostomy, fundoplication), Chapter 9 (drooling, aspiration) and Chapter 20 (decision making for gastrostomy placement).

Oral-motor impairment

Oral-motor impairment or dysfunction is defined by differences in strength, tone and sensation of the oro-pharynx that affect the coordination of motor movements for both speech and eating. It is associated with disorders of swallowing, known as dysphagia. The terms dysphagia and oral-motor dysfunction are frequently used interchangeably but should be differentiated. Both can exist independently of one another but quite often have a reciprocal relationship. Oral-motor dysfunction can result in the mistiming of the swallow leading to aspiration. Dysphagia can exist with or without oral-motor dysfunction, and is sometimes secondary to structural or postural elements that impact the oral, pharyngeal or esophageal phase of the swallow.

Oral-motor impairment often impacts on the efficiency and pleasure of eating, as well as the social dynamics of feeding. Eating is the physical act of biting, chewing and swallowing food, whereas feeding describes eating in the social context. These social factors include caregiver–child relationships as well as the mealtime environment. Feeding is one of the most important initial interactions between a caregiver and a child, and any disruption in this process can have a negative impact on the child and the entire family.

Maturation of oral-motor skills follows an organized hierarchy of steps. This process begins with a reflexive pattern for suckling during early infancy, and proceeds through a series of learned behaviors that result in the ability to bite, lateralize, chew and safely swallow foods. Each step requires practice in a supportive environment so that the child can master efficient, effective and pleasurable eating. Motor and sensory impairments at any stage can affect the process of learning to eat.

The abnormalities in tone and the difficulties with motor coordination common in children with CP negatively impact eating skills. In early infancy, oral-motor dysfunction may be a presenting feature of CP since these children have impairments in coordinating and sustaining the rhythmic sucking pattern needed for feeding. In these young infants, frequent choking is common as well as prolonged feeding time and decreased intake, often leading to poor growth. Some children may have minimal oral-motor dysfunction as young infants (with reflexive suckling), but later struggle when they fail to master the complex voluntary, learned motor movements necessary for safe and efficient biting, chewing and swallowing.

The presence of increased muscle tone can make graded control of mouth position difficult. In effect, opening of the mouth for food entry and chewing is impaired.

Lingual lateralization, which is essential for maneuvering higher textured foods to the molars for proper mastication, is often impaired. In the absence of appropriate lingual manipulation, the child may not be able to transition safely and efficiently to a variety of textures.

Children with hypotonia often have difficulty achieving a closed mouth posture and this alone can make eating difficult. Weakness and decreased tone can result in a sluggish suck/swallow/breathe pattern (reflexive suckling) often associated with choking and a weak cough. Silent aspiration is also a potential problem due to weakness and poor sensory awareness. These difficulties lead to inefficient, prolonged and often unsafe eating. Children who are mostly hypotonic demonstrate significantly slower transition to purees and table foods, but generally progress further in oral-motor skills than children with significant hypertonia.

Assessment of eating

The three stages of eating – oral, pharyngeal and esophageal – are important to consider when assessing oral-motor dysfunction and dysphagia. Box 7.1 shows the American Speech and Hearing Association (ASHA) description of potential difficulties in each stage of eating that may be present in children with CP.

Box 7.1 Potential difficulties in each stage of eating that may be present in children with cerebral palsy

- Oral stage
  - Difficulties with motor coordination for graded movements of the lips, jaw and tongue.
  - Differences in tone impacting efficient motor and or sensory processing of age-appropriate textures and foods.
  - Difficulties with sensory tolerance of tastes, textures and temperatures.
- Pharyngeal stage
  - Difficulties with safe and efficient passage of food/liquids past the airway.
  - Penetration of liquid or food into airway.
  - Aspiration of liquid or food into airway.
  - Pooling or coating of residue.
- Esophageal phase
  - Difficulties with efficient and effective passage of food or liquids to the stomach.
  - Slow transit of food/liquid through esophagus.
  - Reflux of food/liquid back into airway.
  - Spasm or inability of sphincters to open/close appropriately.

Children with CP most commonly experience challenges in the oral stage. Abnormal motor movements and postural alignment of the head, neck and trunk significantly impact presentation of food to the child and their ability to keep food contained in the mouth. The loss of foods frontally can result in inefficient oral intake and unsafe swallow. These difficulties are only optimized by proper positioning and hands-on techniques, and cannot be 'fixed' or cured. Other difficulties during the oral stage include wide jaw excursion, tongue protrusion/thrusting and impaired lingual lateralization. As a result, these children have poor control of the food bolus as they attempt to swallow and this often leads to aspiration.

Assessment of feeding should be completed by a speech-language therapist along with a physical and/or occupational therapist to maximize feeding position. Additional consultation with the nutritionist allows for optimization of the child's diet within the constraints of his/her oral-motor dysfunction. An oral-functional evaluation by the speech-language therapist provides information regarding food texture that is most efficient and safe for a child with oral-motor dysfunction. This evaluation can also determine which utensils might optimize the child's oral-motor potential.

During the oral-functional evaluation, the clinician should be cognizant of potential aspiration. Clinical signs of aspiration include coughing, cessation of breathing, watery eyes, wet/or gurgly vocal quality and oral mucosal color changes. Cervical auscultation is another method that is useful for identifying more subtle signs of aspiration. This method entails the placement of a stethoscope on the median line of the cricoid cartilage and the listener interprets swallowing sounds. Consensus supports cervical auscultation as a good tool to determine if video-fluoroscopic study (VFSS) is necessary (Leslie et al. 2007).

VFSS study is warranted when there are clinical signs of aspiration as listed above, or if, in the absence of clinical signs, a child repeatedly has pneumonia or respiratory issues or a history of structural issues. VFSS is also a useful evaluation tool for the pharyngeal and esophageal stages of swallow that cannot be observed clinically. VFSS is not indicated when a child has 'never' eaten in the past, when there is the complaint of frequent gagging or as a precursor to 'feeding therapy'. These issues can be addressed through a clinical feeding evaluation.

Classification of eating and drinking abilities

The Eating and Drinking Ability Classification System (EDACS) has been developed specifically for children with CP in order to provide a meaningful framework for distinguishing varying eating abilities in everyday life. The EDACS classifies an individual's usual performance rather maximal abilities in ideal circumstances. The classification scheme characterizes eating and drinking abilities at five different levels for children with CP aged 3 years and older. The most useful aspect of this scale is that it correlates with the Gross Motor Function Classification System (GMFCS) used for characterizing independent ambulation. Increasing EDACS level correlates with increasing risk for gastrostomy tube use (Benfer et al. 2017).

- Level I – Eats and drinks safely and efficiently.

- Level II – Eats and drinks safely but with some limitations to efficiency.

- Level III – Eats and drinks with some limitations to safety; there may be limitations to efficiency.

- Level IV – Eats and drinks with significant limitations to safety.

- Level V – Unable to eat or drink safely – tube feeding may be considered to provide nutrition.

Feeding interventions

The goal of feeding therapy is to aid families with providing nutrition in a manner that is manageable, safe, and efficient. Oral-motor therapy is an important part of feeding therapy to help the child develop and maximize eating skills. In order to optimize a child's oral potential in the home the following elements must be determined: safe and comfortable positioning, appropriate diet regarding consistency, and a supportive environment including appropriate applied techniques.

Oral-motor therapy
Oral-motor therapy, also known as sensorimotor treatment, is intended to augment oral-functional skills required for speech and eating. Of note, this is different from oral stimulation (see Applied techniques, on page 113). The skills addressed through oral-motor therapy include: awareness, strength, coordination, movement, and endurance of the lips, cheeks, tongue, and jaw as well as positioning and texture modifications. Oral-motor therapy may be beneficial in children with mild CP, but the scientific literature is equivocal regarding its benefits for children with severe CP (Gisel 1994, Gisel et al. 1995).

Positioning
The optimal position for children with feeding difficulties is one that provides good trunk and head stability with alignment at the hips and knees, and with the feet resting securely on a surface. This ideal positioning is nearly impossible when feeding a child in a lap, but can be achieved in most wheelchairs. It is usually easier to optimally position a child in the morning when he/she is rested; however, this may be more difficult after multiple transitions in and out of the chair throughout the day. Of note, care providers in the school system who are feeding children with oral-motor dysfunction should also have training in optimal positioning and feeding techniques.

Diet consistency

The most appropriate diet consistency for a child with CP will depend on the extent of the oral-motor dysfunction as well as the time of day, positioning, environment and fatigue level of the child. Due to the impact of limited lingual manipulation and chewing abilities, many children will require modified textures. Children with significant oral-motor dysfunction need a pureed diet that does not require any lateralization to the molars for chewing. Others may only require a soft or chopped diet. Most children with oral-motor dysfunction will have significant difficulty with drinking via cup or straw. Some children with severe oral-motor dysfunction may not be safe for any oral intake and require a gastrostomy tube for nutrition and hydration. Children with hypotonia may not transition to age-appropriate diet textures, but may be able to transition to increased textures over time.

It is useful to systematically characterize food and fluid consistency so that health care providers, therapists and caregivers can be consistent in describing a child's diet. The National Dysphagia Diet (NDD) classifies foods based on the following descriptions.

Solid textures:

- NDD level 1 (pureed): These foods require no chewing, are homogenous, very cohesive and are a pudding consistency. It is important to keep in mind that 'pureed' foods are not all equal. Thicker purees are usually recommended in order to prevent aspiration during the swallow as they move in a slow manner. Thicker purees, however, result in increased amount of food residue in the pharynx following the swallow, especially in children with hypotonia.

- NDD level 2 (mechanical altered): These foods require some chewing ability, but are cohesive, moist and semi-solid.

- NDD level 3 (advanced): These foods require some chewing ability, but are rarely multi-layered or mixed consistencies (e.g. vegetable soup).

Drinking is often difficult for children with oral-motor dysfunction because of the speed at which fluid flows. It can also be challenging for a child to pull liquids from a cup or straw. Maintaining adequate hydration can therefore be a slow and tedious process. Just as with solid food textures, a variety of liquid viscosities exist for children with oral-motor dysfunction.

Liquid viscosity:

- Thin liquids: Regular liquids such as water, juice or milk. Milk and chocolate milk as well as some prepared formulas tend to be slightly more viscous than water or juice.

- Nectar liquids: Thickened to the level of 'nectar' as found in canned fruit.

- Honey liquids: Thickened to the level of honey.

- Spoon-thick liquids: Resemble purees.

Environment

The ideal feeding environment is one that is quiet and calm, especially since some children with CP startle easily. Infants in general feed better before reaching extreme hunger, fatigue and related irritability. Infants with CP who become upset may demonstrate increased extensor tone, making feeding even more challenging. In older children the environment should be conducive to safe and efficient oral intake but should not be socially isolating if possible. Sometimes feeding children with complex CP in a crowded and noisy school cafeteria can be particularly challenging.

Applied Techniques

A few hands-on techniques may be utilized during feeding to improve efficiency and safety.

- **Jaw/cheek support** – The thumb and pointer finger of the person feeding are positioned on either side of mouth on the cheek surface and under the chin. This helps the child achieve mouth closure, which aids in triggering a swallow. This technique is most useful in children with hypotonia and/or mild hypertonia. In children with more extensive oral-motor dysfunction, it is not usually effective.

- **Lip closure** – This technique is applied in conjunction with jaw/cheek support to help the lips close. This maneuver assists in achieving a more efficient and effective swallow.

- **Direct food placement** – This technique varies from child to child depending on the level of oral-motor dysfunction. Some children are able to keep pureed foods in their mouths if it is placed on the sides of the tongue/cheek pocket rather than directly on the surface of the tongue. Other children can 'munch' dissolvable foods safely when they are placed directly on their molars.

- **Oral stimulation** – This is a theoretical strategy in which sensory stimulation prepares the child and their mouth for eating more efficiently and safely. For children with sensory processing issues, oral stimulation is another strategy, though the scientific evidence is limited and unclear as to whether it results in more efficient or safe eating for children with severe oral-motor dysfunction (Arvedson 2013).

Hunger and satiety

Hunger/satiety is a complex cycle regulated by numerous different elements including physiologic, developmental and environmental elements. Children with CP are at high risk for disordered hunger/satiety regulation for many reasons. Impairments in motor activity with associated reduced metabolic needs results in decreased hunger. Differences in tone and gastro-intestinal motility cause constipation and gastroesophageal reflux disease (GERD), which negatively affect appetite. Lengthy mealtimes and sensory impairments also detract from the feeding experience. Supplemental feeding, such as with a feeding tube, often make it difficult for a child to have normal regulation of hunger/satiety cycles.

In addition to physiological differences, children with CP may be more easily influenced by the environments in which they eat. School cafeterias, birthday parties, sporting events may be too noisy and result in increased tone or startle responses. Caregiver stress due to concerns about inadequate nutrition and lengthy feeding times impacts feeding dynamics, especially in children with CP who already experience poor growth.

Regulating hunger/satiety patterns in children with CP should be a key component of the intervention plan. Children should be transitioned to age-appropriate feeding regimen if possible, especially when receiving gastrostomy tube feeds. Aggressive management of constipation, GERD and other gastro-intestinal dysmotility is important as well. Lastly, oral-motor skills should be optimized in order improve efficiency and safety.

Growth and nutrition

Many children with severe CP are inefficient eaters. These children may be able to chew and swallow safely, but may take excessive time to feed, and/or fatigue easily doing so. The disproportionate effort required to consume food ultimately limits nutrition and growth. Children who eat inadequate calories and protein at first may continue to gain weight, but at a suboptimal rate. When insufficient nutrition persists, linear growth and body mass composition are compromised as well.

Inadequate nutritional intake resulting in poor growth evolves over months to years (Stevenson and Conaway 2007). Infants with CP and associated oral-motor impairment may grow adequately in infancy as they rely on the primitive feeding reflex of sucking/swallowing. As infants develop, they require more calories but are unable to maintain appropriate growth during the transition to more complex oral-motor skills. Children who are inefficient eaters might also struggle with catch-up weight gain after recurrent illnesses. Other children with hyperkinetic CP might have a mismatch of calorie requirements and nutritional intake.

Although malnutrition can refer to both under- and over-nutrition, for the purposes of this handbook, malnutrition will refer only to under-nutrition. Prolonged malnutrition leads to micronutrient deficiencies, low fat stores and decreased height velocity (Krick et al. 1996, Henderson et al. 2002, Stevenson and Conaway 2007). Inadequate nutrient intake negatively affects growth, development, and other relevant outcomes (Mehta et al. 2013). Other consequences of malnutrition include fatigue, increased illness/hospitalization, and familial stress regarding poor growth.

Oral-motor impairment with associated malnutrition is usually a contributing factor to poor growth among children with severe CP, though various other factors have been identified. (Henderson et al. 2005, Stevenson and Conaway 2007, Kuperminc et al. 2009). Other reasons for poor growth include neuroendocrine abnormalities, muscle-bone interactions, and psychosocial influences. Laboratory assessment may be required to identify medical causes of poor growth. Causes of poor growth to consider include hyper- or hypothyroidism, growth hormone deficiency, delayed puberty, and inflammatory disease.

Despite all known factors that might contribute to poor growth, children with CP overall grow differently compared to their typically developing counterparts. In general, children with CP are shorter and smaller compared to peers, and this trend is positively correlated with severity of GMFCS classification. Children with CP tend to have decreased fat mass, lean muscle mass and bone density (Stallings et al. 1995, Henderson et al. 2005). Poor growth, therefore, may be a marker of severe CP, and may not be modifiable in many cases.

When assessing the growth and nutrition of children with CP it is important to consider the complex interaction of multiple influences. Additionally, the differences in body mass composition, which relate to CP severity, should be taken into account. As such, the best strategy is a combination of tools to determine whether a child with CP is growing appropriately and is well nourished.

Growth assessment

Obtaining typical anthropometric measurements can be challenging due to commonly associated physical differences in children with severe CP. Children with CP often have significant scoliosis and contractures, which affect traditional length/height measurements. Weight can also be difficult to obtain using standard scales if the child is non-ambulatory. BMI is not an appropriate calculation using weight and height because children with CP have lower lean muscle mass. (Kuperminc and Stevenson 2008). This measurement may be helpful to assess trends and patterns, but should not be used alone as an indicator of nutrition status, if used at all (Stallings et al. 1995, Samson-Fang and Stevenson 2000). The criterion standard for assessing body composition (includes fat, water, protein and bone) is a Dual X-Ray Absorptiometry (DXA) scan. However, this is not readily available for clinicians so other anthropometric measures are available and acceptable (Kuperminc and Stevenson 2008).

Table 7.1 Equations for estimating height using segmental measurements in children with cerebral palsy under 12 years of age

Segmental Measure	Prediction equation for height (cm)	Standard error of the estimate (cm)
Upper arm length (UAL)	(4.25 x UAL) + 21.8	± 1.7
Tibial length (TL)	(3.26 x TL) + 30.8	± 1.4
Knee height (KH)	(2.69 x KH) + 24.2	± 1.1

Source: Samson-Fang and Bell 2013

Stature/height

Obtaining a height measurement can be challenging if not impossible due to physical differences (Kuperminc and Stevenson 2008). If the child is unable to stand, but is easily and reliably able to lie on a recumbent board, this is an acceptable alternative. If unable to obtain an accurate standing or recumbent length measurement, other options are available. Segmental measurements include ulnar length, knee height, and upper arm length (see Nutrition assessment, below for equations for estimating stature from these measurements). Knee height is the most reliable (Table 7.1). A flexible tape measure along the patient in a lying position is not a valid, reliable or reproducible method for obtaining a height measurement (Samson-Fang and Bell 2013).

Weight

As mentioned, the body composition of children with CP is different, and therefore weight does not reflect typical distribution of body fat and muscle (Stallings et al. 1995, Samson-Fang and Stevenson 2000, Kuperminc et al. 2010). Children with severe CP often appear low on the typical weight curve, but may have appropriate adiposity. Therefore, monitoring weight increase over time is useful. Consequently, it is extremely important to have accurate weight measurements in order to assess growth trends reliably. The minimal goal for children who are less than the 5th centile for age (CDC or WHO growth charts) is to follow his/her own curve and maintain consistent weight gain. Another useful resource are the California Growth Charts (Brooks et al. 2011).

Accurate weight measurements in infants require a naked weight. For children and adolescents who are non-ambulatory, the ideal is to weigh on a chair scale or wheelchair scale with only a light layer of clothing. If it is not possible to place the child on a scale independently, the child and caregiver can be weighed together and then subtract caregiver's weight (Samson-Fang and Bell 2013).

Triceps skinfold

This measurement provides useful information regarding fat stores and it is thought to be the best screening tool for malnutrition in this population (Samson-Fang and

Stevenson 2000). To obtain an accurate measurement, determine the midpoint between the top of the shoulder and the elbow. Then pinch the skin so that the fold is running vertically. Using a skinfold caliper, obtain the measurement (recommend obtaining 2–3 measurements to ensure accuracy). The CDC provides growth references for children from 1.5 to 20 years of age for plotting these measurements.

Triceps skinfold is a better indicator of fat stores compared to weight for length or BMI, as it measures fat stores directly. The goal is for these measurements to be greater than the 10th centile for age as it has been found that children with measurements less than the 5th centile are at higher risk for malnutrition (Samson-Fang and Stevenson 1998) and associated increased health care utilization and decreased social participation. It is important to note that some children with severe CP may hold their fat stores more centrally (in the abdominal cavity) and may demonstrate lower triceps skinfold measurements (Kuperminc et al. 2010, Gurka et al. 2010). Thus, triceps skinfold may underestimate total body fat stores.

Interpreting anthropometrics

Given the constraints of typical anthropometric measurements in children with CP, it is important to consider each measurement respective to other information and review growth trends. If a child is generally following his/her established curve for weight and length measurements, has adequate triceps skinfold (greater than 10th centile for age), and is not significantly limited in oral intake, it is appropriate to continue monitoring and re-assessing nutrition status every 6 months.

CP-specific growth charts are available (Brooks et al. 2011). It is important to note that these charts portray how children with CP *have* grown and not necessarily what is optimal growth (Kuperminc and Stevenson 2008, Krick et al. 1996). These growth charts are based on severity of gross motor impairment in children with CP, with higher level of impairment correlating with poorer growth. They are extremely useful as a clinical guide for children with complex CP. Another resource is for assessing growth is the online PediTools: Clinical Tools for Pediatric Providers which has growth calculators for weight, length/height, triceps skinfold, and mid-upper arm circumference (CDC and WHO), and provides centiles and Z-scores for age (Chou 2012; Available at www.peditools.org).

Nutrition assessment

When there are concerns about adequate nutrition, more frequent growth and diet assessments may be necessary to monitor trends or changes. Importantly, regardless of initial predictions of caloric needs, it is critical to assess weight gain and skinfolds over time. Consultation by a dietician may result in a calculated estimate of nutrition needs, using a variety of formulas and equations. Regardless, it is essential to monitor weight gain at any given estimate of calorie needs to determine if that level is excessive, inadequate or adequate. If a child is growing along his/her expected curve, this should be considered appropriate growth(Kuperminc et al., 2013). Many equations require a weight, height, or both, and thus accurate measurements are requisite.

Assessing physical status is an important component of a nutritional evaluation. The appearance of hair, skin and nails often provides clues to nutritional state. Pallor or pale skin can indicate iron, folate, or cobalamin deficiency. Lesions or fissures in the oral cavity may show signs of vitamin B deficiencies. Edema can be associated with protein malnutrition. Pressure ulcers and poor wound healing may reflect inadequate calorie

Table 7.2a Harris Benedict equation (using basal energy expenditure + activity/stress level)[a, b]

For males:	B.E.E. = 66.5 + (13.75 x kg) + (5.003 x cm) − (6.775 x age)
For females:	B.E.E. = 655.1 + (9.563 x kg) + (1.850 x cm) − (4.676 x age)

Source: Stallings et al. 1996

[a]Stress factors range from 1.2 to 2 depending on activity level

[b]Comment on stress factor: Tone should be taken into account when factoring in activity level for a child with severe cerebral palsy as hypertonicity can increase energy burned even if activity level or movement is low. For a patient who is wheelchair bound without much movement and without significantly increased tone, a provider may choose to use 1–1.2 as an activity factor, but should monitor weight gain closely. Clinical judgment plays a large role when determining activity factor in patients with severe cerebral palsy.

Table 7.2b Equation using kilocalories per centimeter in estimated or actual height

Children 5–11 years	Ambulatory = 14 kcal/cm
	Non-ambulatory = 11 kcal/cm

Source: Adapted from Weston 2012

Table 7.2c The World Health Organization equations for estimating resting energy expenditures

Age (years)	Resting energy expenditures (REE) (kcal/day)
0–3	Males: (60.9 x weight [kg]) − 54 Females: (61.0 x weight [kg]) − 51
3–10	Males: (22.7 x weight [kg]) + 495 Females: (22.5 x weight [kg]) + 499
10–18	Males: (17.5 x weight [kg]) + 651 Females: (12.2 x weight [kg]) + 746

Source: WHO 1985

and protein intake, or vitamin C, vitamin D and zinc deficiencies. Vitamin A deficiency may take the form of corneal clouding or ocular xerosis, whereas thiamin deficiency may present as nystagmus or ophthalmoplegia. Inadequate fat mass secondary to inadequate calorie intake may result in pubertal delays (2013, Pogatschnik 2011) (Table 7.3).

Laboratory assessment
Blood work may also be indicated as part of a complete assessment for growth and nutrition concerns. First consider other factors that might contribute to poor growth such as celiac disease, endocrine disorders, cystic fibrosis, etc. (Samson-Fang and Bell 2013).

Table 7.3   Physical findings and symptoms associated with malnutrition

	Physical exam and symptoms	Possible nutritional deficiency
Skeletal system	Epiphyseal enlargement of wrists, legs, knees; bowed legs; frontal bossing of the head; bone pain	Vitamin D
Muscular system	Wasted appearance	Protein calorie
	Weakness	Phosphorous
		Potassium
		Vitamin D
		Vitamin C
		Vitamin B6 (pyridoxine)
	Absent deep tendon reflexes, foot and wrist drop	Vitamin B1 (thiamin)
	Muscle cramps	Vitamin D
		Calcium
		Magnesium
		Potassium
		Chloride
	Muscle pain	Vitamin D
		Vitamin B7 (biotin)
Nervous system	Inability to concentrate, memory impairment, disorientation, irritability	Vitamin B1 (thiamin) Vitamin B9 (folic acid) Vitamin B12 (cobalamin)

Table 7.3 (Continued)

	Physical exam and symptoms	Possible nutritional deficiency
	Seizures, behavioral disturbances	Vitamin D
		Calcium
		Magnesium
		Zinc
	Peripheral neuropathy (numbness/tingling and weakness)	Vitamin B1 (thiamin)
		Vitamin B5 (pantothenic acid)
		Vitamin B6 (pyridoxine)
		Vitamin B9 (folic acid)
		Vitamin B12 (cobalamin)
		Phosphorous
		Copper
Eyes	Angular blepharitis (inflammation of the eyelids)	Vitamin B2 (riboflavin)
		Vitamin B6 (pyridoxine)
		Vitamin B7 (biotin)
		Zinc
	Pale conjuctiva	Vitamin B6 (pyridoxine)
		Vitamin B9 (folic acid)
		Vitamin B12 (cobalamin)
		Iron
		Copper
	Keratomalacia (opaque/dull cornea, night blindness), Bitot spots (white or grey spots on conjunctiva)	Vitamin A
	Ophthalmoplegia	Vitamin B1 (thiamin)
		Phosphorous (associated with rickets)

Table 7.3 (Continued)

	Physical exam and symptoms	Possible nutritional deficiency
Integumentary system		
A) Skin	Pallor	Vitamin B9 (folic acid)
		Vitamin B12 (cobalamin)
		Iron
		Vitamin C
	Dark cheeks and under eyes, scaling skin around nostrils	Protein calorie
		Vitamin B2 (riboflavin)
		Vitamin B3 (niacin)
		Vitamin B6 (pyridoxine)
	Pellagra (thick, dry, scaly hyperpigmentation on sun-exposed areas)	Vitamin B3 (niacin)
		Vitamin B6 (pyridoxine)
		Tryptophan
	Yellow pigmentation	
		Vitamin B12 (cobalamin)
	Follicular hyperkeratosis	Vitamin A
		Vitamin C
	Seborrheic dermatitis (scaly, waxy, crusty plaques on scalp, nasolabial folds, lips)	Vitamin B2 (riboflavin)
		Vitamin B6 (pyridoxine)
		Vitamin B7 (biotin)
		Vitamin A
		Zinc
		Essential fatty acid deficiency
	Eczema	Vitamin B2 (riboflavin) Zinc
	Xerosis (abnormal dryness)	Protein calorie Vitamin A

Table 7.3 (Continued)

	Physical exam and symptoms	Possible nutritional deficiency
	Slow wound healing, decubitus ulcers	Protein calorie Vitamin C Zinc
	Petechia (purple/red dots) or purpura (purple spots/patches) on skin	Vitamin C Vitamin K
	Cellophane appearance of skin	Protein calorie Vitamin C
	Edema	Protein calorie
	Poor skin turgor	Dehydration
B) Hair	Alopecia (thin, sparse hair)	Protein calorie Zinc Iron
	Easily plucked without pain, dull/dry/lack of shine	Protein calorie Essential fatty acid
	Depigmentation, color changes	Protein calorie Manganese Selenium Copper
	Flag sign (alternating color on hair strand due to lack of melanin)	Protein calorie
	Lanugo (find, soft hair)	Malnutrition
	Cork-screw hair and/or peri-follicular hemorrhage	Vitamin C
C) Nails	Brittle, soft, thin	Severe calorie Vitamin A Magnesium Selenium
	Central ridges	Protein calorie Vitamin B9 (folic acid) Iron
	Beau's lines (transverse ridges or horizontal grooves)	Protein calorie Zinc Calcium

Table 7.3   (Continued)

	Physical exam and symptoms	Possible nutritional deficiency
	Koilonychia (spoon-shaped or concave)	Protein Vitamin B9 (folic acid) Vitamin B12 (cobalamin) Iron
	Muehrcke lines (transvers white lines)	Malnutrition
Mouth and oral cavity	Soreness, burning mouth, tongue, lips	Vitamin B2 (riboflavin)
	Angular stomatitis or chelitis (redness or fissures at corners of mouth)	Vitamin B2 (riboflavin) Vitamin B3 (niacin) Vitamin B6 (pyridoxine) Vitamin B12 (cobalamin)
	Glossitis (sore, swollen, beefy-red tongue)	Vitamin B2 (riboflavin) Vitamin B3 (niacin) Vitamin B6 (pyridoxine) Vitamin B9 (folic acid) Vitamin B12 (cobalamin)
	Gingivitis (swollen, spongy gums that bleed easily)	Vitamin B3 (niacin) Vitamin B9 (folic acid) Vitamin C Vitamin D Zinc
	Missing teeth or late eruption	Malnutrition
	Dental caries	Fluoride Vitamin D Vitamin B6 (pyridoxine)
Gastro-intestinal system	Anorexia, flatulence, diarrhea	Vitamin B6 (pyridoxine) Vitamin B12 (cobalamin)

Children with severe CP are at-risk for poor bone mineral density and osteoporosis, therefore regular assessment of vitamin D (25-OH), alkaline phosphatase, calcium and phosphorus is recommended (Fehlings et al. 2012). C-reactive protein is a useful indicator of inflammation which may lead to increased calorie requirements (Samson-Fang and Bell 2013). A complete blood count helps with determining anemia. If significant concern for malnutrition and/or dehydration is present, consider a basic metabolic panel to assess for electrolyte disarray and/or renal

Table 7.4 Basic laboratory assessment for malnutrition

Anemia	Complete blood count
Bone health	Vitamin D 25-OH
	Calcium
	Alkaline phosphatase
	Phosphorous
Hydration status and re-feeding syndrome risk	Complete metabolic panel
	Magnesium
	Phosphorous

failure. Decreased albumin may reflect chronic malnutrition; however, albumin levels are affected by inflammation and fluid shifts, thus is not usually useful (Samson-Fang and Bell 2013). If available to a clinician, DXA allows for assessment of body composition including fat and lean mass stores (Samson-Fang and Bell 2013) (Table 7.4).

Interventions for poor growth and malnutrition

Children with severe CP who have malnutrition are often amenable to several fairly simple interventions. It is ideal to involve a dietician or gastroenterologist, but this is not uniformly possible. It is also useful to have a speech/language or occupational therapist assess feeding to ensure the child is consuming a diet of appropriate consistency to be safe and most efficient.

An essential component for increasing daily calorie intake is implementation of a meal schedule in order to provide the child with multiple eating opportunities (3 meals plus 2–3 snacks). The caregiver should incorporate nutrient rich foods at each eating occasion. Sources of nutrient rich foods include proteins (meats, fish, beans, eggs), fruits, vegetables, whole grains and dairy.

Oral nutrition supplements or 'calorie boosters' to increase calorie/protein/micronutrient intake are often necessary. Calorie boosters, such as heavy cream, whole milk, dry milk powder, butter, cheese, peanut butter, avocado and black beans, are easy foods to add to the diet. Caregivers can create 'milkshake' supplements using ice cream, milk, fruits, and vegetables to increase calories in liquid consistency. The other option is to use commercially available oral supplementation. See Table 7.5 for a list of common pediatric and adolescent oral supplementation (not an all-inclusive list). A variety of oral nutritional supplements exist and determining which supplement is most appropriate often requires the expertise of a nutritionist. A growing trend has emerged in the U.S. and elsewhere regarding the use of blended table foods in place of commercial

Table 7.5 Common pediatric and adolescent oral supplementation

Pediatric specific supplements *Generally are interchangeable*	Adult/adolescent supplements
Meal Replacements: Pediasure (children 2–13 years of age) • Multiple flavors • Milk based, but suitable for lactose intolerance Pediasmart • Powdered version of Pediasure • Not as easily found in stores Carnation Instant Breakfast • Multiple flavors • Powder that is to be mixed with 8oz milk • Usually a cheaper option to Pediasure Bright Beginnings Soy Parent's Choice Pediatric Drink (Walmart brand) Store brands that are comparable to the above	**Meal Replacements** Ensure or Boost Products • Variety of calorie levels (150–350 calories per container) depending on the level of support needed from supplement Carnation Instant Breakfast • Multiple flavors • Powder to be mixed with 8oz milk • Usually a cheaper alternative to Ensure/Boost Store brands comparable to the above **Non-nutritionally complete supplements** Ensure Clear or Boost Breeze • Juice-based supplements that provide additional calories and protein, but do not contain fat • Not to be used as a meal replacement, but can be used if diet is below adequate, however patient is able to take most nutrients orally and needs small amounts of supplementation • Can be used in the pediatric population as needed

formulas. To insure the adequacy of macro and micronutrients, we recommend that the use of homemade blended "formulas" be supervised by a nutritionist.

Micronutrient supplementation may be indicated if laboratory assessment indicates deficiency or if intake is obviously below recommended daily intake. Vitamin D and calcium supplementation are frequently necessary in children with CP due to several risk factors for poor bone health. If general nutrition is a concern, providers should recommend a pediatric multivitamin supplement.

The decision to place a gastrostomy tube in a child with CP should be made after careful consideration of safety and efficiency of oral intake, growth patterns, number/severity of respiratory illnesses, and overall quality of life. Many children with CP have oral-motor skills that detract from pleasant mealtime interactions due to concerns for safety and quantity of nutrition. This can result in stress for the family and direct health concerns for the children. Healthcare professionals should work with the family and other service providers to achieve the most pleasant, safe and efficient manner of eating for children with CP. Placement of a gastrostomy tube does not preclude oral feeding but may optimize growth, allow for accurate delivery of medication and fluids, and may offer additional time for other aspects of life.

Obesity

Obesity can occur in children with severe CP, especially in those who are gastrostomy tube-dependent. Children who are fed via gastrostomy do not have the ability to self-regulate intake and often have low metabolic needs. These children might easily receive calories in excess and gain weight rapidly, especially in the immediate period after placement of a feeding tube. Other children may have low resting metabolic needs due to decreased muscle mass in addition to low energy needs from lack of movement. At times it is difficult to provide these children with adequate micronutrients due to substantially low caloric needs.

Consequences of obesity in this population include metabolic syndrome and related issues. Obstructive sleep apnea is another serious consideration since these children are already at higher risk due to their motor impairment. Furthermore, it is more difficult for caregivers to move and care for overweight children with severe CP. To monitor children with severe CP at-risk for obesity, track weight gain velocity and triceps skinfold measurement trends over time, at regular intervals. Concerns should arise with consistent crossing of centiles in weight and triceps skinfolds (specifically when TSF reaches greater than the 85th centile for age).

Recommendations to deter obesity include decreased portion sizes, high-calorie foods, and carbohydrate-laden beverages. If the child receives tube feeds, slowly reduce calories, and closely monitor weight and triceps skinfold changes. Micronutrient supplementation may be required if calorie needs are extremely low. The goal is to maintain adequate linear growth and prevent further weight gain, or promote slow weight loss if no more linear growth is to occur.

Conclusion

Children with severe CP often require an extraordinary amount of basic care, with feeding difficulties and the related nutrition challenges comprising a large portion of their medical needs. It is critical to address feeding difficulties in these children not only to optimize overall health and growth, but also to potentially decrease family stress related to feeding. Although children with severe CP may struggle with oral-motor impairment and related nutrition/growth problems, various strategies exist to help optimize the safety and efficiency of feeding. Ideally, this may potentially result in increased pleasurable mealtime experiences for the child but also improved family harmony overall. Children and their families benefit from positive mealtime socialization and it is the job of the health care team to facilitate this experience by providing appropriate guidance, monitoring and interventions.

Key points

- Most children with complex CP struggle with feeding difficulties, although the degree of oral-motor impairment may vary widely with some children requiring only prolonged feeding times and others a gastrostomy tube.

- It is important to assess for safety and efficiency of eating, as well as the impact of the feeding difficulties on the family dynamic.

- Various strategies for improving safety and efficiency of feeding exist and include oral-motor therapy, diet consistency, positioning and environmental accommodations, and applied techniques.

- Children with severe CP overall grow differently compared to their typically developing counterparts. In general, children with CP are shorter and have decreased fat mass, lean muscle mass and bone density. As such, traditional strategies for assessing growth and nutrition require adaptation.

- Obesity among children with complex CP is commonplace due to multiple factors. Children with a gastrostomy must be monitored closely to prevent unintended obesity.

- For many children with severe CP, consultation with nutrition and a speech-language therapist is recommended and helpful.

References

Academy of Nutrition and Dietetics (2013) Academy of Nutrition and Dietetics Position Paper: Oral Health and Nutrition. *Journal of the Academy of Nutriton and Dietetics* 5: 8.

Arvedson JC (2013) Feeding children with cerebral palsy and swallowing difficulties. *Eur J Clin Nutr* 67 (Suppl 2): S9–S12.

Benfer KA, Weir KA, Bell KL, Ware RS, Davies PSW, Boyd RN (2017) The Eating and Drinking Ability Classification System in a population-based sample of preschool children with cerebral palsy. *Dev Med Child Neurol* 59: 647–654.

Brooks J, Day S, Shavelle R, Strauss D (2011) Low weight, morbidity, and mortality in children with cerebral palsy: new clinical growth charts. *Pediatrics* 128: e299–e307.

Chou J (2012) PediTools: Clinical Tools for Pediatric Providers [Online]. Available: http://ped-itools.org/.

Fehlings D, Switzer L, Agarwal P, et al. (2012) Informing evidence-based clinical practice guidelines for children with cerebral palsy at risk of osteoporosis: a systematic review. *Dev Med Child Neurol* **54**: 106–116.

Gisel EG (1994) Oral-motor skills following sensorimotor intervention in the moderately eating-impaired child with cerebral palsy. *Dysphagia* **9**: 180–192.

Gisel EG, Alphonce E, Ramsay M (2000) Assessment of ingestive and oral praxis skills: children with cerebral palsy vs. controls. *Dysphagia* **15**: 236–244.

Gisel EG, Applegate-Ferrante T, Benson JE, Bosma JF (1995) Effect of oral sensorimotor treatment on measures of growth, eating efficiency and aspiration in the dysphagic child with cerebral palsy. *Dev Med Child Neurol* **37**: 528–543.

Gurka MJ, Kuperminc MN, Busby MG, et al. (2010) Assessment and correction of skinfold thickness equations in estimating body fat in children with cerebral palsy. *Dev Med Child Neurol* **52**: e35–e41.

Henderson RC, Gilbert SR, Clement ME, Abbas A, Worley G, Stevenson RD (2005) Altered skeletal maturation in moderate to severe cerebral palsy. *Dev Med Child Neurol* **47**: 229–236.

Henderson RC, Lark RK, Gurka MJ, et al. (2002) Bone density and metabolism in children and adolescents with moderate to severe cerebral palsy. *Pediatrics* **110**: e5.

Krick J, Murphy-Miller P, Zeger S, Wright E (1996) Pattern of growth in children with cerebral palsy. *J Am Diet Assoc* **96**: 680–685.

Kuperminc MN, Gottrand F, Samson-Fang L, et al. (2013) Nutritional management of children with cerebral palsy: a practical guide. *Eur J Clin Nutr* **67** (Suppl 2): S21–S23.

Kuperminc MN, Gurka MJ, Bennis JA, et al. (2010) Anthropometric measures: poor predictors of body fat in children with moderate to severe cerebral palsy. *Dev Med Child Neurol* **52**: 824–830.

Kuperminc MN, Gurka MJ, Houlihan CM, et al. (2009) Puberty, statural growth, and growth hormone release in children with cerebral palsy. *J Pediatr Rehabil Med* **2**: 131–141.

Kuperminc MN, Stevenson RD (2008) Growth and nutrition disorders in children with cerebral palsy. *Dev Disabil Res Rev* **14**: 137–146.

Leslie P, Drinnan MJ, Zammit-Maempel I, Coyle JL, Ford GA, Wilson JA (2007) Cervical auscultation synchronized with images from endoscopy swallow evaluations. *Dysphagia* **22**: 290–298.

Mehta NM, Corkins MR, Lyman B, et al. (2013) Defining pediatric malnutrition: a paradigm shift toward etiology-related definitions. *JPEN J Parenter Enteral Nutr* **37**: 460–481.

Pogatschnik C, Hamilton C (2011) Nutrition-Focused Physical Examination: Nails, Hair, Eyes and Oral Cavity. *Support Line* **2**: 7.

Reilly S, Skuse D, Poblete X (1996) Prevalence of feeding problems and oral motor dysfunction in children with cerebral palsy: a community survey. *J Pediatr* **129**: 877–882.

Samson-Fang L, Bell KL (2013) Assessment of growth and nutrition in children with cerebral palsy. *Eur J Clin Nutr* **67** (Suppl 2) S5–S8.

Samson-Fang L, Stevenson RD (1998) Linear growth velocity in children with cerebral palsy. *Dev Med Child Neurol* **40**: 689–692.

Samson-Fang LJ, Stevenson RD (2000) Identification of malnutrition in children with cerebral palsy: poor performance of weight-for-height centiles. *Dev Med Child Neurol* **42**: 162–168.

Stallings VA, Cronk CE, Zemel BS, Charney EB (1995) Body composition in children with spastic quadriplegic cerebral palsy. *J Pediatr* **126**: 833–839.

Stallings VA, Zemel BS, Davies JC, Cronk CE, Charney EB (1996) Energy expenditure of children and adolescents with severe disabilities: a cerebral palsy model. *Am J Clin Nutr* **64**: 627–634.

Stevenson RD, Conaway M (2007) Growth assessment of children with cerebral palsy: the clinician's conundrum. *Dev Med Child Neurol* **49**: 164.

Walker JL, Bell KL, Boyd RN, Davies PS (2012) Energy requirements in preschool-age children with cerebral palsy. *Am J Clin Nutr* **96**: 1309–1315.

Weston SC, M P (2012) Academy of Nutrition and Dietetics Pocket Guide to Children with Special Health Care Needs: Nutrition Care Handbook. Chicago, IL: Academy of Nutrition and Dietetics.

World Health Organization (1985) Energy and Protein Requirements. Report of a Joint FAO/WHO/UNU Expert Consultation. *Technical Report Series* 724. Geneva, Switzerland: World Health Organization.

Chapter 8

Gastro-intestinal diseases in pediatric patients with complex cerebral palsy

Beate Beinvogl and Munir Mobassaleh

Gastro-intestinal issues are common in patients with cerebral palsy (CP), with a prevalence as high as 92% in this population, and have significant implications for their nutritional status, care, development, and quality of life (Del Giudice et al. 1999).

Gastro-intestinal motility and function are predominantly regulated by the autonomic nervous system and a mesh-like, intricate and highly complex network of neurons, also termed the enteric nervous system (ENS). While the ENS is capable of functioning autonomously, it also depends on the central nervous system (CNS) and spinal cord for its function by receiving important modulatory input. The etiology of gastro-intestinal dysfunction in patients with neurologic impairment is not fully understood; however, it appears that disorders affecting the CNS result in an abnormal modulatory effect, resulting in gastro-intestinal motor dysfunction with various presentations including feeding difficulties, gastro-esophageal reflux disease (GERD), retching, vomiting and chronic constipation (Elawad and Sullivan 2001). Studies have shown that the degree of gastro-intestinal dysmotility may correlate with the degree of brain damage (Staiano et al. 1991). No specific neuroimaging findings, however, have been correlated (Del Giudice et al. 1999). Some background and practical aspects of common gastro-intestinal issues in patients with severe cerebral palsy will be reviewed here.

Feeding considerations in patients with complex cerebral palsy

Feeding problems (see also Chapter 7) are present in up to 86% of patients with severe cerebral palsy and have significant implications for the patients' pulmonary and digestive health, in addition to their development and growth (Erkin et al. 2010). Feeding difficulties are frequently due to swallowing dysfunction and resultant aspiration. Feeding intolerance can also be due to gastro-esophageal reflux, vomiting or retching, which are at least in part a direct result of the abnormal gastro-intestinal motility. Any of these problems may result in inadequate nutritional intake and malnutrition and often necessitate the use of alternative feeding routes such as gastrostomy or gastro-jejunostomy tubes.

Swallowing and oropharyngeal dysfunction

The act of swallowing is a highly complex interplay of muscles and nerves in the mouth, oropharynx and esophagus and includes several key phases (preparatory, oral, pharyngeal and esophageal). Problems with sensory receptors in the pharynx, brain stem or other regions of the brain, spine, peripheral nerves or muscles can result in abnormal swallowing, decreased protective mechanisms and resultant aspiration (Duncan 2017). Therefore, CNS disorders such as cerebral palsy commonly result in swallowing dysfunction, with a prevalence quoted as high as 60–86% (Del Giudice et al. 1999) (Sullivan et al. 2000). This patient population shows predominantly dysfunction in the oral phase of swallowing (93%) with abnormal formation of the food bolus, due to uncoordinated movements of the tongue or a contracted or rigid tongue. Alternatively, they can also have defective propulsion of food toward the oropharynx, likely due to the lack of finely coordinated movements of the tongue against the palate (Del Giudice et al. 1999).

It is important to note that swallowing dysfunction in patients with cerebral palsy can evolve or worsen over time, and patients should be monitored closely for any need to re-evaluate and/or adjust the feeding route (Duncan 2017). An individualized approach to the diagnosis and management is important and often necessitates a multidisciplinary evaluation in subspecialty aero digestive clinics in addition to the care provided by the general practitioner. Early recognition and treatment is important in order to minimize the high morbidity and mortality associated with feeding difficulties (see also Chapter 7: Feeding and Nutrition).

Presentation of swallowing disorders

The history can provide important clues suggestive of feeding or swallowing problems. Feeds taking longer than 30 minutes on a regular basis, stressful mealtimes, weight loss or poor weight gain and evidence of respiratory problems with feeds should prompt further evaluation (Arvedson 2013). Presenting symptoms of swallowing dysfunction include both gastro-intestinal and extra-intestinal signs and symptoms. Patients can have obvious signs of aspiration including choking, gagging, sputtering, coughing and cyanosis with feeds, but symptoms can also be subtle and nonspecific including delayed swallowing, voice changes, tearing, nasal congestion, wheezing, facial redness, and recurrent respiratory infections. Feeding refusal can be a self-protective mechanism in patients who aspirate. Further, aspiration can be subclinical, referred to as silent aspiration (Duncan 2017). It is also important to note that GERD is associated with aspiration, which is frequently overlooked.

Patients with severe cerebral palsy may have sialorrhea, or increased drooling, as a result of oromotor dysfunction and this may be a significant barrier to social acceptance. Swallowing dysfunction may further result in salivary aspiration, even without being fed by mouth, which in turn may present with chronic or recurrent pulmonary disease. Generally, the more severe the neurologic impairment and swallowing dysfunction are, the higher the risk of salivary aspiration.

Diagnostic evaluation of swallowing disorders

For an adequate evaluation, mealtimes should be observed as part of a clinical feeding evaluation, and a video-fluoroscopic swallow study (VFSS) should be considered. In a VFSS, patients are asked to drink small amounts of liquid barium or eat small amounts of barium-laced food. Various consistencies of fluid thickness are tried (liquid, nectar thick, honey thick) to test a patient's ability to swallow them safely without laryngeal penetration (passage of liquid into the laryngeal vestibule, but not below the vocal folds), or aspiration (passage of liquids below the level of the vocal folds into the trachea). Salivary aspiration can be difficult to diagnose definitively. Salivagrams, in which saliva is labeled with a radionuclide and traced into the lung in cases of aspiration, have low specificity. However, in the presence of risk factors for salivary aspiration as discussed previously (see Presentation of swallowing disorders section), a salivagram can provide important information to guide management.

While swallowing dysfunction and aspiration are common in patients with cerebral palsy, other diagnoses should be considered and ruled out, as this can have significant treatment implications. These include large tonsils, a cleft palate, vocal cord paralysis, a laryngeal cleft, upper esophageal sphincter dysfunction, an esophageal stricture or esophagitis, medications which decrease the level of alertness, other neurologic diseases such as neuromuscular disorders and seizures, or a Chiari malformation (Duncan 2017).

Management of swallowing disorders

Each patient should be considered on an individual basis and treatment should be based on the results of the clinical evaluation, diagnostic testing and severity of the feeding dysfunction and resultant complications. In patients who aspirate but clinically tolerate oral feeds, the least invasive intervention includes the thickening of formula to a consistency that was found safe on VFSS. Thickening of feeds prevents aspiration by slowing down the speed at which a liquid bolus moves from the mouth into the pharynx (Duncan 2017). Rice or oat cereal as well as a variety of commercially available thickeners can be used. A similar effect can be achieved by using a slower-flow nipple if a patient is bottle fed. In patients who are motivated, moderately alert and have some residual swallowing dysfunction, oromotor therapy should be part of the treatment plan which includes a variety of possible interventions such as dietary modifications, positioning, exercises to improve oromotor control including compensatory swallowing techniques. In patients with severe swallowing dysfunction, dysphagia, malnutrition or associated respiratory disease, the implementation of gastrostomy tube feedings is often necessary and recommended (Samson-Fang et al. 2003). Unfortunately, however, early avoidance of oral feeding and prolonged *nil per os* status has been shown to imply a faster decline in swallowing dysfunction (Maeda et al. 2016). Families should therefore be encouraged to continue oral feeds whenever safe and appropriate.

Excessive drooling (see also Chapter 9) can be approached with behavioral therapy (oral motor skills program), medications or surgery. Sometimes it improves with age. Anticholinergic medications such as glycopyrrolate or scopolamine decrease salivary flow, and can be administered as liquid or transdermal patch respectively. Anticholinergic side effects include thickening of secretions making swallowing more difficult, hyperactivity, visual disturbances and urinary retention, which should be monitored closely. Botulin toxin A injections into the salivary glands can also decrease salivary flow. Salivary duct ligation or surgical excision can be performed with the intention to reduce saliva production.

Enteral feeding tubes
Enteral feeding tubes are indicated in patients who aspirate all consistencies, have insufficient fluid or caloric oral intake or progressively worsening swallowing dysfunction (Heuschkel et al. 2015). Nasogastric tubes can be used temporarily. However, if the need for enteral tube feeding is anticipated to be longer than three months, surgical, laparoscopic or endoscopic placement of a gastrostomy (G-tube) or gastro-jejunostomy tube (GJ-tube) should be considered. For GJ-tubes, the tip of the feeding tube is placed in the jejunum (post-pyloric). This should be considered in cases of severe gastro-esophageal reflux and/or esophagitis, repeated aspiration of gastric contents, esophageal dysmotility or delayed gastric emptying. Primary jejunostomy tubes (J-tubes) can be indicated in rare cases. It is important to remember, however, that even patients with post-pyloric feeds remain at risk for aspiration of oral secretions and sometimes even gastric secretions, or may have retching or vomiting of gastric content.

Surgically placed enteral feeding tubes have been shown to improve patient's nutritional status, reduce aspiration, provide a reliable route for medication administration and improve the quality of life for both patients and families (Kong and Wong 2005). However, awareness of the risks and complications related to enteral tube placement is important. These include post-operative complications (perforation, poor wound healing, infections, hemorrhage, gastro-colic fistula), skin irritation from leaking of gastric or bilious secretions, skin infections (cellulitis, phlegmon, abscess), formation of granulation tissue or tube dislodgement. Tubes require replacement if they become clogged. Longer tubes with a smaller diameter, such as gastro-jejunostomy tubes are particularly prone to clogging and require frequent flushing to prevent this. In the case of G-tubes, the tube can be easily replaced by the family at home. GJ-tubes, however, typically need to be changed by radiologists under fluoroscopic guidance. A frequent but often overlooked complication of gastrostomies is overfeeding which can lead to vomiting, and distinguishing overfeeding from gastro-esophageal reflux can be challenging. In such cases, it sometimes becomes necessary to empirically switch to a GJ-tube. Disadvantages specific to jejunal feeds include the lower tolerance of rapid feeding rates, typically necessitating continuous feeds which can further complicate care and social participation, and increase the risk for bacterial overgrowth. Further, a GJ-tube tip can act as a lead point causing small bowel intussusception, requiring immediate attention.

Gastro-esophageal reflux disease

Gastro-esophageal reflux (GER) is defined as the passing of gastric contents into the esophagus with or without regurgitation or vomiting. To a certain extent it is physiologic and can occur multiple times throughout the day. Presence of bothersome symptoms or complications is pathologic and termed gastro-esophageal reflux disease (GERD) (Vandenplas et al. 2009). GERD is common in patients with severe neurologic impairment, with a prevalence cited as high as 60–90% and is often refractory to standard medical therapy (Del Giudice et al. 1999). The increased prevalence in this population appears to be related to abnormal esophageal motility and possibly slowed gastric emptying. Spasticity, prolonged supine position, scoliosis, seizures and decreased amounts of swallowed saliva increase the predisposition for GERD and may be responsible for high failure rate of both medical and surgical treatments. Lifelong interventions and adjustments in therapy are often required and the prognosis depends on the severity of both GERD and the degree of neurologic impairment.

Presentation of gastro-esophageal reflux disease

The most common signs and symptoms of GERD in patients with neurologic impairment include vomiting, irritability, arching, feeding refusal, weight loss or poor weight gain, extra-intestinal symptoms such as coughing between meals and/or recurrent aspiration pneumonias. In case of esophageal injury from prolonged stomach acid exposure, patients can present with blood-tinged emesis, hematemesis, or anemia. It is important to be aware that symptoms can be nonspecific and many conditions mimic GERD. Specifically, aspiration secondary to swallowing dysfunction is frequently overlooked because aspiration is often attributed to aspiration of gastric contents, as seen in GERD. Careful consideration is therefore important. The most common GERD-related complications in patients with cerebral palsy include iron deficiency (51.3%), anemia (41%), malnutrition (33.3%), recurrent upper respiratory tract infections (28.2%), and low body weight (28.2%) (Spiroglou et al. 2004).

Diagnostic evaluation of gastro-esophageal reflux disease

GERD is a clinical diagnosis based on history and physical exam. Diagnostic studies can be helpful to guide treatment in cases of treatment refractory symptoms. A feeding evaluation and modified barium swallow is an appropriate diagnostic step if aspiration is a concern (see the Diagnostic evaluation of swallowing disorders section). Anatomic abnormalities that can predispose to increased GERD include achalasia, hiatal hernia, malrotation, pyloric stenosis, duodenal webs or an annular pancreas, and can be ruled out with an upper gastro-intestinal series (UGI). Further, an esophagram or UGI can delineate complications related to GERD including peptic esophageal strictures. It should be emphasized, however, that a UGI is not useful to diagnose GERD and presence of reflux on an UGI does not imply GERD. Esophageal motility studies in a specialty center may be indicated in selected cases.

An esophago-gastro-duodenoscopy is a helpful study to determine the presence of any GERD-related esophageal injury such as esophagitis, esophageal erosions or ulcerations, or to exclude alternate diagnoses such as infectious esophagitis, eosinophilic esophagitis, Barrett's esophagus, *Helicobacter pylori* gastritis and peptic ulcer disease.

A nuclear medicine scan, also known as gastric emptying scan (GES), uses radioactively labeled (Tc99-m) formula or food to evaluate the adequacy of gastric emptying. Patients with neurologic impairment are at risk for gastroparesis (delayed gastric emptying) secondary to their underlying disease. Adverse medication effects (e.g. anticholinergics), temporary or permanent post-operative vagal nerve injury (e.g. fundoplication), post-viral or autoimmune gastroparesis are other potential causes. The high prevalence of gastroparesis (67%) among children with cerebral palsy who also have GERD gives rise to the assumption that gastroparesis may exacerbate reflux and an empiric treatment trial of gastroparesis may be warranted in selected cases (Del Giudice et al. 1999). However, studies to support a causal relationship are currently lacking (Spiroglou et al. 2004).

An impedance and pH-probe study, typically performed simultaneously, consist of placement of a thin and flexible catheter with sensors in the esophagus for a 24-hour period. This enables the measurement of the frequency and length of acid or nonacid reflux episodes, thereby quantifying the extent and duration of esophageal acid exposure. It is also useful to evaluate the efficacy of therapy and to correlate or disprove correlation between GER and unclear symptoms such as chest pain, arching, or coughing, which can be helpful to guide treatment (Rudolph et al. 2001).

Management of gastro-esophageal reflux disease

The management of GERD in patients with cerebral palsy can be challenging. Management is directed at minimizing peptic injury to the esophagus as well as minimizing full column esophageal reflux which may otherwise result in aspiration. Finding the balance of minimizing aspiration risk, while still providing adequate nutrition, can be challenging. Recent guidelines of the North American and European Societies of Pediatric Gastroenterology, Hepatology and Nutrition (NASPGHAN, ESPGHAN) detail these recommendations, with some specific recommendations for patients with neurologic impairment (Rudolph et al. 2001, Vandenplas et al. 2009).

ACID SUPPRESSIVE THERAPY

Both acute and chronic peptic esophageal injury including esophagitis, esophageal erosions or ulcerations and prevention of peptic strictures can be managed effectively with acid suppressive medications. This anti-secretory therapy should be optimized with Histamine-2 (H2) receptor antagonists such as cimetidine, ranitidine, famotidine, nizatidine, or the more potent proton-pump-inhibitors (PPIs) such as omeprazole, lansoprazole, pantoprazole, esomeprazole, dexlansoprazole or rabeprazole. The advantage of the H2-antagonists is their rapid onset of action and their availability as liquids, which facilitates administration via enteral feeding tubes. H2 blockers have the disadvantage of possibly losing efficacy secondary to tachyphylaxis, a rapid decrease in response with repeated doses, thereby making the medication less effective over time. PPIs are not routinely available as liquids, but can be compounded by specialty pharmacies. Omeprazole and lansoprazole are available as powders, and lansoprazole also as a dissolvable tablet (Rudolph et al. 2001). Because of the efficacy of anti-secretory medications, buffering agents such as magnesium and aluminum hydroxide or carafate are no longer routinely recommended for GERD. However, they continue to be used on an as needed basis for immediate symptom relief. In case of esophageal erosions, mucosal defects related to feeding tubes, or peptic ulcers, carafate may be used temporarily to coat the site of mucosal injury, thereby facilitating healing. The most common medications used in the medical treatment of GERD are listed in Table 8.1.

Long-term treatment with anti-secretory medications are often effective for symptom control and maintenance of remission. Nonetheless, it is important to treat as restrictively as possible, given the growing evidence of significant long-term side effects, specifically of PPI therapy. These include idiosyncratic reactions (headache, diarrhea, constipation, nausea), drug-drug interactions, increased respiratory and gastro-intestinal infections, small bowel bacterial overgrowth, hypomagnesemia, osteoporosis and chronic kidney injury. H2 receptor antagonists require dose adjustment in the setting of renal insufficiency. Risks and benefits need to be weighed carefully. One way to approach treatment is to empirically treat patients with a four week medication trial, and continue the medications only in case of clear benefit. Also, the smallest effective dose should be used at all times.

PRO-MOTILITY AGENTS

Pro-motility agents are not recommended for the routine treatment of GERD (Vandenplas et al. 2009). In case of suspected gastroparesis or an abnormal gastric emptying

Table 8.1 Oral medications used in the treatment of pediatric gastro-esophageal reflux disease[a]

Medication	Dosing
Histamine-2 (H2) receptor-antagonists	
Cimetidine	20–40mg/kg per day divided in 4 doses (maximum 400mg per dose)[b,c]
Ranitidine	6–9mg/kg per day divided in 2 doses (maximum 150mg per dose)
Famotidine	1mg/kg per day divided in 2 doses (maximum 40mg per dose)
Nizatidine	5–10mg/kg per day divided in 2 doses (maximum 150mg per day)
Proton pump inhibitors (PPI)	
Omeprazole	1–2mg/kg per day once daily or divided in 2 doses (maximum 20–40mg per day)
Lansoprazole	1–2mg/kg per day once daily or divided in 2 doses (maximum 30–60mg per day)
Pantoprazole	≥12 years: 20–40mg once daily
Esomeprazole	<0.7–3.3mg/kg per day (maximum 20mg daily)
Rabeprazole	**1–11 years** <15kg: 5mg once daily, ≥15kg: 10mg once daily **≥12 years** 20mg once daily
Dexlansoprazole	**≥12 years** 30mg daily
Prokinetic agents[b]	
Erythromycin	3–5mg/kg/dose 3–4 times daily (maximum 250mg per dose)
Metoclopramide	0.1mg/kg/dose 3–4 times daily (maximum 10mg per dose)
Cyproheptadine	0.1mg/kg/dose 2–3 times daily (maximum 16mg/day)
Buffering agents	
Aluminum and magnesium hydroxide[c]	0.5–1 ml/kg per dose 4 times daily (maximum 20 ml per dose)
Sucralfate[c]	**3 months to <6 years** 500mg/dose up to 4 times daily **≥6 years** 1g up to four times daily

[a]Dosing for symptomatic GERD, different dosing may apply for erosive or ulcerative esophagitis, [b]Prokinetic agents are not recommended for routine treatment of GERD, but can be used in specific circumstances if gastroparesis is a contributing factor to GERD, [c]Limited data available.
GERD, gastro-esophageal reflux disease.

study, treatment with erythromycin can be started. Alternatively, metoclopramide, a D2 Dopamine receptor antagonist, may be used. However, risks and benefits should be weighed carefully given its potentially severe adverse effects including lethargy, irritability, gynecomastia, galactorrhea, diarrhea, extrapyramidal reactions and potentially permanent tardive dyskinesia. The pro-motility agent cisapride, a 5-HT4 serotonin receptor agonist, is effective but has been taken off the market given its significant cardiac side effect profile and is only available restrictively in specialty programs run by pediatric gastroenterologists as part of safety studies (Hill et al. 1998, Dalby-Payne et al. 2003).

Baclofen decreases the frequency of relaxations of the lower esophageal sphincter and can be a useful adjunct to decrease GERD-related symptoms. However, it is not recommended for routine use, largely due to its adverse effects of dyspepsia, drowsiness, dizziness, fatigue, decrease in seizure threshold and constipation (Omari et al. 2006, Vandenplas et al. 2009).

FEEDING METHODS

Enteral feeding regimens can be adjusted to increase feeding tolerance and minimize GERD. While bolus feeds are the most physiologic, in case of poor gastric emptying, these can predispose to worsening GERD and its complications. Switching to continuous feeds can alleviate symptoms. An amino-acid based formula has been shown to decrease refractory esophagitis secondary to GERD in neurologically impaired children (Miele et al. 2002). Whole meal-based formulas or 'blenderized' diet options may also be beneficial and warrant a trial. Cyproheptadine, a first generation anti-histamine, can help with gastric accommodation and a treatment trial can be warranted to improve feeding tolerance. Caretakers should be educated about potential side effects including decreased alertness (Rodriguez et al. 2013).

Transgastric jejunal (post-pyloric) feeds are often effective in patients with clinically significant GERD (Vandenplas et al. 2009). Often jejunal feeding tubes are placed in the form of a GJ-tube, providing a gastrostomy port which can be used for venting and may further relieve symptoms and improve feeding tolerance (see Enteral feeding section).

SURGICAL AND ENDOSCOPIC INTERVENTIONS

Surgical interventions for GERD are directed at minimizing or preventing pathologic gastro-esophageal reflux and/or the improvement of gastric emptying. The risks and benefits of any surgical or endoscopic intervention should always be weighed carefully in this high risk population. A Nissen fundoplication is the most common anti-reflux procedure in which the gastric fundus, or upper part of the stomach, is wrapped and stitched around the lower end of the esophagus. This is typically performed laparoscopically. It is considered in patients with the primary symptom of vomiting and concern for decreased protective airway mechanisms resulting in increased risk for aspiration. Other indications include refractory or nonadherence to medical therapy or dependence on long-term medical therapy. The intention of the fundoplication is to mechanically reinforce the lower esophageal sphincter, thereby eliminating reflux of gastric contents into the esophagus. This can be very effective in patients with refractory GERD, with good results and improved quality of life and successful relief of symptoms in the majority of cases (Esposito et al. 2003). However, it has also been shown to decrease gastric accommodation capacity, increase the rate of gastric emptying, altered distribution of food within the stomach and altered sensory motor function, which may at least in part be responsible for some of the post-operative discomfort and complications.

A failure rate of up to 22% has been described after fundoplications (Vandenplas et al. 2009). Up to two thirds of patients have ongoing or re-develop GERD symptoms despite the fundoplication and require acid suppressive treatment within the first 2–24 months after surgery (Mousa et al. 2006). A tight fundoplication may cause increased difficulties passing oral secretions through the distal esophagus, resulting in pooling of secretions and increased risk of aspiration. Bloating, retching, and abdominal discomfort may occur from an inability to relieve air via burping. This can be alleviated by simultaneous placement of a gastrostomy tube at the time of the fundoplication, if not already in place, to allow for venting. The fundoplication can unwrap, resulting in recurrence of symptoms, explaining re-operation rates of up to 20% (Richards et al. 2000). A post-operative increased rate of gastric emptying may result in diarrhea and/or dumping syndrome, a potentially dangerous derangement of glucose and electrolytes secondary to osmotic fluid shifts related to the fast influx of carbohydrates in the proximal small bowel (Rudolph et al. 2001). Supplementation of gastric feeds with uncooked cornstarch may be beneficial in slowing down gastric emptying (Borovoy et al. 1998). Visceral hypersensitivity resulting in abdominal pain may be due to changes in the gastric sensory motor function.

Endoscopic injections of botulin toxin A into the pylorus, causing paralysis and thereby relaxation, can improve gastric emptying in case of refractory gastroparesis (Rodriguez et al. 2012). A pyloroplasty can be performed as a more permanent intervention. The main complication of the pyloroplasty includes dumping syndrome.

Constipation

Chronic constipation is common in patients with cerebral palsy, with a prevalence estimated to be as high as 74% (Del Giudice et al. 1999). No data exists on normal stooling patterns in patients with cerebral palsy, but defecation frequency of less than once every three days is often considered constipation. Stool caliber, associated symptoms such as abdominal pain or bloating, and physical exam findings play an important role in determining whether or not the stooling behavior is abnormal. It is often underdiagnosed, likely because of the individual's inability to communicate the discomfort, and prioritization by the providers of treatment of other manifestations of neurologic impairment such as seizure disorders. Furthermore, constipation is often considered inevitable in this patient population (Elawad and Sullivan 2001). Constipation can be a significant source of discomfort and result in decreased feeding tolerance, abdominal discomfort, reduced quality of life and adversely affect development.

Understanding the normal physiology of defecation is important in order to understand the pathophysiology of abnormal defecation in patients with neurologic impairment, and will be reviewed here. Normal defecation involves both voluntary (external anal sphincter) and involuntary (internal anal sphincter, enteric nervous system) mechanisms. Normally, sympathetic nerve fibers (L1, L2) are responsible for inhibiting rectal contractions and inhibiting relaxation of the internal anal sphincter, creating ongoing autonomic contraction (also called the resting pressure), thereby enabling us to avoid constant leaking of fecal material. Rectal distension by fecal material is the primary stimulus initiating the defecation triggering the recto-anal inhibitory reflex, mostly mediated by parasympathetic fibers (S2-S4), resulting in contraction of the elongated rectal muscles thereby further pushing forward the fecal material. It also causes relaxation of the internal anal sphincter whereby the anal pressure drops, allowing stool to descend. At the same time, afferent signals are sent to the brain via sensory parasympathetic nerves in the spinal cord, which are perceived by the brain as the need to defecate, thereby allowing the voluntary relaxation of the external sphincter and pubococcygeal muscles. Voluntarily increasing intra-abdominal pressure then further helps to expel stool (Elawad and Sullivan 2001). In patients with neurologic diseases affecting the CNS, abnormal modulation of the autonomic nervous system results in abnormal defecation. Upper motor neuron (UMN) dysfunction, suggested by hypertonia and hyperreflexia, results in overactive pelvic muscle contraction and difficulty or inability to voluntarily relax the external anal sphincter, which is key for normal defecation. On the contrary, lower motor neuron (LMN) dysfunction, as seen in spina bifida and suggested by hypotonia, hyporeflexia and absent sensation can result in poor or no sensation of rectal filling and rectal fullness and/or by the instability of the position of the anus by the levator ani muscle during rectal contraction. Further, these patients have an exaggerated inhibitory reflex of the internal anal sphincter, implying that any stool in the rectum will completely inhibit the anal tone (Elawad and Sullivan 2001).

In addition to the underlying neurologic dysfunction, other predisposing and exacerbating factors are often found: feeding intolerance in this patient population often requires enteral tube feeding, with low fiber formulas and/or pureed foods. Fluid intake is often restricted given concern for aspiration or poor oral intake. Skeletal muscle dyscoordination and abnormalities and poor mobility also contribute to constipation. Another important consideration is the use of polypharmacy necessitated for management of seizures, chronic pain and/or bladder dysfunction. Specifically opioid and anticholinergic medications can have a significant effect of slowing down colonic transit. Anti-seizure and skeletal muscle relaxant medications such as sodium valproate, phenothiazines and baclofen may also contribute to constipation (Elawad and Sullivan 2001).

Presentation of constipation

The most frequent complaints of constipation include infrequent bowel movements (less than once every three days), hard small stools, difficulties or pain with stooling of large-diameter stools. Abdominal pain or diffuse discomfort are important symptoms of constipation in patients with cerebral palsy.

It is important to obtain a complete history in the evaluation of a child with constipation. These should include frequency, consistency and size of the stools, pain or hemorrhage with passing of stools and presence of abdominal pain or discomfort. Other important questions to elicit on history include the timing of first bowel movement after birth, age at onset of the abnormal defection, presence of fecal incontinence, withholding behaviors, systemic symptoms such as fever, vomiting, weight loss, decreased appetite, social history including stressors, details of previous therapies and adherence to these therapies. A thorough physical exam is also essential to evaluate for warning signs of organic disease (Table 8.2).

Diagnostic evaluation in constipation

The diagnosis of constipation is made based on history and physical exam and further work up is not routinely recommended unless alarming features are present on history or physical exam (Table 8.2). The formal criteria for functional constipation per ROME IV, a multi-national working team consensus, include the following: two or fewer defecations per week, at least one episode of fecal incontinence per week, a history of retentive posturing or excessive volitional stool retention, history of painful or hard bowel movements, presence of a large fecal mass in the rectum, or history of large-diameter stools in the absence of another medical condition which could account for symptoms (Hyams et al. 2016). For patients with cerebral palsy, these criteria need to be used in context.

It is important to evaluate for fecal impaction, the presence of a large, dry, solid, typically immobile bulk of stool that can develop in the rectum as a result of chronic constipation. In the presence of fecal impaction, patients can have diarrheal stools, often termed overflow diarrhea, or encopresis, and represents involuntary passing of soft stool around the hard fecal mass in the rectum. It is important to determine whether or not fecal impaction is present, given its implications for treatment.

Because cerebral palsy includes such a heterogeneous group of patients, it is important to consider warning signs and symptoms that may point toward another contributory or alternate diagnosis such as congenital malformations of the anorectum or spine, Hirschsprung disease, food allergies, metabolic or endocrine conditions. Such red flags on history and/or physical exam are summarized in Table 8.2 and should be considered in cerebral palsy patients as much as in otherwise healthy patients, as identification of an alternate cause will have significant treatment implications.

Table 8.2 Warning signs suggestive of an organic cause of constipation[a]

History
Acute signs
• Delayed passage of meconium >48h after birth
• Severe abdominal distension
• Fever, vomiting or diarrhea
• Occult or visible blood in the stools in the absence of anal fissures
Chronic signs
• Onset before 1 month of age
• Ribbon stools (very narrow diameter)
• Intermittent diarrhea and explosive stools
• Urinary incontinence or bladder disease
• Failure to thrive, weight loss, delayed growth
• Family history of Hirschsprung disease
• Congenital anomalies associated with Hirschsprung's disease
• Failure to respond to adequate conventional treatment
• Other associated neurologic symptoms
Physical exam findings
• Sacral dimple: deep, tuft of hair, sinus tract
• Midline pigmentary abnormalities of lower spine
• Abnormal position of the anus, tight anal sphincter
• Empty rectum
• Abnormal neurologic exam (absent anal or cremasteric reflex, decreased lower extremity deep tendon reflexes, tone/strength)
• Gluteal cleft deviation
• Anal scars, perianal fistula

[a]Tabbers et al. 2014

The physical exam should include a review of growth parameters, and abdominal exam looking for fullness or palpable stool, external examination of perineum and perianal area, evaluation of thyroid and spine, and neurologic evaluation for appropriate reflexes (cremasteric, anal wink, patellar). Digital examination of the anorectum is recommended to assess for perineal sensation, anal tone, rectum size, anal wink and amount and consistency of stool in the rectum. Test for occult blood should be performed in all children who have pain, failure to thrive, diarrhea, a family history of colon cancer or polyps. Presence of a hard mass in the lower abdomen combined with a dilated rectum filled with hard stool indicates fecal impaction (Nurko and Zimmerman 2014). It should be noted, however, that the absence of such findings does not exclude constipation, especially in patients that are already treated with stool softeners. Abdominal radiographs can be helpful if fecal impaction is suspected, especially when physical examination and a digital rectal exam is unreliable or not possible, as may be the case in patients with behavioral problems or history of abuse. The use of abdominal films to assess overall stool burden is common but its value is questionable given the poor correlation of radiographic stool burden with clinical symptoms and significant inter and intra-observer variability in the interpretation of radiographs (Tabbers et al. 2014).

Further work up should be considered in the presence of alarm features listed in Table 8.2. Anorectal manometry, for example, can be used to assess the absence of the anorectal inhibitory reflex, indicating Hirschsprung disease. A barium enema can be valuable to evaluate for anatomic abnormalities and colonic motility studies to determine coexistence of a colonic neuropathy. Any suggestion of LMN dysfunction in patients with cerebral palsy, particularly if associated with urinary symptoms, should prompt obtaining a spinal magnetic resonance image (MRI)to rule out spinal abnormalities such as tethered cord or occult spina bifida.

Management of constipation
Medical therapy

Early recognition of constipation is very important for effective treatment and should include parental education, dietary measures and medications. Regular follow up is essential. Parents should be educated on the signs and symptoms concerning for constipation including abdominal discomfort, pain with stooling, feeding intolerance, or abdominal distension. Fiber should be added to the diet, either as a supplement or in the form of commercially available formulas containing fiber, formulas with real food ingredients or blenderized diets. As guidance, the goal fiber intake in grams can be calculated by adding 5–10g to the patient age in years (maximum 30g per day).

There is little risk in anticipatory treatment of constipation and there should be a low threshold to do so. Many consider that time spent upright in a stander or walker/gait trainer can be helpful in promoting bowel movements. Prophylactic treatment with a stool softener should be considered. If fecal impaction is present, it needs to be resolved before initiation of maintenance therapy. The goal of maintenance therapy is to prevent accumulation of stool by maintaining soft bowel movements, preferably once daily. Though equally effective, a rectal clean out may be faster, and can be used as adjunct to an oral clean out. The Peristeen® anal irrigation system instills water into the colon through a rectal catheter and incorporates an inflatable balloon which is inserted into the rectum to promote evacuation of the contents of the lower colon. It can be helpful for a more efficient bowel evacuation, resulting in decreased fecal incontinence and discomfort. Rarely, manual disimpaction may be necessary in cases of severe refractory constipation and requires general anesthesia. Table 8.3 gives an outline of treatment recommendations for both disimpaction and maintenance therapy. Lubiprostone, linaclotide and prucalopride are newer medications that have been found effective in adults with constipation, but evidence in children is limited.

Table 8.3   Common oral and rectal laxatives used for disimpaction and maintenance treatment in pediatric constipation[a,b]

Disimpaction therapy
Enteral

Osmotics

- Polyethylene glycol 3350

  - 1–1.5g/kg per day, divided in three doses for 2–4 days (maximum 256g per day for 1 day or 100g per day for 5 consecutive days)

- Polyethylene Glycol Electrolyte Solution (GoLYTELY®)

  - 25ml/kg per hour by mouth or via nasogastric/gastrostomy tube

- Magnesium citrate (1.745g/30 ml)

  - **2–5 years** 60–90 mL per day, single or divided doses

  - **6–12 years** 150-200 mL per day, single or divided doses

  - **>12 years** 150–300ml per day, single or divided doses

- Magnesium hydroxide (400mg/5ml or 800mg/5ml)

  - **<2 years** 80–160mg/kg per day, single dose at bedtime or divided doses for 3–6 day (maximum 4800mg per day)

Stimulants

- Senna (8.8mg/5ml syrup or 8.6mg/tablet)

  - **2–5 years** 2.5–7.5ml (0.5–1.5 tablets) per day, single or divided doses for 2–4 days

  - **6–12 years** 5–15ml (1–2 tablets) per day, single or divided doses for 2–4 days

  - **>12 years** 10–15ml (2–4 tablets) per day, single or divided doses for 2–4 days

- Bisacodyl (5mg /tablet)

  - **≥2 years** 5–15mg (1–3 tablets) per day, single dose for 2–4 days

Table 8.3 (Continued)

Disimpaction therapy

Rectal

Suppositories

- Glycerin

  - **<2 years** 0.5 pediatric suppository per day

  - **2–5 years** 1 pediatric suppository per day

  - **≥6 years** 1 adult suppository per day

- Bisacodyl (10mg/suppository)

  - **2–10 years** 5mg (0.5 suppository) per day for 2–4 days

  - **>10 years** 5–10mg (0.5–1 suppository) per day for 2–4 days

Enemas

- Sodium chloride (NaCl)

  - **>1 year** 6ml/kg once or twice daily

- Mineral oil (133 ml/enema)

  - **2–10 years** 30–60ml once daily

  - **≥11 years**: 60–150 ml once daily

- Sodium docusate (100mg/5ml or 283mg/5mL)

  - **2–12 years** 100mg (1 unit) once daily

  - **≥12 years** 283mg (1 unit) once daily

- Sodium Phosphate (66ml or 133ml enema)[c]

  - **>2 years** 2.5 ml/kg per day (maximum 133 ml per day)

- Bisacodyl enema (10mg/30ml)

  - **≥12 years** 10mg once daily

Manual disimpaction

Maintenance therapy

Enteral

Osmotics

- Polyethylene Glycol 3350

  - 0.2–1g/kg per day as single or divided dose

Table 8.3 (Continued)

Maintenance therapy
• Lactulose
• 1–2g/kg once or twice daily as single or divided dose
• Magnesium hydroxide (400mg/5ml or 800mg/5ml)
• 40–80mg/kg per day, single or divided doses (max 2 400mg–4 800mg daily)
Stimulants
• Senna (Syrup 8.8mg/5ml or 8.6mg/tablet)
• **2–5 years** 2.5–3.75 ml (0.5 tablet) daily at bedtime (max 3.75ml or 1 tablets twice daily)
• **6–12 years** 5–7.5 ml (1 tablet) daily at bedtime (maximum 7.5ml or 2 tablets twice daily)
• **>12 years** 10–15 ml (2 tablets) daily at bedtime (maximum 15ml or 3 tablets twice daily)
• Bisacodyl (5mg/tablet)
• **3–10 years** 5mg daily
• **>10 years** 5–10mg daily
Rectal
• Rectal therapy as needed (see Disimpaction therapy and Rectal therapy sections)
• Peristeen® anal irrigation system

[a]Tabbers et al. 2014, [b]Nurko and Zimmerman 2014, [c]Should not be used in children <2 years given risk of electrolyte abnormalities.

Generally, all laxatives can have the adverse effect of potentially causing cramping, abdominal distension, increased flatulence or diarrhea. More specifically, magnesium hydroxide can cause hypermagnesemia, hyperphosphatemia or hypocalcemia, especially in infants. Bisacodyl has been associated with hypokalemia, proctitis and urolithiasis. Idiosyncratic hepatitis and melanosis coli, nephropathy and hypertrophic osteoarthropathy have been described as rare complications of senna (Nurko and Zimmerman 2014). While mineral oil can be an effect rectal laxative, it should not be used as an enteral laxative in neurologically impaired children, given its risk for lipoid pneumonia in case of aspiration (Bandla et al. 1999).

SURGICAL THERAPY

Unfortunately, the medical treatment failure rate of constipation in patients with severe neurologic impairment is high at 40%, re-emphasizing the importance of early and aggressive treatment. For medically refractory constipation, surgical interventions can be considered.

The antegrade continence enema (ACE) procedure has been shown to be effective and improves quality of life. It is performed by bringing the reversed appendix to the skin to act as a stoma that allows easy access to the cecum. Through the appendicular stoma, a catheter can be introduced and saline, bisacodyl phosphate enema or polyethylene glycol solutions can be administered at regular intervals to ensure adequate antegrade evacuation. Alternatively, a cecostomy is performed when the cecum is surgically attached to the abdominal wall and a non-latex tube can be placed directly in the cecum for easier access. Rarely, de-functioning ileostomy or colostomy is necessary in the management of extreme megacolon secondary to chronic constipation.

Abdominal pain

Abdominal pain is described in 32% of patients with cerebral palsy (Del Giudice et al. 1999). Patients with severe cerebral palsy have varying degrees of communication difficulties which can make the evaluation of pain and its etiologies more difficult. It is therefore important to keep in mind the broad differential diagnosis of acute and chronic abdominal pain in order to promptly and efficiently address the causes. Gallstones can cause abdominal pain, especially in the case of gallstone-related complications including acute cholecystitis, choledocholithiasis with or without cholangitis, and/or gallstone pancreatitis. Prolonged parenteral nutrition, which is rarely necessary in this patient population, poses a significant risk for gallstone formation. However, gallstones are often an incidental finding and asymptomatic. Care should be taken not to miss alternate diagnoses by attributing pain to gallstones. The need for surgical removal of gallstones and cholecystectomy is indicated for patients with symptomatic cholelithiasis or related complications. Pancreatitis can cause severe abdominal pain, and seizure medications predispose to this in the cerebral palsy population. Peptic ulcer disease or gastritis can present with acute abdominal pain as well, especially in the context of recent use of non-steroidal anti-inflammatory drugs (NSAID). In rare cases, the post-pyloric positioning of the gastro-jejunostomy tubes can act as a lead point, resulting in intussusception, typically presenting as severe abdominal pain with bilious vomiting or increased gastrostomy output. This requires removal of the gastro-jejunostomy tube in order to prevent further complications such as perforation. In infants, the gastrostomy balloon can sometimes cause a gastric outlet obstruction and should be considered as a potential cause of vomiting.

Causes of chronic abdominal pain include esophagitis, gastritis, celiac disease, food allergies, lactose intolerance, small bowel bacterial overgrowth and constipation. Feeding tube cutaneous entry sites, if present, should be carefully evaluated, as complications related to them can cause abdominal pain or discomfort. Inspection of the skin for erythema, swelling or fluctuance, the fit of the tube, the balloon, and any drainage from the tract need to be assessed. Table 8.4 lists common causes specifically of both acute and chronic abdominal pain in patients with cerebral palsy. Table 8.5 lists common etiologies of abdominal discomfort related to feeding tubes. Extra-intestinal causes of abdominal pain should also be considered, but go beyond the scope of this chapter.

Table 8.4 Diagnostic considerations in suspected or evident abdominal pain

Differential diagnosis	Diagnostic clues/ risk factors	Initial evaluation	Empiric or initial treatment
Gallstones	Pain or discomfort related to feeds Fevers (cholangitis) Obesity (overfeeding) Parenteral nutrition	CBC Liver panel Amylase/lipase RUQ US	Emergency room referral if initial evaluation is abnormal
Pancreatitis	Seizure medications Presence of gall stones Family history of pancreatitis	CBC Liver panel Amylase/lipase RUQ US	NPO Emergency room referral if evaluation is abnormal
Esophagitis – peptic vs allergic	Dysphagia Vomiting Increased oral secretions	Empiric treatment EGD	Medication trial with H2 blocker or PPI[a] Dietary modification in case of allergy
Gastritis and PUD: chemical, *H. pylori*	Pain related to feeds Vomiting Recent administration of NSAIDS	Empiric treatment (gastritis) EGD H. pylori stool antigen (may be falsely low if patient on PPI) Hemoccult	Gastritis: PPI[a] PUD: high dose PPI *H. pylori*: double antibiotic therapy and PPI
Bacterial overgrowth	Abdominal distension Diarrhea, malabsorption Continuous or postpyloric feeds	Empiric treatment Hydrogen breath test	Metronidazole or rifaxamin
Constipation	Infrequent bowel movements (less than once every 3 days) Hard, small stools Difficulties or pain with large-diameter stools	Abdominal exam Consider DRE Abdominal radiograph to evaluate for fecal impaction if DRE not possible	Addition of fiber to formula/feeds Acute: • Disimpaction Chronic: • Maintenance laxative therapy[b]
Celiac disease	Gluten exposure	Total IgA Tissue-transglutaminase IgA CBC	Gluten-free diet

Table 8.4 (Continued)

Differential diagnosis	Diagnostic clues/ risk factors	Initial evaluation	Empiric or initial treatment
Food allergy	Bloody stools Feeding intolerance Vomiting, diarrhea Younger age	Hemoccult Specific food allergy testing if indicated	Trial of semi-elemental or elemental formula Dietary restriction Allergist/ Gastroenterologist consultation
Visceral hypersensitivity	Exclusion of other pain etiologies	Diagnosis of exclusion	Empiric treatment with periactin or gabapentin

[a]See Table 8.1 for details, [b]See Table 8.2 for details.
RUQ US: right upper quadrant ultrasound, CBC, complete blood count; NPO, *nil per os,* EGD: Esophago-gastro-duodenoscopy, PPI: proton-pump-inhibitor, NSAID: Non-steroidal-anti-inflammatory drug, PUD: Peptic ulcer disease, DRE: Digital rectal exam.

Table 8.5 Causes of enteral feeding tube related discomfort or abdominal pain

Differential diagnosis	Diagnostic clues	Initial evaluation	Empiric or initial treatment
Feeding tube site infection (cellulitis, phlegmon or abscess)	Erythema, swelling or drainage may suggest infection Scaly erythema may suggest candidal rash	Consider ultrasound to evaluate for an abscess Check for appropriate size and fit of feeding tube	Optimize skin care Topical antifungals Topical or systemic antibiotics May require surgical evaluation
Feeding tube site leakage	Leakage Extensive skin breakdown	Check balloon volume Check fit/size (should be easy to rotate)	Adjust balloon volume Change tube if defective, or change to larger size/ length if needed
Granulation tissue	Visible granulation tissue (care should be taken to consider ectopic gastric mucosa)	Visual and clinical diagnosis	Topical triamcinolone Cauterization
Bleeding at feeding tube site	Inappropriate tube fit (very tight or very loose)	Visual and clinical diagnosis	Avoid mechanical irritation Tape to avoid excessive mobility of the feeding tube

Table 8.5 (Continued)

Differential diagnosis	Diagnostic clues	Initial evaluation	Empiric or initial treatment
Gastric outlet obstruction	Infants with relatively large gastrostomy balloon Vomiting	Deflate gastrostomy balloon and assess if vomiting improves/ subsides Contrast study	Deflation of the balloon Consider surgical evaluation
Intussusception	GJ-feeds Bilious vomiting or G-tube output Acute onset of abdominal pain Abdominal distension	Abdominal radiograph Ultrasound Contrast study	Conversion from GJ to G-tube

GJ: gastro-jejunostomy, G-tube: gastrostomy tube

Conclusion

Gastro-intestinal issues are common in patients with cerebral palsy and are thought to be secondary to the dysfunctional modulation of the autonomic and enteric nervous system by the CNS, resulting in gastro-intestinal motor dysfunction such as feeding difficulties, dysphagia, aspiration, retching, vomiting, GERD, gastric and intestinal dysmotility and chronic constipation. This often has significant implications for the nutritional status, comfort, development and care in patients with cerebral palsy. The variable degrees of communication ability in this patient population can make it very difficult for patients to express their discomfort, emphasizing the importance of being aware of the common gastro-intestinal issues for which they may be at risk and of taking a pro-active approach to address them for optimization of growth, development, well-being and quality of life of each and every patient.

Summary points

- Gastro-intestinal issues are common in patients with cerebral palsy and thought to be secondary abnormalities in the modulation by the CNS of the autonomic and enteric nervous system, resulting in gastro-intestinal motor dysfunction such as dysphagia, aspiration, retching, vomiting, GERD, gastric or intestinal dysmotility, visceral hypersensitivity and chronic constipation. Additionally, anti-seizure medications, muscle-relaxants, and pain medications can further adversely affect the gastro-intestinal function.

- When unrecognized, gastro-intestinal morbidity in this population results in malnutrition, poor growth, development and decreased quality of life.

- Feeding difficulties related to oromotor dysfunction can be overt or subtle and present as gastro-intestinal or extra-intestinal symptoms such as coughing or lung disease. Enteral tube feeding often becomes necessary to ensure adequate nutrition.

- GERD is highly prevalent among patients with cerebral palsy and often refractory to medical therapy. Surgical interventions can be considered.

- Nearly all patients with cerebral palsy have chronic constipation. Early and aggressive treatment of constipation is recommended.

- Patients with severe cerebral palsy have varying degrees of communication difficulties, which can make the evaluation of bothersome symptoms and abdominal pain difficult and often delayed, emphasizing the importance of knowing the common gastro-intestinal issues and taking a pro-active approach to address them.

References

Arvedson JC (2013) Feeding children with cerebral palsy and swallowing difficulties. *Eur J Clin Nutr* **67**(Suppl 2): S9–S12.

Bandla HP, Davis SH, Hopkins NE (1999) Lipoid pneumonia: a silent complication of mineral oil aspiration. *Pediatrics* **103**: E19.

Borovoy J, Furuta L, Nurko S (1998) Benefit of uncooked cornstarch in the management of children with dumping syndrome fed exclusively by gastrostomy. *Am J Gastroenterol* **93**: 814–818.

Dalby-Payne JR, Morris AM, Craig JC (2003) Meta-analysis of randomized controlled trials on the benefits and risks of using cisapride for the treatment of gastroesophageal reflux in children. *J Gastroenterol Hepatol* **18**: 196–202.

Del Giudice E, Staiano A, Capano G, Romano A, Florimonte L, Miele E, et al. (1999) Gastrointestinal manifestations in children with cerebral palsy. *Brain Dev* **21**: 307–311.

Duncan DRR (2017) Swallowing and oropharyngeal disorders. In Faure CTN, Di Lorenzo C (eds.) *Pediatric Neurogastroenterology*, 2nd edn. Switzerland: Springer.

Elawad MA, Sullivan PB (2001) Management of constipation in children with disabilities. *Dev Med Child Neurol* **43**: 829–832.

Erkin G, Culha C, Ozel S, Kirbiyik EG (2010) Feeding and gastrointestinal problems in children with cerebral palsy. *Int J Rehabil Res* **33**: 218–224.

Esposito C, Van Der Zee DC, Settimi A, Doldo P, Staiano A, Bax NM (2003) Risks and benefits of surgical management of gastroesophageal reflux in neurologically impaired children. *Surg Endosc* **17**: 708–710.

Heuschkel RB, Gottrand F, Devarajan K, Poole H, Callan J, Dias JA, et al. (2015) ESPGHAN position paper on management of percutaneous endoscopic gastrostomy in children and adolescents. *J Pediatr Gastroenterol Nutr* **60**: 131–141.

Hill SL, Evangelista JK, Pizzi AM, Mobassaleh M, Fulton DR, Berul CI (1998) Proarrhythmia associated with cisapride in children. *Pediatrics* **101**: 1053–1056.

Hyams JS, di Lorenzo C, Saps M, Shulman RJ, Staiano A, Van Tilburg M (2016) Functional disorders: children and adolescents. *Gastroenterol* **150**: 1456–68.e2.

Kong CK, Wong HS (2005) Weight-for-height values and limb anthropometric composition of tube-fed children with quadriplegic cerebral palsy. *Pediatrics* **116**: e839–e845.

Maeda K, Koga T, Akagi J (2016) Tentative *nil per os* leads to poor outcomes in older adults with aspiration pneumonia. *Clin Nutr* **35**: 1147–1152.

Miele E, Staiano A, Tozzi A, Auricchio R, Paparo F, Troncone R (2002) Clinical response to amino acid-based formula in neurologically impaired children with refractory esophagitis. *J Pediatr Gastroenterol Nutr* **35**: 314–319.

Mousa H, Caniano DA, Alhajj M, Gibson L, di Lorenzo C, Binkowitz L (2006) Effect of Nissen fundoplication on gastric motor and sensory functions. *J Pediatr Gastroenterol Nutr* **43**: 185–189.

Nurko S, Zimmerman LA (2014) Evaluation and treatment of constipation in children and adolescents. *Am Fam Physician* **90**: 82–90.

Omari TI, Benninga MA, Sansom L, Butler RN, Dent J, Davidson GP (2006) Effect of baclofen on esophagogastric motility and gastroesophageal reflux in children with gastroesophageal reflux disease: a randomized controlled trial. *J Pediatr* **149**: 468–474.

Richards CA, Carr D, Spitz L, Milla PJ, Andrews PL (2000) Nissen-type fundoplication and its effects on the emetic reflex and gastric motility in the ferret. *Neurogastroenterol Motil* **12**: 65–74.

Rodriguez L, Diaz J, Nurko S (2013) Safety and efficacy of cyproheptadine for treating dyspeptic symptoms in children. *J Pediatr* **163**: 261–267.

Rodriguez L, Rosen R, Manfredi M, Nurko S (2012) Endoscopic intrapyloric injection of botulinum toxin A in the treatment of children with gastroparesis: a retrospective, open-label study. *Gastrointest Endosc* **75**: 302–309.

Rudolph CD, Mazur LJ, Liptak GS, Baker RD, Boyle JT, Colletti RB, et al. (2001) Guidelines for evaluation and treatment of gastroesophageal reflux in infants and children: recommendations of the North American Society for Pediatric Gastroenterology and Nutrition. *J Pediatr Gastroenterol Nutr* **32**(Suppl 2): S1–S31.

Samson-Fang L, Butler C, O'Donnell M, AACPDM (2003) Effects of gastrostomy feeding in children with cerebral palsy: an AACPDM evidence report. *Dev Med Child Neurol* **45**: 415–426.

Spiroglou K, Xinias I, Karatzas N, Karatza E, Arsos G, Panteliadis C (2004) Gastric emptying in children with cerebral palsy and gastroesophageal reflux. *Pediatr Neurol* **31**: 177–182.

Staiano A, Cucchiara S, Del Giudice E, Andreotti MR, Minella R (1991) Disorders of oesophageal motility in children with psychomotor retardation and gastro-oesophageal reflux. *Eur J Pediatr* **150**: 638–641.

Sullivan PB, Lambert B, Rose M, Ford-Adams M, Johnson A, Griffiths P (2000) Prevalence and severity of feeding and nutritional problems in children with neurological impairment: Oxford Feeding Study. *Dev Med Child Neurol* **42**: 674–680.

Tabbers MM, di Lorenzo C, Berger MY, Faure C, Langendam MW, Nurko S, et al. (2014) Evaluation and treatment of functional constipation in infants and children: evidence-based recommendations from ESPGHAN and NASPGHAN. *J Pediatr Gastroenterol Nutr* **58**: 258–274.

Vandenplas Y, Rudolph CD, di Lorenzo C, Hassall E, Liptak G, Mazur L, et al. (2009) Pediatric gastroesophageal reflux clinical practice guidelines: Joint Recommendations of the North American Society for Pediatric Gastroenterology, Hepatology, and Nutrition (NASPGHAN) and the European Society for Pediatric Gastroenterology, Hepatology, and Nutrition (ESPGHAN). *J Pediatr Gastroenterol Nutr* **49**: 498–547.

Chapter 9

Overview of pulmonary and sleep disorders in children with complex cerebral palsy

Sebastian K. Welsh and Umakanth Katwa

Introduction

Children with complex cerebral palsy are at high risk for increased morbidity and mortality from respiratory and sleep-related complications; these complications often lead to reduced quality of life both for children and their families, and to increased health care costs. These children need to be evaluated and managed by a multidisciplinary team consisting of various specialists. In this chapter we discuss the role of the pulmonologist and the pathophysiologist, the evaluation and management of pulmonary and sleep disorders in children with complex cerebral palsy, including chronic aspiration, reactive airways disease, and recurrent respiratory infections, with special emphasis on pulmonary airway clearance. We will also review pulmonary considerations in the perioperative evaluation of these children to prevent postoperative adverse outcomes.

Pathophysiology of lung disease in cerebral palsy

Chronic lung disease in children with cerebral palsy has several etiologies: it can be restrictive or obstructive in nature, or both. Restrictive lung disease in cerebral palsy arises due to the mechanical disadvantage created by muscle contractures, scoliosis, and progressive changes to the chest wall mechanics that impair normal lung growth, respiration and, subsequently, gas exchange. With improved enteral nutrition, some children with cerebral palsy are at risk of developing obesity that could also cause resistive load which leads to worsening restrictive lung component. Surgical correction of scoliosis has been shown to slow the rate of pulmonary function decline but does not necessarily correct the restrictive lung disease. Therefore, indications for surgical correction are usually not strictly pulmonary. Obstructive lung disease occurs secondary to chronic aspiration, poor pulmonary clearance, recurrent infections, and eventual development of irreversible bronchiectasis. Also, children may have upper airway obstruction at the level of the nasopharynx, oropharynx and tongue, vocal cords, or supra- or subglottic areas.

Long-term pulmonary and sleep-related complications
The long-term sequelae of lung disease in cerebral palsy include chronic/recurrent infection, impaired gas exchange, and central or obstructive sleep apnea. The goal of early maintenance and preventive therapy is to stop or delay lung injury and impaired gas exchange.

Disease progression
Progression of pulmonary disease in cerebral palsy follows the pathway of chronic inflammation, often times associated with longitudinal aspiration of secretions and/or malnutrition or obesity, with acute exacerbations leading to gradually decreasing lung function. An obstructive pathology of bronchiectasis develops with further impairment of pulmonary clearance and chronic colonization with organisms such as *Pseudomonas*. Children will eventually develop worsening pulmonary restrictive lung disease over time either through severe scoliosis, muscular weakness or contractures. This impaired ventilation coupled with decreased gas exchange results in worsening carbon dioxide retention and oxygenation during sleep and wakefulness. At end-stage disease, the reduction in lung function will lead to severe illness or death from a pulmonary infection or exacerbation. Indeed, this is one of the leading causes of morbidity among individuals with complex cerebral palsy, and likely contributes to early mortality (Reddihough et al. 2001).

Evaluation for pulmonary and sleep disorders
Care and coordination with a pulmonologist should occur early in the life of a patient with severe cerebral palsy to assist with preventive strategies and optimization of pulmonary regimens. Common reasons for referral include recurrent respiratory infections, hospital admission for respiratory causes, sleep disturbances and aspiration risk. Evaluation for infection or chronic changes can often be completed with a chest X-ray but may require chest CT scans for more subtle findings of bronchiectasis. As children may not be able to report reflux symptoms, a pH/impedance probe may be considered. Blood gasses are useful in the setting of evaluating impaired ventilation during wakefulness as well as sleep. If evaluating for sleep hypoventilation, a venous blood gas immediately upon awakening is recommended. For chronic hypoventilation, serum chemistry to

monitor for increased bicarbonate is also useful. A polysomnogram can be utilized to determine the type and degree of sleep-disordered breathing, but overnight oximetry and venous blood gas may be used in settings where a polysomnogram is unavailable.

Sialorrhea

Causes
Children with severe cerebral palsy are at risk for both increased oral secretions and impaired clearance. The secretions may be increased by the normal salivary response during enteral feeds as a result of stomach stretch and hormonal response to feeds or gastro-esophageal reflux. Poor oral hygiene can also create irritation of the oral mucosa resulting in increased salivation. Sometimes self-stimulatory behaviors of putting hands or objects into the mouth can also contribute to increased salivation. Most importantly, however, the normal swallow mechanism is impaired which causes impaired swallowing, pooling of secretions in the pharynx, and potential aspiration of oral secretions.

Complications
Chronic aspiration of secretions can continue to cause respiratory complications, even when a patient no longer takes feedings by mouth. Chronic aspiration of secretions contributes to recurrent infections leading to bronchiectasis, more frequent hospital admissions, and diffuse interstitial changes. The oral flora and bacterial overgrowth of anaerobes in the oropharynx can potentially lead to necrotizing pneumonia.

Evaluation
Clinical observation can account for the majority of the evaluation. If the patient has obvious difficulty tolerating secretions, or families are having trouble with the frequency of suctioning required, then interventions are clearly indicated. Additionally, a sensitive test for salivary aspiration is a salivagram that can show ongoing aspiration (Fitzgerald et al. 2009, Gerdung et al. 2016, Khatwa and Dy 2015).

Management
A stepwise approach is recommended in escalating interventions for children with persistent aspiration or difficult to control sialorrhea (AACPDM 2017). Children with mild or moderate sialorrhea frequently respond well to the use of anticholinergic medications. In children with more severe sialorrhea or that do not show improvement with medical intervention (or who have intolerable side effects, such as significant worsening of constipation or urinary retention) botulinum toxin (Botox) injections and salivary duct ligation or removal may reduce the amount of oral secretions. However, Botox injections need to be repeated, salivary ducts can reroute after ligation, and outcomes can vary widely between children. In children with substantial and persistent intolerance of secretions, a laryngotracheal separation can be performed; however, this is an extreme

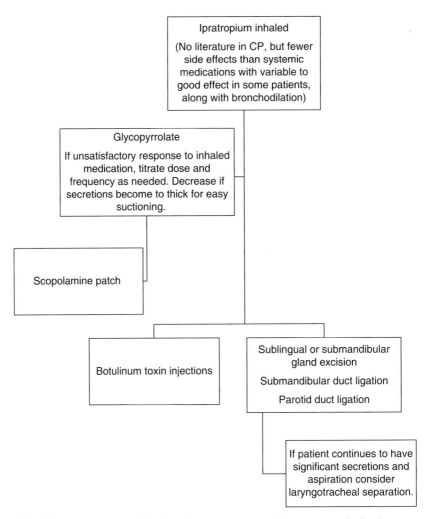

Figure 9.1 Step-wise approach to sialorrhea management in severe cerebral palsy

intervention and should be reviewed with the surgical team and family only after failure of other proven methods for managing sialorrhea (Fig. 9.1) (Formeister et al. 2014, Manrique and Sato 2009, Porte et al. 2014, Reddihough et al. 2010, Shima et al. 2010).

Chronic pulmonary aspiration
Aspiration of secretions and oral feeds
The impaired mechanism of swallowing leads to oropharyngeal contents both liquid and solid, including saliva, potentially contaminating the airway. This form of aspiration can be mitigated by thickening liquids; however, if severe swallowing dysfunction is present, children may be forced to forego oral feeding and switch to gastrostomy tube

feeding. Management of sialorrhea (see Sialorrhea – Management section) can further mitigate the potential for aspiration.

Aspiration of gastric reflux
Children with cerebral palsy can have varying degrees of gastro-esophageal reflux. Due to impaired swallowing mechanism and decreased airway protective reflex, children with complex cerebral palsy are frequently at risk of developing silent aspiration and exposure of their upper airways to acidic gastric contents. The acidic contents and enteric organisms create an environment of inflammation and chronic persistent airway infection. Treatment options include thickening feeds, proton pump inhibitors, postpyloric feeding (e.g. gastro-jejunal tube or jejunostomy), or Nissen fundoplication.

Presentation
Aspiration can present in multiple ways depending on the frequency, type, and volume of aspiration. Chronic, intermittent aspiration of oral feedings may or may not manifest with coughing during an aspiration event but can lead to chronic congestion or wet cough and chronic bronchitis or recurrent pneumonia. This typically improves when treated with antibiotics. Chronic aspiration of reflux is often difficult to determine in children with severe cerebral palsy as cough, throat clearing, or complaint of foul or sour taste may not be present or cannot be communicated. Empiric treatment is appropriate if aspiration of reflux is suspected. Large acute aspiration events are less subtle and frequently lead to rapid clinical decompensation with possible need for admission to the hospital or critical care unit.

Evaluation
Clinical assessment should focus on symptoms of coughing, choking, and gagging with feeding or with oral secretions. Additionally, an assessment of the consistencies of foods or liquids that make the symptoms worse is critical to understanding which types of food may be considered safe for feeding. A modified barium swallow study or video-endoscopic evaluation of swallowing can provide evidence of aspiration and identify which portion of the swallow mechanism is most impaired, guiding speech pathology intervention and feeding management. A normal barium swallow study does not rule out aspiration of oral feeding, as the aspiration may be intermittent. Children may also be unable to fully participate in swallowing studies, limiting their usefulness in determining the degree of aspiration. A salivagram can be used to evaluate aspiration in children who do not take oral feedings.

Management
Clinical evidence of aspiration of oral feeding can be treated empirically with thickening liquids (see Chapter 7: Feeding and Nutrition). Many children require enteral feeding and limited oral feedings due to severe impairment of the suck/swallow mechanism.

Mild reflux can be treated with thickening feeds and proton pump inhibitors. Many children with refractory reflux and severe cerebral palsy benefit from postpyloric feeds via a gastrojejunal tube (see also Chapter 8). Surgical interventions include Nissen fundoplication, direct jejunostomy and pyloroplasty (Lansdale et al. 2015). Fundoplication has been shown to be effective, but can have a significant failure rate with repeat surgery rates reported between 6–14% within 20–36 months.

Complications

Children may have episodes of aspiration of gastric contents, large volume gastrostomy tube feeds, or oral liquids resulting in acute signs of aspiration such as respiratory distress, fever, cough, and new pulmonary infiltrate or atelectasis on chest radiograph. This represents a medical emergency and frequently requires hospital admission or intensive care.

Aspiration, both acute and chronic, contributes significantly to pulmonary disease in children with cerebral palsy. Chronic aspiration of food, liquids, and secretions results in a chronic inflammation of the lower airways. This chronic bronchitis creates a setting in which colonization with *Pseudomonas aeruginosa*, Gram-negative rods, and other organisms can occur.

Reactive airways disease

Symptoms

Children with cerebral palsy may have reactive airway disease or asthma in addition to lung disease secondary to cerebral palsy. If children have wheezing or pulmonary exacerbations more than what is expected from underlying disease, or if symptoms persist after optimization and control of other common causes of wheeze and cough, then asthma should be suspected and treated accordingly. Chronic bronchitis or persistent airway inflammation from chronic aspiration is the most commonly seen cause of wheezing and chronic cough in this population of children.

Treatment

As children may not have typical reporting of symptoms, inhaled corticosteroids should be utilized with the goal of treatment to reduce the number of pulmonary exacerbations. Inhaled steroids can be increased and decreased based on the number of exacerbations, and degree of cough and wheezing. In addition to controller medications, families should have inhaled bronchodilators for use in the setting of increased cough, wheeze, or work of breathing. In the setting of pulmonary exacerbations, children should have the inhaled bronchodilators increased to every 4-hour treatments at the first signs of illness. Many children utilize nebulized medications; however, inhalers can be used with an appropriately sized mask, thus reducing treatment time and burden of disease. Orally administered systemic steroids can be utilized in the setting of an exacerbation to help control airway inflammation.

Table 9.1 Considerations in the treatment of chronic and acute pulmonary symptoms

Chronic therapies	Infection	Acute exacerbations
Manual chest physiotherapy	Immunizations	Increase frequency of pulmonary clearance
High frequency chest wall oscillation (Vest)	Inhaled antibiotics	Early use of treatment antibiotics with longer course (4–6 weeks)
Intrapulmonary percussive ventilation	Prophylactic oral antibiotics	Frequent suctioning as needed
Assisted coughing (manually assisted cough/ air stacking or mechanical insufflation-exsufflation)		Increased bronchodilators if associated with wheezing
Normal or hypertonic saline		Consider steroids
Mucolytics (n-acetylcysteine and dornase alfa)		If on NIV, extend duration of use
Inhaled corticosteroids		Make patient NPO
Inhaled bronchodilators		

NIV: non-invasive ventilation, NPO: *non per os* (no oral intake).

Chronic bronchitis exacerbation

Inflammation and colonization will result in recurrent infections that require acute treatment and long-term control of the inflammation and colonizing organisms (see Table 9.1). Children will frequently require longer courses of antibiotics than typical individuals. They may also benefit from chronic inhaled antibiotics such as tobramycin or inhaled corticosteroids to control the underlying inflammation. Triggering events include allergies, viral infections, or aspiration events. Due to poor oral hygiene and aspiration of secretions, colonizing organisms include anaerobes, Gram-negative enteric rods, and *Pseudomonas*. Empiric antimicrobial therapy should target these organisms with antibiotics such as ampicillin-clavulanate, ampicillin-sulbactam, or clindamycin. Duration of antimicrobials should be increased to 2–6 weeks depending on clinical improvement due to chronic inflammation, impaired mucociliary clearance, and underlying lung disease in these children.

Role of enhanced pulmonary airway clearance in children with complex cerebral palsy

Pathophysiology of impaired airway clearance in cerebral palsy

Unlike diseases such as cystic fibrosis and primary ciliary dyskinesia, the secretions and mucociliary function of children with cerebral palsy are normal. However, pulmonary airway clearance defects can be significant through other mechanisms. These mechanisms include decreased cough, lack of normal lung recruitment maneuvers, poor general mobility and impaired swallowing of secretions. The secretions may remain in the airway allowing bacterial overgrowth, chronic inflammation, and recurrent infections. The secretions mobilized to the upper airway may not be swallowed and can be aspirated.

Complications of impaired airway clearance

Impaired airway clearance results in chronic inflammation, risk for recurrent infection, and, over time, bronchiectasis. The development of bronchiectasis then causes even further impairment of secretions, thus establishing a cycle of ever worsening exacerbations and lung injury.

Assessment

The most important airway clearance component that is likely to be impaired in children with severe cerebral palsy is cough. A cough can be evaluated in several ways. If the patient can, they may be asked to cough voluntarily and the effectiveness of a cough monitored in that way. Many times the patient will need to have cough induced. This can be done with suctioning or inhaled hypertonic saline of 3% to induce cough. Children without an inducible gag reflex will almost always have an insufficient cough. Observing chest wall motion can also give an indication of whether the patient can perform lung recruitment maneuvers, such as incentive spirometry. The frequency of suctioning can also indicate how well a patient can swallow secretions normally mobilized by mucociliary clearance. Children often require increased pulmonary clearance during times of illness, and changes in secretions such as increased volume, viscosity, color change, or purulence can be used to dictate the need for additional therapies.

Management

Airway clearance comprises secretion mobilization followed by assisted coughing or suction. Impaired pulmonary airway clearance leads to recurrent chest infections, bronchiectasis, and eventually respiratory failure (Fitzgerald et al. 2009, Khatwa and Dy 2015). In addition to chest physiotherapy to mobilize secretions, inhaled medications can be added to assist by altering secretion viscosity.

Suctioning

Suctioning plays a critical role in the clearance of secretions, both following physiotherapy throughout the day to remove secretions that exceed a patient's ability to safely manage. Proper suctioning should occur in home management and inpatient settings. Suctioning can be performed with a flexible catheter passed through the nasopharynx or rigid (i.e. Yankauer suction tip) suction of the oropharynx. The suction catheter should only be passed far enough to induce a cough followed by slow withdrawal of the catheter while suctioning. The caregiver should also follow infection precautions, such as wearing gloves and hand washing. Due to the risk of vomiting, the patient may need to be positioned in a lateral recumbent position if gagging during suctioning. The suction pressure should be sufficient to draw up secretions but should not exceed 10–20kPa (75–150mmHg) (Crow 1986, Fitzgerald et al. 2009).

Mucolytics and hypertonic saline
Nebulized treatments can assist with secretion clearance by altering the viscosity of secretions. Once the secretions are mobilized these must be cleared either by a patient cough, assisted cough, or suctioning. Available treatments include normal saline, 3% saline, 7% saline, N-acetylcysteine, and dornase alfa (Khatwa and Dy 2015). In theory, mucociliary clearance should be unaltered by cerebral palsy; however, comorbid conditions such as bronchiectasis, chronic aspiration, and purulent bronchitis may require inhaled treatments to promote clearance with physiotherapy and assisted cough. Mucolytics and hypertonic saline should be used with caution, as they can be irritating to the airways, which can increase coughing or secretions. Thus, the patient's response to these therapies should be monitored after initiation, or used only in the setting of acute exacerbations.

Manual chest physiotherapy
Manual chest physiotherapy or postural drainage remains a mainstay of airway clearance techniques. However, this method may pose certain risks in children with cerebral palsy due to reflux and aspiration in certain positions. Severe motor impairment, presence of severe scoliosis, and impaired respiration caused by the mechanical disadvantage in these positions may preclude children from receiving manual chest physiotherapy as the primary mode of airway clearance. Alternative methods for providing airway clearance such as flutter valves, incentive spirometry, and coughing measures (huff cough or deep cough) can frequently not be performed by children with cerebral palsy due to degree of intellectual disability, voluntary motor control, the inability to make a seal with device or complexity of technique.

High-frequency chest wall oscillation
In children unable to tolerate manual chest physiotherapy due to positioning, high-frequency chest wall oscillation (Vest) therapy allows for provision of high-quality pulmonary clearance. Vest therapy has been shown to decrease admissions and total cases of pneumonia in children with cerebral palsy. The authors have been successful in justifying Vests for insurance providers using the following references in letters of medical necessity (Fitzgerald et al. 2014, Plioplys et al. 2002).

Cough assist device
Children with an inadequate cough are at risk for chronic *Pseudomonas aeruginosa* or other Gram-negative rod colonization. The use of mechanical insufflation-exsufflation

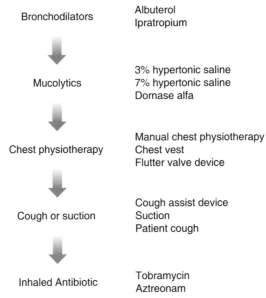

| Bronchodilators | Albuterol
Ipratropium |

| Mucolytics | 3% hypertonic saline
7% hypertonic saline
Dornase alfa |

| Chest physiotherapy | Manual chest physiotherapy
Chest vest
Flutter valve device |

| Cough or suction | Cough assist device
Suction
Patient cough |

| Inhaled Antibiotic | Tobramycin
Aztreonam |

Figure 9.2   Pulmonary clearance regimens

devices (cough assist) can allow for clearance of secretions mobilized by pulmonary clearance techniques. Suctioning during a clinic visit can often reveal efficacy of cough. If a patient has minimal cough, or does not have an inducible cough, they may benefit from a cough assist device. Pressure settings should be evaluated in conjunction with a respiratory therapist to determine optimal response by a patient, but pressures frequently range from 15 to 45cm H_2O (Khatwa and Dy 2015). Manual maneuvers with a bag-valve-mask device or abdominal thrust can be performed, however, the risks of aspiration should be considered in children with cerebral palsy. See Fig. 9.2 for examples of pulmonary clearance regimens.

Sleep-related breathing disorders
Obstructive sleep apnea/central sleep apnea/sleep hypoventilation/sleep hypoxemia
Sleep-disordered breathing in children with cerebral palsy can consist of obstructive sleep apnea, central apnea, or both. Central apnea can be the result of disordered control of breathing or oxygen desaturations with normal pauses in respiration caused by decreased pulmonary reserve. The lung diseases described in the previous sections can all result in impaired gas exchange that would appear as central apnea on polysomnogram. The most notable abnormalities will occur during REM sleep when the mechanical disadvantage created by scoliosis, chest wall abnormalities, and contractures will be exacerbated by normal paralysis associated with REM. Obstructions will also be most notable during REM sleep and may occur at any level of the upper airway. Treatment of

obstructive sleep apnea can consist of surgical (i.e. adenoidectomy), CPAP, or even BiPAP if severe obstruction or resulting from weakness. Central apnea may respond to oxygen therapy alone but frequently will require BiPAP to attempt to normalize gas exchange.

Evaluation

A focused history of sleep-disordered breathing should contain an assessment of snoring, gasping in sleep, morning headache, and daytime sleepiness. Physical examination may reveal large tonsils, stertor or inspiratory stridor that can indicate airway obstruction. A serum chemistry and venous blood gas can be used to evaluated chronic or sleep hypoventilation. Overnight oximetry can indicate sleep hypoxemia with or without nocturnal hypoventilation. Polysomnograms can be utilized to determine the pathology, possible seizure activity, and phase of sleep that is most affected.

Management

A discussion with the patient's family regarding goals for patient care is an important facet of treatment, particularly if gas exchange is impaired while both awake and asleep. Families at this time may opt for a palliative approach instead of the significant escalation of respiratory support, such as BiPAP more than 16 hours a day or tracheostomy (See Chapter 20: Difficult Topics). Indications for tracheostomy include: need for ventilator support for 16 hours a day or more, respiratory exacerbations resulting in invasive ventilation, extubation attempts that are unsuccessful despite optimal management, non-invasive ventilation that is ineffective to correct gas exchange abnormalities, or the necessity for frequent and intensive airway clearance (Khatwa and Dy 2015).

Pulmonary considerations in the perioperative period

Preoperative

A pulmonary evaluation should be performed with adequate time before surgery to allow for pulmonary optimization. This evaluation includes investigation of sleep-disordered breathing, impaired airway clearance, aspiration, sialorrhea, and reactive airway disease.

Concerns/risk

Commonly in the postoperative period, pulmonary clearance is reduced due to pain and decreased movement. The use of sedative and narcotic medications can also result in exacerbation of sleep-disordered breathing. Chronic colonizing organisms may proliferate resulting in pulmonary exacerbation.

Common recommendations

Evaluate for underlying lung disease and untreated sleep-disordered breathing before undergoing surgical procedures. Consider non-invasive positive pressure ventilation or need for increased settings for adequate gas exchange and pulmonary recruitment during the postoperative period. Longer procedures, such as spinal fusions, prolonged recovery time, decreased mobility, and pain with respiration may necessitate use of NIPPV or increased settings compared to other procedures. Antibiotics targeted at known colonizing organisms may be utilized if the patient develops changes in secretions or evidence of pulmonary exacerbation perioperatively.

Conclusion

Children who have severe cerebral palsy are at risk of lung disease of multiple etiologies as well as sleep-disordered breathing. Monitoring and preventive therapies can improve quality of life and slow progression of pulmonary disease in this population of children.

Summary points

- Pulmonary complications of cerebral palsy are the most common causes of significant morbidity and mortality.

- Ongoing pulmonary aspiration often plays a role in chronic airway disease, recurrent respiratory infection and progression of pulmonary disease in children with cerebral palsy.

- Aspiration of oral feeds, salivary secretion and gastro-esophageal reflux should be evaluated and treated.

- Enhanced pulmonary airway clearance is an integral part of any respiratory management strategy in decreasing bacterial burden and progression of chronic lung disease.

- Sleep-related breathing disorders are common, can be multifactorial, and need to be actively evaluated and treated.

- Initial screening of sleep-disordered breathing consists of blood gas, chemistry, overnight oximetry and/or capnometry. If abnormal, polysomnogram is indicated.

- Children with severe cerebral palsy should be evaluated by a pulmonologist in the preoperative period to assess for underlying pulmonary disease before sedation and surgery for optimization of treatment and to reduce postoperative complications.

References

AACPDM (2017) *Sialorrhea Care Pathway* [Online]. Available at: https://www.aacpdm.org/publications/care-pathways/sialorrhea.

Crow S (1986) Tips for successful respiratory suctioning. *RN* **49**: 31–3.

Fitzgerald DA, Follett J, Van Asperen PP (2009) Assessing and managing lung disease and sleep disordered breathing in children with cerebral palsy. *Paediatr Respir Rev* **10**: 18–24.

Fitzgerald K, Dugre J, Pagala S, Homel P, Marcus M, Kazachkov M (2014) High-frequency chest wall compression therapy in neurologically impaired children. *Respir Care* **59**: 107–12.

Formeister EJ, Dahl JP, Rose AS (2014) Surgical management of chronic sialorrhea in pediatric patients: 10-year experience from one tertiary care institution. *Int J Pediatr Otorhinolaryngol* **78**: 1387–92.

Gerdung CA, Tsang A, Yasseen AS 3rd, Armstrong K, McMillan HJ, Kovesi T (2016) Association between chronic aspiration and chronic airway infection with *Pseudomonas aeruginosa* and other gram-negative bacteria in children with cerebral palsy. *Lung* **194**: 307–14.

Khatwa UA, Dy FJ (2015) Pulmonary manifestations of neuromuscular diseases. *Indian J Pediatr* **82**: 841–51.

Lansdale N, McNiff M, Morecroft J, Kauffmann L, Morabito A (2015) Long-term and 'patient-reported' outcomes of total esophagogastric dissociation versus laparoscopic fundoplication for gastroesophageal reflux disease in the severely neurodisabled child. *J Pediatr Surg* **50**: 1828–32.

Manrique D, Sato J (2009) Salivary gland surgery for control of chronic pulmonary aspiration in children with cerebral palsy. *Int J Pediatr Otorhinolaryngol* **73**: 1192–4.

Plioplys AV, Lewis S, Kasnicka I (2002) Pulmonary vest therapy in pediatric long-term care. *J Am Med Dir Assoc* **3**: 318–21.

Porte M, Chaléat-Valayer E, Patte K, D'Anjou MC, Boulay C, Laffont I (2014) Relevance of intraglandular injections of Botulinum toxin for the treatment of sialorrhea in children with cerebral palsy: a review. *Eur J Paediatr Neurol* **18**: 649–57.

Reddihough D, Erasmus CE, Johnson H, McKellar GM, Jongerius PH, Institute CP (2010) Botulinum toxin assessment, intervention and aftercare for paediatric and adult drooling: international consensus statement. *Eur J Neurol* **17**: 109–21.

Reddihough DS, Baikie G, Walstab JE (2001) Cerebral palsy in Victoria, Australia: mortality and causes of death. *J Paediatr Child Health* **37**(2):183–6.

Shima H, Kitagawa H, Wakisaka M, Furuta S, Hamano S, Aoba T (2010) The usefulness of laryngotracheal separation in the treatment of severe motor and intellectual disabilities. *Pediatr Surg Int* **26**: 1041–4.

Chapter 10

Speech and communication

John M. Costello and Elizabeth N. Rose

We never know when the words and phrases we try so hard to make with our disobedient lips, tongues, soft palates and diaphragms, all having to function simultaneously, will come out in a breathy, inaudible whisper or a terrifying roar. And in neither case, is it certain that what we are trying to say will be understood at all (Roe 1948).

Introduction

Globally, there are over 17 million people diagnosed with cerebral palsy (CP) (Cerebral Palsy Foundation, n.d.). While reports vary, in general it is agreed that one in five individuals with CP have significant difficulty producing speech (Watson, 1999, Pennington 2005, Andersen 2010). To understand communication more broadly, as defined by the International Classification of Functioning, Disability, and Health (ICF; see Chapter 1 for description), we must consider the frameworks that support communication. These include, but are not limited to: body structure and function (anatomy and physiology), activity (opportunities in home, school, community), participation (involvement in daily life), environmental factors (the physical, social and attitudinal environment of the child including communication partner's engagement), and personal factors (age, sex, personal style, coping style). With such complex interconnected frameworks, it is understandable that some studies find as many as 80% of individuals with CP have communication difficulties (Pellegrino 2002, Parkes 2010, Cerebral Palsy Foundation 2016). The exact nature of these communication problems has not been systematically studied or classified in children with CP; however, research indicates that communication difficulties can have a variety of adverse effects on children with CP and can result in differences in social interaction patterns (Light, Collier, & Parnes, 1985a, 1985b, 1985c; Pennington & McConachie, 2001b) and in quality of life (Dickinson et al. 2007). Moreover, within the ICF Framework, one must recognize that communication is more than speech production alone (Hidecker 2010), and includes reading, writing, texting, and all forms of sending and receiving messages. Finally, coexisting factors play a role in the severity, diagnosis, and treatment of communication difficulties. Hearing, in particular, has a significant effect on communication abilities. Cognition, including social cognition, memory, attention, problem solving, and executive function, plays a complex role in an individual's ability to communicate (American Speech-Language-Hearing Association, [ASHA] 2003).

Speech, language, communication

Communication is any act by which one person gives to or receives information about that person's needs, desires, perceptions knowledge or effective state. Communication may be intentional or unintentional, may involve conventional or unconventional signals, may take linguistic or nonlinguistic forms and may occur through spoken or other modes (National Joint Committee for the Communication needs of Persons with Severe Disabilities 1992).

In this process of giving and receiving information, there are two overarching areas to consider: speech and language.

Speech refers to verbal message production and is a coordination of respiration, phonation, articulation, prosody, and resonance. Individuals with CP who have a communication difficulty often present with a motor speech disorder called dysarthria. Dysarthria consists of 'problems in oral communication due to paralysis, weakness, or incoordination of the speech musculature' (Darley 1969, ASHA 2016). Exact prevalence of the presence and severity of dysarthria is not currently available, as speech is not currently measured in CP surveillance registers (Pennington 2012).

Dysarthria affects motor speech production and speech intelligibility at several levels. Recently, research has revealed that intelligibility of dysarthric speech in very young children with CP is most impacted by the articulatory speech subsystem (Lee 2014). Hustad et al. (2012) report that 4-year-old children with dysarthria due to CP (both with and without a concomitant language disorder), have significantly reduced intelligibility when producing spoken language, often 20% intelligible or lower as compared to their typically developing peers who are intelligible in nearly 90% of utterances. In individuals with CP, the type, presentation, and severity of dysarthria is often directly linked to the type, presentation, and severity of their CP (Duffy 2005, Hidecker et al. 2011). As a result, those who present in Gross Motor Function Classification System (GMFCS) level IV or V (see Chapter 1 for description of GMFCS) may experience the most severely dysarthric speech (Duffy 2005, Hidecker 2011, Pennington et al. 2013). Due to decreased intelligibility and limited effect of traditional methods of therapeutic intervention to improve natural speech (Pennington 2013), alternative methods of communication may be required to help children achieve functional communication goals across communication partners and communication settings.

Language refers to the comprehension and/or use of a spoken, written, or other graphic symbol system. Language is characterized as receptive language (i.e. understanding language input), expressive language (i.e. producing language through any means), and pragmatic language (i.e. social abilities). Language disorders range from the ability to understand or produce language form (e.g. using verb tenses), content (e.g. encoding or retrieving new words), or function (e.g. conversational turn-taking) (ASHA 1993). Social and cultural rules govern language and provide a framework for understanding and use of language skills. Language can exist independently of speech, for example, American Sign Language is a rich and full language in the absence of verbal message production. For individuals with CP, language skills may remain intact, or relatively increased as compared to the individual's speech production abilities.

Augmentative and alternative communication

Approximately 20–25% of children and young people with CP have a communication impairment so significant that they are unable to speak (Andersen 2010, Pennington 2005). For these children, augmentative and alternative communication (AAC) strategies are the only solution to assure the opportunity for successful expressive communication, participation in daily life, and social connectedness independent of the full support of their most familiar communication partners. The term 'smart partner' is often used to describe communication partners who are so familiar that they can interpret a child's needs and reoccurring messages based on vocalizations or nonverbal cues such as facial expressions or changes in posture. Unfortunately, relying on smart partner interpretation limits the opportunity for children to self-determine by independently communicating intended messages. It severely limits the range of successful communication partners, social opportunities, language-learning opportunities, and authentic participation in life.

Children and adults typically communicate through myriad methods including spoken language, written language, drawing, gestures, facial expressions, and body posture, as well as a range of technologies from high-tech (computers, smart phones, tablets) to low-tech solutions (photographs and symbols). This 'total communication approach,' also known as 'multimodal communication,' is often not readily recognized for children with CP and other non-speaking conditions. While peers will choose the communication medium(s) that most effectively meets the context and the skills and familiarity of their communication partners, children who use AAC are often required to 'use their device'. Children and youth with CP must be afforded the same opportunity to choose freely from a variety of communication options. In fact, children who use augmentative communication most often try to use a multimodal approach (Light 2007) which includes both unaided and aided strategies.

Unaided communication is any mode of expressive communication that does not require a tool, aid, or piece of equipment. Examples of unaided communication methods include vocalizations, gestures and body movements, sign language, head movements, eye pointing, facial expressions, verbal approximations, and speech production. Unaided methods of communication may involve unconventional or unexpected signs and/or signals that are only recognized by a smart partner and therefore require other communication partners to be explicitly taught its meaning. For example, a child may look up to indicate 'yes,' vocalize to protest, use a unique hand gesture to indicate toileting needs, or touch his/her wheelchair tray to ask for 'more.' Further, established rule-based sign languages such as American Sign Language or any of the other 140 or more formal sign languages across the world (Simons 2017) are also unaided methods of communication. Pure form American Sign Language is rarely used with people who have communication difficulties that are not primarily caused by hearing impairment. This is owing to both the linguistic differences between spoken versus signed languages as well as the need for communication partners to be familiar with the signed language itself. Further, for children with CP, fine motor accuracy and precision to produce sign language may be an additional complicating factor. Nonetheless, a review of studies focused on encouraging simultaneous sign language and speech production for children with varied disabilities and little or no spoken language behavior, revealed a positive effect on the speech and oral language production of the children (Dunst 2011). Consequently, unaided methods are beneficial in that they are available to individuals at all times and across all physical positions; however, they may not be successful strategies with all communication partners.

Aided communication refers to the use of communication symbols, strategies, or techniques that use something external to the body to represent, select, or transmit messages (Lloyd 1986). Aided methods include low-tech, mid-tech, and high-tech options. Low-tech is typically non-electronic and includes photographs, real objects, symbols or letter boards. Mid-tech communication aids may be electronic, but are typically not computer-based. These can include simple voice output devices that play recorded messages and may be single message systems or tools that support multiple messages. For example, a child may access a voice output device to gain attention with a pre-recorded message such as, 'Come over here, mom,' or may indicate a preference when being presented with a number of options by activating a pre-recorded message such as, 'That's it! That's the one I want.' It could even include a device with multiple pre-recorded messages related to a specific context. For example, during a reading activity a child may have pre-recorded messages such as, 'Please read me a book,' 'Let's read a different one,' 'Turn the page,' 'Read in a silly voice,' etc.

High-tech communication aids, often referred to as speech-generating devices or SGDs, are typically computer or tablet-based. Because motor control and physical access can be a substantial challenge for children and youth with CP, many communication aids may be accessed through a variety of methods such as switch scanning, head stick pointing, manual direct selection, mouse/joystick, or eye gaze control. For some children, large and colorful symbols with a few symbols per page will be most meaningful. Other children benefit from a menu-driven language organization with a large grid of vocabulary available on each page. Still others are most successful when a large photograph that represents a familiar visual scene is used to support communication. For children with established literacy skills, a high-tech system may be used to allow for generative communication by creating and speaking any message desired using a keyboard for text-to-speech production. For children who are not yet literate or who demonstrate emerging literacy skills, messages may be stored as whole sentences and/or phrases.

To best match the skills, strengths, and needs of a child to all available augmentative communication tools and technology, a 'feature matching' process (Shane and Costello 1994) must be completed by the child's multidisciplinary team. This process provides a framework for clinical decision making based on a set of rules and pertinent questions that cut across several assessment domains including: child, family, medical, motor, cognitive, sensory, linguistic, social, cultural, educational, behavioral, and financial areas. When successfully executed, this process yields clearer insight into AAC tools and strategies needing further investigation through functional evidence-based clinical trials. Table 10.1 highlights unaided communication strategies as well as many aided tools available at the time of this writing.

Augmentative and alternative communication: candidacy,
timeframe, and misconceptions

Augmentative communication should be considered whenever there is a divergence between what a child wants to communicate and what he/she can successfully communicate. This 'communicative dissonance' (Shane 1986) is the disparity between a child's communication needs and the child's ability to successfully communicate those needs. Yet, regardless of increased societal acceptance of technology and the mainstream availability of mobile devices, for some, a negative perception of non-standard methods of communication creates an adverse stigma toward AAC strategies and devices. Often, AAC is thought of as a 'last resort' for communication and seen as 'less than' natural communication methods. Parents and other caregivers question whether AAC strategies will inhibit verbal speech development (Romski 2005, Miller 2006, Light 2007). Providers hesitate to introduce AAC until children reach a certain age, exhibit specific cognitive skills, or prove a level of skill-readiness such as literacy skills (Romski 2005, Light 2007). Research reveals, however, that AAC improves spoken language development in many children (Cress 2003, Miller 2006, Light 2007) and should be introduced as soon as possible to support language development and provide children with

Table 10.1 Communication strategies and tools[a]

Unaided strategies Strategies that do not require a tool, aid, or piece of equipment		
Naturalistic strategies	Facial expressions	
	Body language	
	Vocalizations, verbal attempts, verbal approximations	
	Physical communication (e.g., pulling a parent to a preferred item)	
	Common gestures (e.g., pointing, reaching, nodding, shaking head)	
Learned Strategies	Partner assisted scanning	
	Sign language	
	Informal signs (e.g., child touches pants to indicate toileting needs)	
	Pre-determined signals (e.g., child looks up to indicate 'yes')	
Aided strategies Strategies that require specialized tools, aids, or equipment		
Low-tech	Objects	Child points to or looks at real objects to make choices, to generate sentences, to answer questions
	Photographs	Child points to or looks at photographs of objects to make choices, to indicate wants/needs, to answer questions
	Symbols	Child points to or looks at picture symbols to make choices, to generate sentences, to answer questions. Examples include:

PCS (Boardmaker/Mayer-Johnson)   Symbol Stix (N2Y)

Yes/No symbols (positioned on wheelchair tray)

	Communication board	Examples include:

Table 10.1 (Continued)

	Communication book	Examples include:		
		Personalized book	Flip n' Talk (Mayer-Johnson)	Pragmatic organisation dynamic display (PODD)
	Letter boards	Examples include:		
		Vowel-start (positioned on wheelchair tray)		QWERTY-based
	Other	Examples include:		
		Pain scale		
		Visual schedule/ADL support		Yes/No bracelets (child moves arm to indicate answer)
Mid-tech	Voice-output devices and voice-output communication aides	Examples include:		
		LITTLE Step-by-step (Ablenet)	Partner/Plus (AMDi)	iTalk2 (Ablenet)

Table 10.1 (Continued)

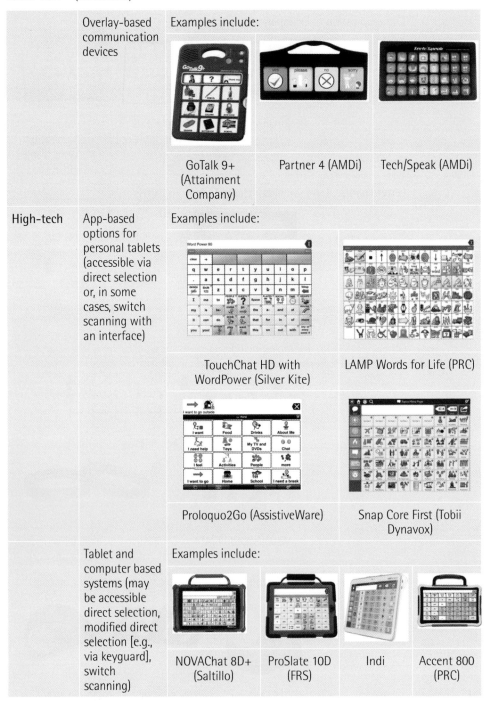

	Overlay-based communication devices	Examples include:
		GoTalk 9+ (Attainment Company) — Partner 4 (AMDi) — Tech/Speak (AMDi)
High-tech	App-based options for personal tablets (accessible via direct selection or, in some cases, switch scanning with an interface)	Examples include: TouchChat HD with WordPower (Silver Kite) — LAMP Words for Life (PRC) — Proloquo2Go (AssistiveWare) — Snap Core First (Tobii Dynavox)
	Tablet and computer based systems (may be accessible direct selection, modified direct selection [e.g., via keyguard], switch scanning)	Examples include: NOVAChat 8D+ (Saltillo) — ProSlate 10D (FRS) — Indi — Accent 800 (PRC)

Table 10.1   (Continued)

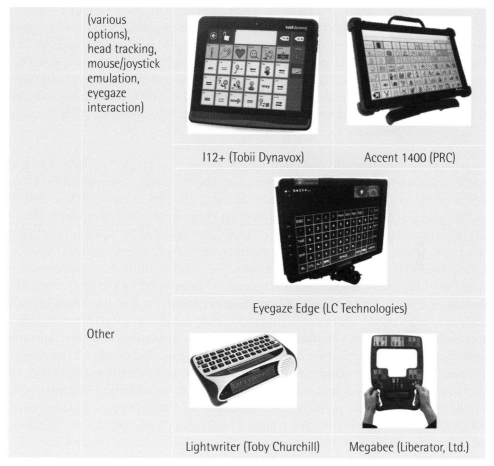

(various options), head tracking, mouse/joystick emulation, eyegaze interaction)		
	I12+ (Tobii Dynavox)	Accent 1400 (PRC)
	Eyegaze Edge (LC Technologies)	
Other	Lightwriter (Toby Churchill)	Megabee (Liberator, Ltd.)

[a]Not all systems, formats, layouts, software options or brands are represented. Devices are not to scale.

communicative success (Cress 2003, Romski 2005). Further, AAC not only serves as a primary means of expressive communication, but can help equalize the gap between comprehension and production, promote greater participation in school, promote interpersonal/social interactions, reduce frustration associated with communication failure, facilitate speech development, enhance vocational opportunities, provide supports for receptive language (Shane 1986), and serve as a language intervention strategy (Cress 2003, Romski 2005, Miller 2006, Light 2007).

Understanding communication performance and goal setting
All language learning requires many learning opportunities including formal instruction, informal observation and functional models. As previously referenced, the ICF

recognizes this by emphasizing opportunity, participation and a social environment. If an augmentative communication strategy is employed, then to develop effective communication skills the child with CP must be provided with opportunity to learn language and appropriate language stimulation using the tools and symbols of the child. The practice of using the actual tools, symbols, and strategies the child is expected to master in the presence of the child is known as 'aided language stimulation.' Without these formal and informal language learning opportunities, the child must independently scaffold use of tools and symbol set to the spoken words he/she hears but is not able to functionally produce.

To determine the most effective communication supports for a child with CP, one must clearly understand current performance. The Communication Function Classification System (CFCS) focuses on activity and participation levels as described in the ICF and was developed to describe everyday communication performance. While initially created to focus on individuals with CP, the utility of the CFCS is now being used to describe the communication performance of any person with a disability (Hidecker 2011). The CFCS is used to classify daily communication performance into one of five levels. It considers both communication sending and receiving skills, noting that in an authentic communication exchange, each partner fulfills both rolls. It focuses on the pace of the communication, recognizing that the most effective exchanges occur at a comfortable pace with few communication breakdowns and minimal wait time between communication turns. The degree of familiarity between the communication partners is considered, as it recognizes the benefit of previous knowledge and personal experience in the communication exchange with familiar partners ('smart partners' as previously described) as opposed to the added effort necessary with unfamiliar partners. Finally, the CFCS considers all methods of communication when measuring successful communication. For children who use multimodal communication with a range of communication partners, this tool is particularly valuable as it acknowledges and documents the interrelatedness of skill, communication partners, opportunities, and context. Since the very nature of communication is the 'establishment of joint attention' wherein meaning is jointly established or co-constructed through simultaneous use of common modalities such as speech, gestures, manual signs, facial expressions, electronic, and nonelectronic technologies (von Tetzchner 2000) and, to be truly effective, communication requires a two-way process (expressive and receptive) in which messages are negotiated until the information is correctly understood by both parties (Blackstone 2007, The Joint Commission 2010) the CFCS may be used to clearly understand effective communication for children and youth with CP and may help identify areas for meaningful intervention.

In reviewing the CFCS classification system (Table 10.2), note that distinctions between the levels are based on the performance of sender and receiver roles, the pace of

Table 10.2   Communication function classification system[a]

Level 1 Effective sender and receiver with unfamiliar and familiar partners	The child independently alternates between sender and receiver roles with most people in most environments. Communication is easy and moves at a comfortable pace with both unfamiliar and familiar communication partners. Communication misunderstandings are quickly repaired and do not interfere with overall effectiveness of the child's communication.
Level 2 Effective but slower paced sender and/or receiver with unfamiliar and/or familiar partners	The child independently alternates between sender and receiver roles with most people in most environments, but the conversational pace is slow and may make the communication interaction more difficult. The child may need extra time to understand messages, compos messages, and/or repair misunderstandings. Communication misunderstandings are often repaired and do not interfere with the eventual effectiveness of the person's communication with both unfamiliar and familiar partners.
Level 3 Effective sender and receiver with familiar partners	The person alternates between sender and receiver roles with familiar conversational partners in most environments. Communication is not consistently effective with most unfamiliar partners but is usually effective with familiar partners.
Level 4 Inconsistent sender or receiver with familiar partners.	The person does not consistently alternate sender and receiver roles. The child may occasionally be an effective sender and receiver, may be an effective sender but limited receiver or may be a limited sender but limited receiver. Communication is sometimes effective with familiar partners.
Level 5 Seldom effective sender and receiver even with familiar partners	The child's communication is difficult for most people to understand and the child may appear to have limited understanding of messages from most people. Communication is seldom effective even with familiar partners.

[a]Hidecker et al. 2011, 2017

communication, and the type of conversational partner (Hidecker et al. 2011). It is important to note that this classification system does not rate the child's competence as a communicator; rather, it reflects everyday functional communication performance.

According to Light (1989), communicative competence is a relative and dynamic, inter-personal construct based on functionality of communication (the skills needed to initiate and maintain daily interactions within the natural environment), adequacy of communication (possessing an adequate level of communication skills to function within the environment), and sufficiency of judgment, knowledge, and skill to perform as required given the partner, the environment, and the intent in the areas of linguistic competence, operational competence, social competence and strategic competence. For children and youth with CP who rely on aided augmentative communication strategies, demonstrating communicative competence requires mastery of tools (operational competence); use of a language symbol system such as objects, symbols, or text (linguistic competence); effective coping strategies to most effectively communicate an intended message (strategic competence), and finally use of appropriate social rules and pragmatics (social competence).

Patient profiles

Candidates for AAC intervention, strategies, and devices, can be broadly classified into three communication profiles: emergent communicator, context-dependent communicator, and independent communicator (Dowden 1999). It is essential to note that these classifications are not representative of an individual's cognitive status, their ability to understand language, or their potential for language learning.

An *emergent* communicator does not yet have a consistent or reliable use of symbols for communication. This person uses facial expressions, body language, gestures, vocalizations, and other non-symbolic modes of communication, which may be idiosyncratic and not immediately apparent to unfamiliar partners. This group of communicators relies on communication partners, especially familiar or 'smart' partners, to interpret their messages about the 'here and now'. Emergent communicators are most successful when in a familiar environment and when engaged in familiar, routine, or motivating tasks.

A *context-dependent* communicator uses reliable symbolic communication modes, but communication may still be limited to certain partners, topics, or contexts. Familiar or 'smart' partners are best able to interpret complex messages. Context-dependent communicators can achieve basic communication tasks in non-familiar settings, but are the most successful either when in a familiar setting, with a familiar person, or highly motivated. Context-dependent communicators may have developing literacy skills, such as print awareness.

An *independent* communicator has a tried and true communication system (or collection of systems) that he/she seems to know better that his family or therapists. The independent communicator can participate in real-time (or close to real-time) conversations with others, and uses a variety of language functions in multiple ways. Communication breakdowns are rare, and when they occur, the independent communicator is able to recast and repair the conversation. Communication is successful with familiar and unfamiliar partners, across settings, and even in novel situations. Spelling and/or literacy skills are often at age-level.

Patient examples

Lucy is a 3-year-old girl with spastic quadriplegic CP, in GMFCS level V. She has cortical visual impairment (CVI), refractory seizures and receives all nutrition via a gastrostomy tube. Lucy communicates with family using smiles, squeals, happy or angry vocalizations, and changes in physical positioning to indicate her mood. She communicates preferences between two objects or two large photos using eye pointing. Partners interpret her smile as a 'yes' response and she is learning the power of communication through consistent exposure to simple voice output tools that she incidentally activates, resulting in partners immediately responding so she learns the cause-effect connection. Lucy is an emergent communicator.

Andrew, age 9 years, has spastic and athetoid type CP and functions at a GMFCS level V. He has medically controlled seizures, receives nutrition both orally and through his gastrostomy tube and wears bilateral hearing aids due to moderate sensorineural loss. Andrew uses vocalizations and facial expressions to communicate emotion, mood and predictable needs with familiar partners. He has a low-tech picture communication book, requiring his partners to manually point to symbols on each page and Andrew will signal 'yes' by raising his right arm/hand. Andrew also uses a high-tech speech-generating device, accessed through eye tracking to create sentences such as 'I want – Wheels on the Bus song!' and to speak single word messages that his partner must interpret based on context, such as 'out'. Andrew demonstrates frustration characterized by tantrums when his communication needs are not immediately understood by others, or when his communication attempts are interpreted incorrectly. Andrew is a context-dependent communicator.

Meghan, age 12 years, presents with athetoid type CP and functions at a GMFCS level IV. While Meghan's speech is characterized by moderate to severe dysarthria, she communicates with the most familiar partners primarily using speech. Less familiar partners do not successfully understand Meghan's speech so she successfully employs a variety of strategies based on the context. Meghan points to words and symbols in a multipage communication notebook to comment, request, ask questions, share information and turn-take in conversation, requiring her partner to look over her shoulder and speak out each word/phrase as she indicates it or Meghan creates novel sentences using a robust language page set in an app on her personal tablet/SGD. Meghan's literacy skills are emerging and she has recently begun to use her SGD to phonetically spell novel words and combine those with stored words and phrases marked with symbols. With access to multiple communication tools, Meghan is an emerging-independent communicator.

Paul is a 10-year-old boy with spastic quadriplegic CP and functions at a GMFCS level V. He has a tracheostomy, requires vent support overnight, and is learning to drive his power wheelchair using a joystick control with his right hand. Paul was referred at age 3 months to an AAC specialist and has been working on low-, mid-, and high-tech strategies at home, with his nurses, and at school ever since. He moves his head and eyes to the left to indicate 'yes' and to the right to indicate 'no.' Paul has a communication system that he accesses via 2-step switch scanning, with a scan switch at his right temple and a select switch at his left temple. He can scan through pre-programmed messages and phrases to request, direct, and comment on activities. He loves to tease his older brother and he creates messages on his device to participate in real-time arguments with his brother. Paul's literacy is developing at the same pace as his classmates, and he uses a keyboard on his device to add novel vocabulary to his messages. He advocates for himself (e.g. 'my left wrist splint is on wrong'). Paul is an independent communicator.

Conclusions

Children and young people with CP must be afforded every opportunity possible to be successful and independent communicators. Perhaps the single most positive influence on communicative success for a child who demonstrates any difficulty with effective communication is an early referral to a qualified speech and language pathologist (SLP). Recognizing that communication development is both an expressive and a receptive task, caregivers of children with CP who are 6 months or younger should be supported to engineer an environment that supports a rich language learning and expressive communication environment.

The communication development of children with CP is highly at risk due to the mismatch between their receptive language skills (understanding language) and expressive language abilities (producing language). Knowing that even newborn infants may someday require AAC intervention, immediate referral to a qualified speech-language pathologist (SLP) is key. Rather than the 'wait and see' method, in which traditional means of communication or traditional interventions are allowed to fail before AAC is considered, children and young people with CP must be afforded every possible opportunity to be successful and independent communicators, regardless of the form their communication takes. Providing education to caregivers of children age 6 months or younger will help to develop a language-rich environment in which to learn communication. Allowing a young child with CP to develop alternative communication naturally, at the same time and in the same settings in which their age-matched peers are learning language, can allow for matched growth across receptive, expressive, and social/pragmatic language skills. In this way, a child can be provided with a natural, consistent method of communication that works with, rather than against, his/her physical status from a very early age.

Key points

- Expressive communication is multimodal for all people and includes speech, vocalizations, facial expressions, posture, gestures and signs as well as pictures, symbols, text and use of low, mid and high-tech technology.

- Successful communication development is based on many factors including; body structure and function, medical status, sensory status, cognition, level of activity, opportunities to participate and environmental factors including modeling and formal instruction. These areas all need to be assessed individually and as a whole to determine appropriate augmentative methods of communication.

- There is no hierarchy to augmentative methods of communication. Low-tech methods may be more successful for some people or in some contexts. Providing individuals with CP with an arsenal of successful strategies allows them to use the best option for the context – just as typical speakers do.

- AAC should be considered whenever there is a difference between what a child wants to communicate and what he/she can successfully communicate.

- Introducing back-up communication strategies as early as possible to someone who is suspected to be communication vulnerable is critical. Do not wait for communication to fail before providing intervention.

References

Andersen GM (2010) Prevalence of Speech Problems and the Use of Augmentative and Alternative Communication in Children with Cerebral Palsy: A Registry-Based Study in Norway. *Perspect Augment Altern commun* **19**: 12–20.

American Speech-Language-Hearing Association [ASHA] (1993) Definition of Communication Disorders and Variations. Available at www.asha.org/policy/ RP1993-00208/

ASHA (2003) Evaluating and Treating Communication and Cognitive Disorders: Approaches to Referral and Collaboration for Speech-Language Pathology and Clinical Neuropsychology. Available at www.asha.org/policy/TR2003-00137/

ASHA (2016) What is Dysarthria? Available at www.asha.org/public/speech/disorders /dysarthria/#what_is_dysarthria

Blackstone SW (2007) Key principles underlying research and practice in AAC. *Augment Altern Commun* **23**: 191–203.

Cerebral Palsy Foundation (2016) Communication Classification. Available at http://yourcpf .org/communication-issues/

Cerebral Palsy Foundation (2017) Key Facts. Available at http://yourcpf.org/statistics/

Cress C (2003) Responding to a common early AAC question: 'Will my child talk?'. *Perspectives on Augment Altern Commun* **12**: 10–12.

Darley FA (1969) Differential diagnostic patterns of dysarthria. *J Speech Lang Hear Res* **12**: 246–269.

Dowden P (1999) Lesson 2C: The impact of current communication skills on intervention. In P Dowden, *Communication Augmentation for Non-Speaking Individuals.* Seattle, WA: University of Washington Educational Outreach.

Duffy J (2005) *Motor Speech Disorders: Substrates, Differential Diagnosis and Management* (vol. 2). St. Louis, MO: Elsevier Moby.

Dunst CJ (2011) Influence of sign and oral language intervention on the speech and oral language production of young children with disabilities. *CELL Reviews* 4(4). Available at www.earlyliteracylearning.org/cellreviews/cellreviews_v4_n4.pdf.

Hidecker M (2010) Communication activity and participation research. *Dev Med Child Neurol* **52**: 408–409.

Hidecker M et al. (2017) Communication Function Classification System (CFCS). Available at http://cfcs.us/wp-content/uploads/2014/02/CFCS_universal_2012_06_06.pdf

Hidecker MJ, Paneth N, Rosenbaum PL, et al. (2011) Developing and validating the Communication Function Classification System (CFCS) for individuals with cerebral palsy. *Dev Med Child Neurol* **53**(8): 704–10.

Hustad LS (2012) Intelligibility of 4-year old children with and without cerebral palsy. *J Speech Lang Hear Res* **55**: 1177–1189.

Lee JH (2014) Predicting speech intelligibility with multiple speech subsystems approach in children with cerebral palsy. *J Speech Lang Hear Res* **57**: 1666–1678.

Light J (1989) Toward a definition of communication competence for individuals using Augmentative Alternative Communication. *Augment Altern Commun* **3**(3): 137–144.

Light J (2007) AAC technologies for young children with complex communication needs: State of the Science and Future Directions. *Augment Altern Commun* **23**: 204–216.

Lloyd L (1986) Toward an augmentative and alternative communication symbol tasonoly: proposed superordinate classification. *Augment Altern Commun* **2**: 165–171.

Miller DL (2006) The impact of augmentative and alternative communication intervention on the speech production of individuals with developmental disabilities: A research review. *J Speech Lang Hear Res* **49**: 248–264.

National Joint Committee for the Communication needs of Persons with Severe Disabilities (1992) Guidelines for meeting the communication needs of Persons with Severe Disabilities. *ASHA* **34** (Supp) 7: 1–8.

Parkes JN (2010) Oromotor dysfunction and communication impairment in children with cerebral palsy: A register study. *Dev Med Child Neurol* **52**: 1113–1119.

Pellegrino L (2002) Cerebral palsy. In ML Batshaw (ed), *Children with Disabilities*, 5th edn. Baltimore, MD: Paul Brookes Publishing Co, pp. 443–466.

Pennington L (2012) Speech and Communication in cerebral palsy. *East J Med* **17**: 171–177.

Pennington L (2005) Direct speech and language therapy for children with Cerebral Palsy: findings from a systematic review. *Dev Med Child Neurol* **47**: 57–63.

Pennington L, Roelant E, Thompson V, Robson S, Steen N, Miller N (2013) Intensive dysarthria therapy for younger children with cerebral palsy. Dev Med Child Neurol 55: 464–471.

Roe FH (1948) The Evolution of My Walkie-Talkie. *Lecture, Parent Association for Spastic Childrens Aid.*

Romski M (2005) Augmentative and alternative communication: myths and realities. *Infant and Young Children* **18**: 174–185.

Shane HC (1986) Goals and Uses. In SW Blackstone (ed), *Augmentative Communication: An Introduction.* Rockville, Maryland: American Speech Language and Hearing Association.

Shane, HC and Costello, JM (1994) *Feature Matching and Domains of Assessment.* New Orleans, LA: American Speech Language Hearing Association.

Simons GF (2017) *Ethnologue: Languages of the World*, 20th edn. Available at www.ethnologue.com

The Joint Commission (2010) *Advancing Effective Communication, Cultural Competence, and Patient- and Family-Centered Care: A Roadmap for Hospitals.* Oakbrook terrace, IL: The Joint Commission.

von Tetzchner S (2000) *Introduction to Augmentative and Alternative Communication.* London: Whurr.

Watson LSF (1999) *Report of the Western Australian Cerebral Palsy Register – to the Birth Year* 1994. Perth: Register.

World Health Organization (2007) *International Classification of Functioning, Disability and Health: ICF.* Geneva: World Health Organization.

Chapter 11

Cognitive and sensory impairment

Katheryn F. Frazier

Introduction

Cognitive and sensory impairments are common in children with complex cerebral palsy (CP) and often as the level of severity of the motor impairment increases, so does the severity of the comorbid impairments. While it can be difficult to accurately assess children with complex CP for these comorbidities, it is imperative to do so as they frequently have more of an impact on daily activities and participation than the child's motor limitations. Screening for hearing, vision, and cognitive impairments are Level A recommendations (those that are established as useful for the given population based on scientific evidence) from the American Academy of Neurology and should be part of the initial assessment after a new diagnosis of CP, regardless of the severity of motor impairment. Once evaluated, appropriate supports, therapies, and interventions can then be put into place for the child both at home and at school.

Cognitive impairment

Overview

About half of children with CP have some level of cognitive impairment or intellectual disability (Ashwal et al. 2004, Pruitt and Tsai 2009). This can range from mild deficits in specific cognitive domains such as language and visual perception to more severe and global intellectual disabilities.

Typically, the diagnosis of intellectual disability is not given until a child enters elementary school, around age 6–7 years. Until that time, a child may have the more general diagnosis of 'global developmental delay'. A diagnosis of intellectual disability requires an intelligence quotient (IQ) of less than 70 on standardized intelligence testing along with deficits in adaptive functioning. Historically, intellectual disability has been broken down in to the following descriptive categories based on IQ: mild (IQ 55–70), moderate (IQ 40–55), severe (IQ 25–40), and profound (IQ<25); however, DSM-5 (American Psychiatric Association 2013) instructs providers to base severity on the person's level of adaptive functioning.

Standardized intelligence testing is usually completed by a trained psychologist and includes standardized tests such as the Wechsler Preschool and Primary Scale of Intelligence (WPPSI-III) or the Wechsler Intelligence Scale for Children (WISC-V). In the United States, this is typically done through the Department of Education but can also be done privately in an outpatient setting. Depending on the country or region, other avenues for testing may be available. Standardized intelligence tests rely on aurally and visually processing information, manipulating testing objects such as puzzle pieces, and then providing verbal or written responses. For those children who have severe motor impairments, speech/language delays, or hearing/vision impairments, this type of testing may lead to underestimation of true cognitive abilities. Testing should be modified appropriately when possible to do so and test results should be interpreted carefully, taking into account the child's specific impairments.

As mentioned, along with intelligence testing, impairments in adaptive functioning need to be documented as well. Examples of the standardized tools to assess adaptive functioning include the Vineland Adaptive Behavior Scales (VBAS-III) or the Adaptive Behavior Assessment System (ABAS-III) among others.

Risk factors
In general, children with spastic quadriplegia tend to have more impairment than those with hemiplegia or diplegia and the severity of motor deficits in spastic CP often correlates with the severity of cognitive impairment. However, this is not true with dyskinetic CP in which motor abilities tend to be more impaired than cognition (Fennell and Dikel 2001, Ashwal et al. 2004, Pruitt and Tsai 2009). Particularly in children with dyskinetic CP and dysarthria it is important not to underestimate cognition; however, accurate assessment can be challenging. History of comorbid epilepsy or abnormal neuroimaging increases the risk of cognitive impairment.

Assessment/management
In the United States, children under the age of 3 years old should be referred to Early Intervention providers for assessment and treatment or to a developmental pediatrician or psychologist for evaluation. This should include assessment of speech/language development, problem-solving abilities, and social/cognitive skills. Based on these results, appropriate

therapies can be initiated, either privately as an outpatient or through the creation of an Individual Family Service Plan (IFSP) with Early Intervention.

On or around their third birthday, children with disabilities transition their care from Early Intervention services to their local school system. Children undergo an assessment, based on their needs, to determine appropriate educational placement and supports and therapy services and an Individualized Education Plan (IEP) is created. This process involves a team of people including the parents or caregivers, special education team, school therapy providers, and school psychologist.

Once children are school-age (around 6–7 years old), if it has not already been done, they should have a full psychological assessment as reviewed above as part of their triennial IEP re-evaluation. The results of this larger assessment should be used to determine most appropriate educational placement, therapy services, and need for adaptive equipment or assistive technology in the classroom. Additionally, the diagnosis, if appropriate, of intellectual disability should be given to help with determining eligibility for certain lifetime supports, such as insurance waivers.

This assessment can be more difficult to complete in children with more severe cognitive and motor impairments and these children may carry the more generic diagnosis of 'global developmental delay' into adolescence. This can be an issue when addressing concerns such as guardianship, post-secondary education, or eligibility for services as an adult, which all require more specific diagnoses. Therefore, it is important for those working with the child, regardless of their complexity, to provide the most specific and accurate diagnoses as early as possible. This will allow everyone on the child's team, including medical, educational, and community providers, to best prepare and plan for the child's future.

Vision impairment

Overview

Thirty-five percent of children with CP have some degree of visual impairment (Colver et al. 2014). Severe visual impairment occurs in about 8% of children with CP and occurs mostly in those children classified in Gross Motor Function Classification System (GMFCS, see Chapter 1) levels IV–V (Guzetta et al. 2001). Children with severe CP are more likely to have visual impairments that do not typically occur or are never seen in typically developing children such as high myopia or dyskinetic strabismus (Pruitt and Tsai 2009).

Risk factors

Risk factors for visual impairment include prematurity, hypoxic-ischemic encephalopathy, congenital infections, respiratory distress requiring high oxygen supports, and cerebral malformations, among others.

Types of visual impairment

While some children with CP have visual impairments caused by problems in the eye itself, such as retinopathy or cataracts, most children have abnormalities related to damage of the central visual pathway. This latter type is often referred to as cerebral (or cortical) visual impairment (CVI) and refers to any visual abnormality due to lesions in the retrochiasmatic visual pathway and other areas associated with processing of visual stimuli such as the occipital cortex and visual associative areas. CVI is a broad term and includes problems with visual acuity, visual field deficits, oculomotor disorders, and visual-perceptual impairments (VPI). Children with spastic diplegia or whose CP is secondary to periventricular leukomalacia are more likely to have VPI (Guzzetta et al. 2001, Fazzi et al. 2010, Ego et al. 2015).

Assessment

Children with severe CP should have a thorough evaluation by a pediatric ophthalmologist or neuro-ophthalmologist at time of diagnosis and then be followed yearly. If there are no providers in your area, then recommend an evaluation with an optometrist who is experienced in working with children. This includes assessment of refraction, eye motility, and fundoscopy.

Management

Along with regular follow-up by a pediatric ophthalmologist, those children with low vision may also need a functional vision assessment (FVA) to help determine their functional visual abilities. This assessment can evaluate a child's acuity, visual fields, and sensitivity to colors, contrast, and light. In the United States, one resource for obtaining a FVA is through the Department of Education. This assessment can be helpful in determining what supports and tools are best for children with low vision. These results are then used to modify a child's therapeutic and educational plans. Examples of accommodations could include large print or high-contrast images or the need for orientation and mobility assistance. The goal is to allow for maximal participation by the child within the classroom and the school.

Children with low vision may also have stereotypic or self-stimulating behaviors such as body rocking, eye pressing or poking, or prolonged gazing at lights. This can often be very distressing to the family and, in the case of eye poking, may cause damage to the eye. These behaviors are more prominent in children who also have comorbid intellectual disability and often improve some as the child gets older. Management typically involves behavioral modification and finding more acceptable ways to provide sensory input for the child (Molloy and Rowe 2011).

Hearing impairment

Overview

Between 10–15% of children with CP have some level of hearing impairment, with an estimated 2% having moderate-to-severe bilateral hearing loss (Ashwal et al. 2004). Those children who do have hearing impairments are often more likely to have more severe motor impairments (GMFCS IV–V), visual or cognitive impairments, or have hypotonic, dyskinetic or spastic quadriplegic types of CP. Children with CP can have conductive hearing loss, sensorineural hearing loss, or a combination of both. It is crucial to diagnose hearing loss as it can have a dramatic impact on speech/language and cognitive development.

Risk factors

Children who have a history of congenital infections, neonatal meningitis, kernicterus, severe hypoxic-ischemic injury, or those with very low birthweight have the highest risk of developing a hearing impairment. Other risk factors include use of ototoxic drugs (i.e. gentamicin, furosemide) during the neonatal period, prolonged respiratory support after birth, or history of requiring extracorporeal membrane oxygenation.

Assessment

While all should undergo neonatal hearing screening, children with CP should have a repeat audiology evaluation at time of diagnosis. Of note, pure tone audiometry or other types of behavioral audiometry that are typically used to detect hearing loss may not be a viable option for children with severe CP. This is because these children may not have the physical or cognitive abilities to respond to these types of behavioral assessment. Oto-acoustic emissions may provide useful assessment without the need for behavioral compliance or sedation. If these measures are inadequate, the audiologist may need to do the evaluation using auditory brainstem response which may require sedation, adding risk to the procedure.

Management

If hearing loss is detected, children should be referred to an otolaryngologist, audiologist, and speech/language therapist for further evaluation and management. Depending on the type and severity of hearing loss, different interventions such as amplification devices (FM systems), hearing aids, specialized hearing therapies or the addition of sign language may be necessary. In some cases, cochlear implantation should be considered. Having the appropriate supports and services in place early can help with long-term speech/language and cognitive outcomes as well as improve a child's ability to interact with the world around them.

Tactile impairment

Overview

Tactile discrimination is defined as the ability to perceive, organize, and interpret incoming touch information, including both the spatial and temporal aspects of that sensation. Children with CP often have an impairment of this type of sensory perception and may under-react or over-react to various tactile stimuli. Examples of over-reaction to stimuli include being sensitive to certain food or clothing textures, irritability when being touched by parents or caregivers, or oral aversions. Under-reaction to incoming tactile information may include lack of response to painful injuries. Children may also have self-stimulating or self-injurious behaviors that are reinforced by the type of sensory input they provide.

Assessment/management

Assessment of tactile impairment can be complicated in children with severe CP as they may not be able to verbalize what sensations they are feeling. As a result, evaluations are often based on observations of behavioral reactions to various stimuli gathered by parents, occupational therapists, physicians, or others that work closely with the child. If abnormal responses to tactile stimulation are identified, parents can work with occupational and behavioral therapists to find ways to incorporate sensory integration techniques, modify the child's environment, and lessen their discomfort.

Conclusion

The range of sensory and cognitive impairment in children with severe CP is broad and can be difficult to assess and diagnose. The role of the primary care provider is to be aware

Table 11.1   Resources for families (organized by concern)

Cognitive	• Early Intervention (in the United States, 0–3 years)
	• Special education services through the Department of Education (in the United States, 3 years and older)
	• Testing through private psychologists or neuropsychologists
Hearing	• Audiology
	• Otolaryngology
Vision	• Ophthalmology
	• Optometry
	• Functional visual assessment (in the United States, often done through the Department of Education)
Tactile	• Occupational therapists

of the range of cognitive and sensory impairments, address concerns with families, and know the resources and services available in the area (Table 11.1). As the trusted contact for the family, providers can help identify and address concerns early, allowing for early intervention and potentially better outcomes for children with severe CP.

Key points

- Cognitive and sensory (hearing, vision, tactile) impairments are common in children with severe CP.

- Discussions with families about potential cognitive and sensory impairments are an important aspect of the long-term management of complex CP.

- Screening is strongly recommended and should be done at the time of diagnosis and then as needed when concerns arise, including hearing, vision and cognitive testing.

- Children can receive services and interventions through both medical and educational providers, optimally combining efforts to allow for maximum supports for the child.

- Primary care providers should know the appropriate resources in their area, including pediatric subspecialists, audiologists and therapy providers. Additionally, primary care providers should know how families can contact their local special education offices.

References

American Psychiatric Association (2013) Neurodevelopmental disorders. In *Diagnostic and Statistical Manual of Mental Disorders*. DSM Library. American Psychiatric Association. Available at: http://dx.doi.org/10.1176/appi.books.9780890425596.dsm01

Ashwal S Russman BS, Blasco PA, Miller G, Sandler A, Shevell M, Stevenson R (2004) Practice parameter: diagnostic assessment of the child with cerebral palsy: report of the Quality Standards Subcommittee of the American Academy of Neurology and the Practice Committee of the Child Neurology Society. *Neurology* 62: 851–863.

Clayton K, Fleming JM, Copley J (2003) Behavioral responses to tactile stimuli in children with cerebral palsy. *Phys Occup Ther Pediatr* 23: 43–62.

Colver A, Fairhurst C, Pharoah POD (2014) Cerebral palsy. *Lancet* 383: 1240–1249.

Dufresne D, Dagenais L, Shevell MI (2014) Epidemiology of severe hearing impairment in a population-based cerebral palsy cohort. *Pediatr Neurol* 51: 641–644.

Ego A, Lidzba K, Brovedani P, et al (2015) Visual-perceptual impairment in children with cerebral palsy: A systematic review. *Dev Med Child Neurol* 57: 46–51.

Fazzi E, Signorini S, Bianchi P (2010) Visual impairment in cerebral palsy. In G Dutton, M Bax (eds.) *Visual Impairment in Children Due to Damage to the Brain.* London; Mac Keith Press, pp. 194–204.

Fennell EB, Dikel TN (2001) Cognitive and neuropsychological functioning in children with cerebral palsy. *J Child Neurol* 16: 58–63.

Guzzetta A, Mercuri E, Cioni G (2001) Visual disorders in children with brain lesions: 2. Visual impairment associated with cerebral palsy. *Eur J Paed Neurol* **5**: 115–119.

Molloy A, Rowe FJ (2011) Manneristic behaviors of visually impaired children. *Strabismus* **19**: 77–84.

Pruitt DW, Tsai T (2009) Common medical comorbidities associated with cerebral palsy. *Phys Med Rehab ClinNorth Am* **20**: 453–467.

Reid SM Modak MB, Berkowitz RG, Reddihough DS (2011) A population-based study and systematic review of hearing loss in children with cerebral palsy. *Dev Med Child Neurol* **53**: 1038–1045.

Straub K, Obrzut JE (2009) Effects of cerebral palsy on neuropsychological function. *J Dev Phys Disabil* **21**: 153–167.

Chapter 12

Challenging behaviors, sleep and toileting

Alisa B. Bahl and Kurt A. Freeman

Advances in the understanding of challenges faced by individuals with cerebral palsy (CP) and their families have often focused on the motoric and developmental impact of cerebral palsy. Extant evidence supports that individuals with severe cerebral palsy often display comorbid behavioral sequelae in a variety of domains (e.g., sleeping, feeding, toileting). The biopsychosocial model of understanding cerebral palsy highlights the importance of focusing on the functional capacity of individuals in their home, school, work, and community (World Health Organization 2001). It is important to not just acknowledge that comorbid challenges may occur, but to also give proper consideration to the psychosocial contributions to an individual's experience with cerebral palsy. An awareness of behavior problems that may occur and an understanding of interventions that are likely to be most effective at ameliorating those problems are important issues for families. Given the heightened medical complexity of children with cerebral palsy, assessment and intervention often involves a family-centered, team approach to address the physical, social and behavioral needs.

In this chapter, select behavioral issues experienced by individuals with cerebral palsy are discussed, including a brief introduction to effective intervention based on empirical evidence. In many situations, a behavioral clinical psychologist is critical to the evaluation and treatment of children with complex cerebral palsy and behavioral problems.

Challenging behavior

Challenging behavior displayed by young people with and without disabilities can take many forms. For those with neurodevelopmental disabilities such as cerebral palsy, common examples including aggression (e.g., hitting, kicking), self-injury (e.g., head banging, self-biting, self-hitting), and disruption (e.g., throwing objects). Other challenges may include tantrums and noncompliance.

Several risk factors exist for increased frequency of challenging behavior in young people. Specifically, presence of a neurodevelopmental disability increases risk, with young people with neurodevelopmental disabilities displaying higher rates of challenging behavior than those without disabilities (Ageranioti-Belanger et al. 2012). Having cerebral palsy appears to increase risk, with the prevalence of challenging behavior in individuals with cerebral palsy being as high as 26% of individuals (Novak et al. 2012). Odding et al. (2006) reported estimates of challenging behavior in children with cerebral palsy as being five times the rate of reported challenging behavior in children without cerebral palsy or other neurodevelopmental disabilities. Rates of behavior problems are typically higher in children with moderate to severe intellectual impairment compared to those with intellectual abilities in the average to mildly impaired range (Parkes et al. 2008). Thus, when considering risk for behavioral challenges, the severity of physical and intellectual disability is important (McDermott et al. 1996). Further, it is important to note that children who are in pain have higher levels of behavioral problems than children without pain (Russo 2008), a finding that is pertinent to children with cerebral palsy given high rates of reported pain (Novak et al. 2012). Pain can be associated with a range of issues. Medical issues associated with pain (e.g. spasticity, fracture, constipation, reflux) should be considered. Further, children with disabilities like complex cerebral palsy are at increased risk for abuse and neglect and challenging behaviors can also arise as a result of such abuse or neglect. Finally, high rates of challenging behavior are displayed by individuals with limitations in their nonverbal and verbal communication, and approximately 25% of individuals with cerebral palsy do not talk (Novak 2006).

Behavioral interventions for challenging behavior

While pharmacological treatment of challenging behavior is possible and can be helpful (Ageranioti-Belanger et al. 2012), the implementation of behavioral intervention is often more effective at impacting long-term changes in behavioral functioning. The following is a review of the components that should be part of any plan so that pediatricians can assist families in determining whether the supports being provided represent best practices.

Behavioral interventions are grounded in the perspective that the vast majority of challenging behaviors displayed by individuals with neurodevelopmental disabilities, including those with cerebral palsy, are learned through experience and are influenced by contextual variables. Further, intervention planning includes assessment and intervention strategies that are designed to better understand and address the *function* of behavior (meaning the outcomes accomplished), rather than focusing on its *form* (what the behavior looks like). The focus of such interventions is therefore to understand (a) the contextual factors that may increase the likelihood of behavior, (b) the outcomes of behavior that may inadvertently reinforce its occurrence, and (c) the skills that can be taught or strengthened so that individuals are best prepared to accomplish a desired outcome using more acceptable prosocial behavior. Appropriate intervention goes beyond simply targeting amelioration of challenges and includes an emphasis on promoting access to community and social engagement.

Broadly speaking, there are three possible functions of challenging behavior that are influenced by contextual and social factors: (1) to gain attention or reactions from others (social positive reinforcement), (2) to gain access to preferred activities or objects (non-social positive reinforcement), and (3) to escape or avoid undesired situations or experiences (social negative reinforcement). Behavior may also be 'automatically reinforced,' meaning that engaging in the act itself causes some type of reinforcing outcome (e.g., producing reinforcing physical sensations).

From this perspective, comprehensive and effective intervention plans should contain a minimum of three components. First, plans should examine contextual factors that seem to increase the likelihood of challenging behavior and propose strategies for minimizing exposure to or altering those factors. For example, if a child starts hitting each time a specific educational tasks is presented, the plan may involve eliminating that task from the curriculum (if possible) or changing the manner in which it is presented (e.g., present one step of the task at a time rather than presenting the entire task).

Second, the plan should address inadvertent reinforcement for the negative behavior. Using the example of educational tasks above, perhaps the hitting results in a break from the task, and thus the hypothesized function of the behavior is to escape an undesired situation. With this hypothesis, the plan should include approaches that minimize the likelihood that tasks are ended in response to hitting.

Finally, appropriate plans should focus on skills development for the individual with cerebral palsy. Two categories of skills should be emphasized. First, the plan should teach or strengthen prosocial skills that result in the same outcome as the challenging behavior. Thus, if hitting results in escape from tasks, the plan should strengthen appropriate behavior that results in the same outcome such as touching a break sign, saying the word 'break,' or other similar behaviors. Second, the plan should emphasize teaching skills for being more successful in the challenging situations, for example breaking down educational tasks into achievable component parts.

Sleep

Up to 80% of children with neurodevelopmental disorders experience problems with sleep (e.g., sleep onset and maintenance, excessive somnolence, seizures, sleep–wake transition difficulties, hyperhidrosis) (Newman 2014, Blackmer and Feinstein 2016). In contrast, parental reports indicate that only 25% of typically developed children experience sleep disorders (Owens 2008). The higher prevalence of sleep disorders in children with cerebral palsy is likely multifactorial in origin. Multiple biological factors (e.g. visual impairment, pain, seizures, altered circadian rhythms) likely play a role in combination with complicating environmental (e.g. physical, social) factors (Lélis et al. 2016).

Sleep difficulties are problematic because they impact functioning for both children and their families across several realms. Rates of daytime behavior problems – such as disruptive behavior, excessive daytime sleepiness, academic underachievement, and mood and anxiety disorders – are significantly higher in children with sleep disturbance (Owens et al. 2012). In addition, disruptions in child sleep negatively impact the quantity and quality of caregiver sleep, the rates of parental depression, parental fatigue, and family satisfaction. Mothers of children who have sleep disorders are more likely to report higher rates of sleep disturbance and maternal depression (Wayte et al. 2012).

Assessment of sleep problems

It is important for practitioners to have a thorough assessment of the sleep disorder to determine whether there are medical or behavioral sleep problems (or both) and to provide a tailored and effective sleep intervention. Most commonly, assessment of sleep difficulties relies upon caregiver report during a clinical interview, but there are also standardized measures that are useful tools to screen for sleep problems.

Parent-report forms are useful for determining whether a child has clinically significant sleep disturbances. Further, most published measures also provide information about overall sleep disturbances as well as specific domains of disturbance (e.g., initiation, maintenance, parasomnias).

A comprehensive review of available parent-report forms is beyond the scope of this chapter, but there are a few standardized measures for evaluating sleep problems in pediatric populations, such as the Sleep Disturbance Scale for Children (SDSC; Bruni et al. 1996) and the Children's Sleep Habits Questionnaire (CSHQ; Owens et al. 2000). While developed for use with typically developing children, extant literature also demonstrates their utility with children with a variety of special health needs. However, caregivers may find that some of the questions are not relevant for their children with cerebral palsy, in that they rely on a child's recall and verbal report (e.g., nightmares) or independent mobility (e.g., sleepwalking). In addition, neither of these measures takes into consideration factors that may be impacting sleep in children with psychomotor impairment such as factors present in cerebral palsy (e.g., spasticity, pain).

Prospective information gathering via completion of a sleep diary is common when pursuing interventions for sleep disturbance. The sleep diary has been shown to be an accurate representation of a child's sleep-wake cycle when compared to objective measures such as actigraphy, but has the advantage of being more clinically accessible and useful (e.g., Corkum et al. 2001). Information obtained via a sleep diary typically includes sleep onset latency, duration of sleep, night awakenings, possible triggers or associated symptoms at the time of awakenings, and sleep–wake patterns within a 24-hour period. In conjunction with parental report, specific patterns of sleep associations can be identified and linked to the child's sleep data. This provides the basis for development of individualized sleep intervention.

A detailed assessment of sleep problems requires an understanding of the variables that maintain the sleep difficulty. It is useful to gather information regarding the antecedents of the sleep situation (e.g., noises from the television or others in the home, divided attention among other children with parental needs, anxiety or family stress contributing to problems falling asleep, lack of separate sleeping space, napping during the day interfering with nighttime sleep onset, nighttime tube feedings, muscle spasm or other medical problems or interventions) as well as information regarding what occurs when the sleep problem presents (e.g., immediate attention to behaviors to prevent waking others in the home, sleep associations, lack of consistency on insistence on same routine each night). A child's responses to these actions can also lend insight to whether they are waking as a result of pain or the need for a positional change versus factors related to overall sleep hygiene. It is important that pediatricians are aware of extraneous issues that may have an effect on sleep as part of this assessment, such as cultural differences in sleeping arrangements, and unrealistic expectations.

Medical intervention for sleep disorders
There are no Food and Drug Administration (FDA) approved medications for treating sleep disorders in children and many pharmacological sleep aides are prescribed for off-label uses. Commonly used agents include melatonin, clonidine, trazodone, and amitriptyline. Use of these agents requires consideration of general medical status and potential exacerbation of obstructive sleep apnea. Also, some of these agents may lead to or worsen daytime drowsiness. While pharmacological interventions may be helpful, particularly when pain, spasticity, seizure disorders, gastro-esophageal reflux or other interfering medical variables are at the root cause, they may not adequately address environmental, psychosocial, or behavioral variables contributing to sleep challenges. However, once the medical variables have been ameliorated, sleep challenges often persist due to nighttime routines and environmental factors. With some individualized adaptations as needed, children with cerebral palsy can benefit from the same

evidence-based behavioral interventions that are effective for children without neurodevelopmental disorders.

Behavioral intervention for sleep disorders

Numerous studies indicate that behavioral interventions effectively address many pediatric sleep disorders (e.g. Mindell et al. 2006). While the majority of research has been conducted on individuals without neurodevelopmental disorders, increasingly more applications of behavioral sleep intervention with children with neurodevelopmental disorders have been documented (e.g. Allen et al. 2012, Vriend et al. 2011). Systematic reviews of published sleep interventions for young people with neurodevelopmental disabilities support the effectiveness of behavioral interventions (e.g. Vriend et al. 2011), although it is noted that more research is necessary to ensure that these interventions are well-established. In particular, sleep studies with children with neurodevelopmental disabilities tend to use small-n designs with individualized sleep protocols which are excellent for demonstrating functional control of treatment effects but do not establish external validity to larger populations. Further, little has been published with regard to interventions for sleep problems in children with cerebral palsy. Despite the limitations on sleep interventions with young people with cerebral palsy specifically, and neurodevelopmental disabilities more generally, it follows that individualized sleep programs based on well-established interventions for pediatric sleep disorders should be considered.

Pediatric behavioral sleep interventions generally involve three primary components that require caregivers to be the agent of change across multiple dimensions that affect sleep problems. First, a consistent routine that prepares the young people and an environment that is conducive to sleep must be established (e.g., quiet, dark/low light). Second, a sleep–wake cycle that is predictable and consistent must be established and closely managed to ensure maintenance over time. Third, caregivers must learn to respond to their child in a manner that promotes desired child sleep behaviors related to independent sleep initiation and avoids inadvertent reinforcement for undesired behavior (e.g., calling out from room).

Prior to intervention, a baseline of average daily sleep should be obtained by having caregivers maintain a sleep diary for 1 to 2 weeks (Figure 12.1). Sleep diaries are useful because they typically provide a more accurate report of nightly sleep as opposed to caregiver report which tends to focus on the most difficult nights or the most recent nights. In addition, maintaining a sleep diary throughout intervention is also important because it (a) provides objective data regarding improvements or ongoing challenges, and (b) can be used to demonstrate positive improvements that might not be noticed otherwise due to the gradual nature of the change.

After evaluation of the sleep diary information with caregivers, an individualized intervention plan can be developed. It is important to note the total time slept in a given

Two-Week Sleep Record

1. Mark time child goes into bed. →   2. Mark time child gets out of bed. ←   3. Shade in times when child is asleep. ▢   4. W= wakened (parents, alarm)

       S = child awakened on own

Day	Date	12am	1am	2sm	3am	4am	5am	6am	7am	8am	9am	10am	11am	Noon	1pm	2pm	3pm	4pm	5pm	6pm	7pm	8pm	9pm	10pm	11pm
Wed	4/17							S←														→			
Thur	4/18									←W													→		

Day	Date	12am	1am	2am	3am	4am	5am	6am	7am	8am	9am	10am	11am	Noon	1pm	2pm	3pm	4pm	5pm	6pm	7pm	8pm	9pm	10pm	11pm

Figure 12.1   Example of a two week sleep record

day/night cycle and to use the average total time slept as a baseline for the intervention. From these individualized data, optimal sleep onset times and wake times can be derived and recommended. Pediatricians should support families in preventing sleep at other times during the day/night, as this will interfere with the intervention.

Oftentimes, middle-of-the-night challenges are improved by first addressing sleep onset difficulties and interfering sleep associations.

Unmodified extinction is an evidence-based intervention that ameliorates bedtime problems as well as night-waking (e.g. Mindell et al. 2006). Caregivers are instructed to not respond to a child's behaviors (e.g., crying, yelling), while monitoring for safety or illness, for the duration of the night from bedtime until an established wake time. A consistent sleep schedule is maintained for bedtime, wake time, and daytime sleep, and typically children exhibit improvement in sleep problems within a few days. However, caregivers find this strategy to be quite stressful, and as a result, adherence can be difficult. Some research suggests that children who take medication in addition to caregivers using the unmodified extinction procedure exhibit the fastest results.

Graduated extinction, also referred to as time-based visiting, is an alternative to unmodified extinction that involves caregivers checking on their child at pre-determined intervals that gradually increase within and across nights. This may be preferable for caregivers who find unmodified extinction too difficult to implement. For children with complex medical needs, the core feature of regular checks allows parents to have frequent monitoring to ensure that their child's safety, positioning needs, or medical needs are fully addressed. Many families may wish to use a video monitoring system so that they can watch their child between scheduled checks. For some children, it may be necessary for the caregiver to remain in the room but not engage with the child. The parent may pretend to read or sleep. Over the course of a few nights, caregivers may gradually move themselves out of the room. Time-based graduated extinction is explained in Table 12.1.

It is important for caregivers and pediatricians to understand if sleep problems are resulting from factors that require medical attention. For example, if a child is crying but soothes immediately upon parental presence and interaction, it may be that the behavior is maintained by attention. If, however, a child does not soothe when provided with parental presence, it is likely that other factors, including pain, need for position change, or other physiological discomfort are the reason for the night waking.

Sleeping positions that provide optimal comfort as well as safety may address the underlying causes of sleep problems for children with cerebral palsy. Medical issues, such as overnight feedings, gastro-esophageal reflux, spasticity, and obstructive sleep apnea (see Chapter 9) can also interfere. Again, having families keep a sleep log can drive the schedule for nighttime intervention to occur prior to the occurrence of disrupted sleep and nighttime distress due to medical issues.

Table 12.1   Time-based graduated extinction

Visit child based on time, regardless of behavior, at increasingly longer intervals within and across nights.

- Be brief, less than 15 seconds
- Provide quiet positive attention and reassurance for child in bed
- Tuck in again if necessary
- Say goodnight and leave
- Return quickly enough to catch child still in bed (if child able to get out alone)
- Gradually increase time between visits until child falls asleep

Day	First visit	Second visit	Third visit	Fourth visit	Fifth visit	Sixth visit	Seventh visit
1	10 sec	1 min	1 min	3 min	5 min	10 min	30 min
2	30 sec	3 min	3 min	5 min	10 min	30 min	
3	30 sec	3 min	5 min	10 min	30 min		
4	1 min	5 min	10 min	30 min			
5	1 min	10 min	30 min				
6	5 min	30 min					
7	5 min						

Adapted from Hanley (2015)

Toileting

Several factors likely contribute to the high prevalence rate of elimination disorders among children with cerebral palsy. Approximately 25% of individuals with cerebral palsy experience enuresis (frequent diurnal or nocturnal wetting in locations other than the toilet) (Novak et al. 2012). Bladder control is delayed in children with cerebral palsy (Roijen et al. 2001), and the likelihood of developing bladder control decreases over time. Children with spastic quadriplegia and intellectual disability may be less likely to obtain bladder control, and the greater level of intellectual disability is correlated with a greater likelihood of diurnal enuresis (Singh et al. 2006). In addition, 85% of children with cerebral palsy who were nonambulatory had diurnal enuresis, compared with 15% of children who could walk (Singh et al. 2006). Similarly, nocturnal enuresis occurred in 77% of children who were non-ambulatory in contrast with 23% of children who were ambulatory.

Assessment

A simple scatterplot is an easy, effective tool to use to track toileting prior to initiating a toileting training intervention (Table 12.2). Data obtained this way provide a clear

Table 12.2   Simple scatterplot to track toileting baseline and intervention progress

Time	Sun	Mon	Tues	Wed	Thur	Fri	Sat
7:00–7:30							
7:30–8:00							
8:30–9:00							
9:00–9:30							
9:30–10:00							
10:00–10:30							
10:30–11:00							
11:00–11:30							
11:30–12:00							
12:00–12:30							
12:30–1:00							
1:00–1:30							
1:30–2:00							
2:00–2:30							
2:30–3:00							
3:00–3:30							
3:30–4:00							
4:00–4:30							
4:30–5:00							
5:30–6:00							
6:00–6:30							
6:30–7:00							
7:00–7:30							
7:30–8:00							
8:30–9:00							

Complete this chart using the following abbreviations as appropriate: EAT (meal or snack); SIT (time on toilet); U (successful void in toilet); BM (successful bowel movement in toilet)

visual picture of a child's natural toileting schedule and can be used for the development of a toileting intervention plan.

Medical intervention

Because issues with motility and constipation are prevalent in children with cerebral palsy, it is important to consider a medical evaluation prior to implementing a behavioral toileting intervention, depending on age, cognitive ability, and suspicion for underlying medical contributors (see Chapters 8 and 16).

Behavioral intervention

Although many of the components of an effective toileting training plan are consistent with those recommended for any comprehensive plan to teach children independent toileting, it is important to keep in mind that toilet training is likely to be more challenging for children with cerebral palsy due to potential barriers related to cognitive, motoric, and communication abilities. Specific motor challenges such as balance or weakness may require specialized equipment and physical support. Removing clothing for toileting may pose additional motor challenges. Before initiating training, pediatricians should help families determine whether their child is showing developmental readiness signs. Caregivers should be encouraged to delay toilet training if their child is not ready so as to avoid frustration for everyone involved.

The characteristic motor impairments of children with complex cerebral palsy that result in additional challenges for toilet training include (1) dependence on adaptive equipment and care assistance to get to the bathroom, (2) dependence on others for clothing removal needed for toileting, and (3) muscular control for functional voiding. Interventions that focus on promoting communication with others who can assist with mobility and physical manipulation of clothing for toileting success may be the best choice.

The initial attempt at toilet training is often focused on schedule training. This allows children to learn toileting skills without the added demand of recognizing the biological cues (e.g., sensation of a full bladder) indicating that they need to either request toileting or move to the toilet. Schedule training requires caregivers to be responsible for a child's toileting, but this introduction is a starting point for leading a child to develop independent toileting in the future. It is important for children to wear underwear during the day while toilet training so that they can feel when they are wet. It is fine to wear rubber pants over the underwear, if necessary. Pullups and diapers should not be worn, with the exception of during naps and bedtime, if deemed developmentally appropriate.

Once data have been collected on the scatter plot, caregivers can determine the typical pattern of toileting for their child throughout the day. Scheduled sits can be implemented at the times just before when urination or defecation most often occurs. Often, these times occur postmeal and postactivity. A good starting point for families is to recommend sitting about 5–10 minutes after meal and snack times for approximately 5–10 minutes.

For children who have given indications of interest in toilet training or who have fewer motoric interferences, families may want to consider a toileting protocol that teaches independent initiation. The most effective way to teach children independent toileting is by implementing an intensive toilet training program (Azrin and Foxx 1974) with modifications to address an individual's motoric needs. For an intensive toilet training program, it is important to include a planned schedule for sitting, positive consequences for successful urination, increased fluids, communication training, and positive practice for accidents (LeBlanc et al. 2005). Related, the use of urine alarm can increase awareness and success more quickly (Levato et al. 2016).

The sample protocol in Table 12.3 assumes that the child takes food orally.

Table 12.3   Intensive Toilet Training Protocol[a]

1. Get prepared: extra underpants, towels, supported seat/step stool for toilet, salty snacks, lots of fluids/juice.
2. Write a list of 'people who care' to call when child is successful.
3. Have child wear a shirt and underpants only.
4. Teach child to check and identify dry pants/wet pants. Reward and praise for having dry pants. Perform checks every 3 to 5 minutes.
5. Give child as much to drink as desired to create a strong, frequent desire to toilet (at least 8 oz/hr). Salty snacks increase thirst. Use as a positive reinforcement.
6. Teach child to request 'potty' before going to the toilet using either a vocal response, a hand sign, or an electronic or paper picture exchange.
7. Help child to get to the potty, lower pants, sit down quietly for several minutes. Watch to see if urination begins and praise/ reward immediately. Physical assistance, including specialized toilet seating, is needed for many children with complex cerebral palsy.
8. After urination takes place, have the child wipe him or herself and leave the toilet; if no urination occurs after 10 minutes have child stand up and independently raise pants.
9. Prompt child to 'go potty' every 15 minutes in the beginning, decrease frequency as child acquires skill.
10. Conduct 'dry pants' checks every 5 minutes, and help child to feel for dry pants as well.
11. If there is an accident, say something like 'Oh no, wet pants,' and help the child with clean up and putting wet clothes where they belong. Remind the child, 'remember pee goes in the potty' and have the child practice signaling or requesting 'potty' and going with a caregiver to the potty (also known as Positive Practice).

Table 12.3 (Continued)

12. At first, have child sit on the potty about 10 minutes; after two to three successful urinations into the potty and much praise, the child will begin to understand and prompting and sit time can be reduced.

13. Gradually change from directing child to 'Go potty' to asking child if he or she 'Needs to go potty?' to general questions such as 'Are your pants dry?'

14. Continue praising for dry pants throughout the day.

15. For next several days, do dry pants checks at meals, naps, bedtimes, etc., and praise each time pants are dry.

16. Anytime there is an accident, say something like 'Oh no, wet pants', help the child to clean up, change clothes, and put the wet clothes where they belong.

[a]Additional adaptations may be needed, depending on functional/cognitive status

Conclusion

The challenging behaviors exhibited by children with severe cerebral palsy are unique as a result of the motoric involvement, varying levels of cognitive functioning, medical complexity including seizure activity, and environmental variables such as family support factors. Behavior challenges can significantly interfere with the quality of life for the individual as well as for family members. An individualized approach to assessment and the development of uniquely tailored function-based interventions will be the best strategies for developing sustainable, pro-active support for these individuals and their families. Behavioral psychologists have expertise in systematically integrating functional information obtained from assessment and clinical interview into evidence-based interventions, and can be essential team members in addressing behavioral challenges in children with complex cerebral palsy.

Summary points

- There are three possible functions of challenging behavior that are influenced by contextual and social factors: (1) to gain attention or reactions from others (social positive reinforcement), (2) to gain access to preferred activities or objects (non-social positive reinforcement), and (3) to escape or avoid undesired situations or experiences (social negative reinforcement). Behavior may also be 'automatically reinforced', meaning that engaging in the act itself causes some type of reinforcing outcome (e.g., producing reinforcing physical sensations).

- Evaluation of sleep problems begins with sleep diary and identification of all the medical, musculoskeletal, and household factors that may be impacting on sleep.

- Schedule training is a good starting place to teach children the skills and steps required for toileting while not requiring them to recognize the physiological cues that indicate the need for requesting the toilet.

- The most effective way to teach children independent initiation of toileting (when they are ready) is by implementing an intensive toilet training program with modifications to address an individual's motoric needs.

- Pediatricians will usually work in concert with behavioral psychologists (among others) to address challenging behaviors, complex sleep problems, and toileting.

References

Ageranioti-Belanger S, Brunet S, D'Anjou G, Tekkuer Gm Boivin J, Gauthier M (2012) Behaviour disorders in children with an intellectual disability. *Paediatr child health* **17**(2): 84–88.

Allen KD, Kuhn BR, DeHaai KA, Wallace DP (2013) Evaluation of a behavioral treatment package to reduce sleep problems in children with Angelman Syndrome. *Res Dev Disabil* **34**: 676–686.

Azrin NH, Foxx RM (1974) *Toilet training in less than a day*. New York: Simon & Schuster.

Blackmer AB, Feinstein JA (2016) Management of sleep disorders in children with neurodevelopmental disorders: A review. *Pharmacotherapy* **36**(1): 84–98.

Brehaut JC, Kohen DE, Raina P, Walter SD, Russell DJ, Swinton M et al. (2004) The health of primary caregivers of children with cerebral palsy: how does it compare with that of other Canadian caregivers? *Pediatrics* **114**:e182–e191.

Brossard-Racine M, Hall N, Majnemer A, Shevell MI, Law M, Poulin C, Rosenbaum P (2012) Behavioural problems in school age children with cerebral palsy. *Eur J Paediatr Neurol* **6**(1): 35–41.

Bruni O, Ottaviano S, Guidetti V, Romoli M, Innocenzi M, Cortesi F et al. (1996) The Sleep Disturbance Scale for Children (SDSC). Construction and validation of an instrument to evaluate sleep disturbances in childhood and adolescence. *J Sleep Res* **5**: 251–261.

Corkum P, Tannock R, Moldofsky H, Hogg-Johnson S, Humphries T (2001) Actigraphy and parental ratings of sleep in children with attention-deficit/hyperactivity disorder (ADHD). *Sleep* **24**(3): 303–312.

Elsayed RM, Hasanein BM, Sayyah HE, El-Auoty MM, Tharwat N, Belal TM (2013) Sleep assessment of children with cerebral palsy: Using validated sleep questionnaire. *Annals Indian Acad Neurol* **16**(1) 62–65.

Hanley G (2015) Understanding and treating sleep problems of children. Presented at the Berkshires Association for Behavior Analysis Annual Conference.

Kuhn BR (2014) Practical strategies for managing behavioral sleep problems in young children. *Sleep Med Clin* **9**: 181–197.

LeBlanc LA, Carr JE, Crossett SE, Bennett CM, Detweiler DD (2005) Intensive outpatient behavioral treatment of primary urinary incontinence of children with autism. *Focus Autism Other Dev Disabil* **20**: 98–105.

Lélis ALPA, Cardoso MVLM, Hall WA (2016) Sleep disorders in children with cerebral palsy: an integrative review. *Sleep Med Rev* **30**: 63–71.

Levato LE, Aponte CA, Wilkins J, Travis R, Aiello R, Zanibbi K et al. (2016) Use of urine alarms in toilet training children with intellectual and developmental disabilities: A review. *Res Dev Disabil* **53–54**: 232–241.

Majnemer A, Shevell M, Rosenbaum P, Law M, Poulin C (2007) Determinants of life quality in school-age children with cerebral palsy. *J Pediatr* **151**: 470–475, 475.e1–475.e3.

McDermott S, Coker AL, Mani S, Krishnaswami S, Nagle RJ, Barnett-Queen LL et al. (1996) A population-based analysis of behavior problems in children with cerebral palsy. *J Pediatr Psychol* **21**: 447–463.

Meltzer LJ, Mindell JA (2014) Systematic review and meta-analysis of behavioral interventions for pediatric insomnia. *J Pediatr Psychol* **39**: 932–948.

Mindell JA, Kuhn B, Lewin DS, Meltzer LJ, Sadeh A, American Academy of Sleep Medicine (2006) Behavioral treatment of bedtime problems and night wakings in infants and young children. *Sleep* **29**: 1263–1276.

Mindell JA, Telofski LS, Wiegand B, Kurtz ES (2009) A nightly bedtime routine: impact on sleep in young children and maternal mood. *Sleep* **32**: 599–606.

Newman CJ (2014) Sleep: the other life of children with cerebral palsy. *Dev Med Child Neurol* **56**: 610–611.

Newman CJ, O'Regan M, Hensey O (2006) Sleep disorders in children with cerebral palsy. *Dev Med Child Neurol* **48**: 564–568.

Novak I, Hines M, Goldsmith S, Barclay R (2012) Clinical prognostic messages from a systematic review on cerebral palsy. *Pediatrics* **130**: e1285–e1312.

Odding E, Roebroeck ME, Stam HJ (2006) The epidemiology of cerebral palsy, incidence, impairments and risk factors. *Disab Rehabil* **28**(4): 183–191.

Owens J (2008) Classification and epidemiology of childhood sleep disorders. *Primary Care* **35**: 533–546, vii.

Owens JA, Spirito A, McGuinn M, Nobile C (2000) Sleep habits and sleep disturbance in elementary school-aged children. *J Dev Behav Pediatr* **21**: 27–36.

Roijen LE, Postema K, Limbeek VJ, Kuppevelt VH (2001) Development of bladder control in children and adolescents with cerebral palsy. *Dev Med Child Neurol* **43**: 103–107.

Romeo DM, Brogna C, Musto E, Baranello G, Pagliano E, Casalino T et al. (2014) Sleep disturbances in preschool age children with cerebral palsy: a questionnaire study. *Sleep Med* **15**: 1089–1093.

Romeo DM, Bruni O, Brogna C, Ferri R, Galluccio C, DeClemente V et al. (2013) Application of the sleep disturbance scale for children (SDSC) in preschool age. *Eur J Paediatr Neurol* **17**(4): 374–382.

Sandella DE, O'Brien LM, Shank LK, Warschausky SA (2011) Sleep and quality of life in children with cerebral palsy. *Sleep Med* **12**: 252–256.

Singh BK, Masey H, Morton R (2006) Levels of continence in children with cerebral palsy. *Paediatr Nurs* **18**: 23–26.

Tietze AL, Blankenburg M, Hechler T, Michel E, Koh M, Schlüter B et al. (2012) Sleep disturbances in children with multiple disabilities. *Sleep Medicine Rev* **16**: 117–127.

Vriend JL, Corkum PV, Moon EC, Smith IM (2011) Behavioral interventions for sleep problems in children with autism spectrum disorders: current findings and future directions. *J Pediatr Psychol* **36**(9): 1017–1029.

Wayte S, McCaughey E, Holley S, Annaz D, Hill CM (2012) Sleep problems in children with cerebral palsy and their relationship with maternal sleep and depression. *Acta Paediatrica* **101**: 618–623.

World Health Organization. The International Classification of Functioning, Disability and Health (ICF). 2001; Geneva, WHO (http://www.who.int/classifications/icf/en/).

Chapter 13

Mental health in children and adolescents with cerebral palsy

Kerim M. Munir and Ikram Rustamov

Introduction

Cerebral palsy (CP), one of the most common neurodevelopmental disorders, manifests with persistent motor impairments beginning before, during, or immediately after birth and affects every aspect of the child's future development. The nature, timing, and extent of a brain injury, as well as the effectiveness of any remediation, will determine how the given damage impacts a child's motor function and associated impairments in cognition, adaptation and behavior. CP represents a highly heterogeneous set of neurodevelopmental conditions with more than half of affected children and adolescents also presenting with co-occurring intellectual disability/intellectual developmental disorder (ID/IDD) or borderline intellectual functioning (Munir et al. 2015, 2018, Reid et al. 2016). As in children and adolescents with other chronic health conditions, neurological disorders and ID/IDD, there is elevated risk of co-occurrence of mental disorders (Einfeld and Emerson 2011, Munir 2016, Downs et al. 2018).

Each child with CP is unique, which means that any general description should take individual cognitive/adaptive or emotional/behavioral functioning into account, with particular attention to the affected child's specific circumstance. In this chapter, we highlight an overarching framework in order to improve the identification and provision of services to reduce the mental health burden on individuals diagnosed with CP (Table 13.1). As has been learned in the case of autism spectrum disorders (ASD), alleviation of co-occurring mental health burdens is likely to pay dividends in reducing direct medical and nonmedical costs, as well as improving societal care for individuals with CP across their lifetimes (Ganz 2007).

Table 13.1 A framework for action: improving the mental well-being of individuals with cerebral palsy

1. Unique nature of each child with cerebral palsy

2. Developmental and lifespan course

3. Importance of awareness of mental health concerns and health promotion

4. Implementation of early screening and diagnosis of emotional and behavioral problems and specific disorders

5. Surveillance of mental health across the lifespan at each transition: childhood, adolescence through adulthood

6. Multidisciplinary pediatric and medical team orientation inclusive of mental health and also physical, cognitive, communicative impairments, as well as epilepsy and pain

7. Holistic approach in the provision of evidence-based mental health therapies and delivery of services, rather than exclusive psychopharmacology approach

8. Implementation of family support systems and community networking, including mental health, especially in addressing stigma and bullying and other public health concerns currently more prevalent in low-resource regions

9. Access to the least restrictive, inclusive public education, carefully planned transition to vocational training and assisted employment – collaborations across health, education and social sectors

10. Need for training of multiple-tiers of mental health expertise in cerebral palsy and disabilities including psychiatry, psychology, counseling and guidance, social work, community health across various modalities of proven mental health interventions

11. Opportunity to participate in high quality research and program development.

Prevalence of CP

Registries of persons with CP have proven to be highly valuable tools for addressing questions regarding prevalence and disability needs assessment.

The prevalence of CP in the general population ranges from 1.5–4 per 1 000 live births (Surveillance of Cerebral Palsy in Europe 2002; Winter et al. 2002, Bhasin et al. 2006, Odding et al. 2006 Paneth et al. 2006 Andersen et al. 2008, Arneson et al. 2009, Durkin et al. 2016, Reid et al. 2016). According to the Autism and Developmental Disabilities Monitoring (ADDM) Network of the Center for Disease Control and Prevention (CDC), prevalence estimate for CP among 8-year-old children for the 4 out of 14 sites that track CP (Alabama, Georgia, Missouri and Wisconsin) was noted to be 1 in 323 children (CDC 2012). The CP prevalence figure in the United States has remained relatively constant, based on ADDM reports since 1996, ranging from 3.1 to 3.6 per 1000. The ADDM Network surveillance also provides characteristics of children identified with CP: the majority (77%) was reported to have the spastic bilateral or unilateral type of CP; over half (58%) of the children could walk independently.

The public health goal for prevention of CP in the United States has been to reduce the percentage of children born with low birthweight (LBW; <2 500g) by 10%, as measured for 8-year-old children between the surveillance years 2006 and 2020 (Durkin et al. 2016). The relative risks for associations between CP and LBW declined, though not significantly, during the 2006 and 2010 surveillance years, in terms of both the prevalence of CP and the percentage of children with CP born with LBW (Durkin et al. 2016).

In Europe, there are 18 population registers for CP that represent an important research network (Cans et al. 2004). The CDC has also been collaborating with the Danish National Cerebral Palsy Register as part of the CDC–Denmark Program to examine potential contributory factors: including multiple births, preterm birth, assisted reproductive techniques, asphyxia or reduced oxygen before or during birth.

The magnitude of the problem is very poorly understood in resource-poor settings and especially in low-income developing countries where the majority of children with CP are born. The prevalence and incidence rates of childhood disability, and particularly of childhood CP, is not known. Using the Ten Question Questionnaire for 2–9-year-old children, rates of CP were noted to range from 82–160 per 1 000 among children with disability, to 19–61 per 1 000 among children with neurological impairment (Gladstone 2010). Rates of CP in population-based settings in middle-income developing countries such as China and India have given figures of 2–2.8 per 1000, figures very similar to those in the United States, Canada and throughout Europe.

Methods of identifying children with CP, and causal factors, in resource-poor settings have been difficult to determine. Hospital-based studies in resource-poor countries showed CP with increased rates of spastic quadriplegia rather than diplegia or hemiplegia, and possibly increased rates of meningitis, jaundice and asphyxia, and lower rates of low LBW and prematurity.

Co-occurrence of challenging problem behaviors

Whether the type and severity of underlying CP influences the distribution of challenging problems remains an unanswered question. Questionnaires such as the Child Behavior Checklist (CBCL) (Achenbach and Ruffle 2000) and the Strengths and Difficulties Questionnaire (SDQ) (Goodman et al. 2000) have both been used to describe the prevalence of mental health symptoms in children with CP (Parkes et al. 2008, Sigurdardottir et al. 2012). More research is clearly needed to untangle the topography of mental health in children with CP. Nevertheless, the co-occurrence of challenging problem behaviors in children and adolescents with CP are likely to be influenced by the same factors that influence mental health in general, i.e., age, sex, familial/genetic and psychosocial circumstances. CP is more common among boys than girls, with an overall male/female ratio of 1:3 (Surén et al. 2012), and externalizing problem behaviors and attention-deficit–hyperactivity disorder (ADHD) are likely to be overrepresented in CP populations.

A study of preschool age children with CP in Iceland found elevated rates of inattention, aggressiveness, as well as social withdrawal, anxiety/depression compared to children without CP (Sigurdardottir et al. 2012). The emotional and behavioral measures were assessed with the CBCL (ages 1½–5) and Caregiver-Teacher Report Form (C-TRF). The children with CP had higher scores on all subscales of the CBCL (1½–5) and the C-TRF.

A population register-based study of school-aged 8–12-year-old children with CP in eight European countries found a significant proportion of children with psychological problems and social impairments necessitating referral to specialist mental health care (Parkes et al. 2008). About a quarter of the children had Total Difficulties Scores (TDS) on the SDQ (P4–16) indicating significant psychological problems, most common in the Peer Problems domain. Children with the most severe versus least functional limitations, children with intelligence quotient (IQ) scores less than 70 versus 70 or above, and children in pain versus others, and children with another disabled sibling versus no disabled siblings and others, were more likely to have elevated TDS more than 16. Among parents who reported their children to have psychological problems, 95% said they persisted over a year, with 37% reporting parental distress, and 42% describing the family burden as 'quite a lot' (Parkes et al. 2008).

A study involving a national sample of Canadian adolescents, aged 11–16 years, examined the psychosocial issues related to growing up with a physical disability such as CP, using the Health Behaviors in School-Aged Children (HBSC) of the World Health Organization Cross-National Survey. Despite reporting good self-esteem, strong family relationships and many close friends, the adolescents in the national sample with physical disabilities were noted to participate in fewer social activities, had less intimate relationships with friends, and fewer plans for postsecondary education. The adolescents with physical disabilities also reported that they had not received information on parenthood, birth control, or sexually transmitted diseases (Stevens et al. 1996).

A study in Bergen, Norway, reported an elevated rate of challenging emotional and behavioral problems among school age children with CP, compared to participants in the epidemiological Bergen Child Study (Bjorgaas et al. 2013). The investigators used the complex symptom presentation approach of the Early Syndromes Eliciting Neurodevelopmental Clinical Examination (ESSENCE) model developed by Gillberg

(2010). The mental health problems were screened through the SDQ and the children were interviewed using the DSM-IV Kiddie-SADS semi-structured diagnostic interview. CP was classified according to ICD-10 criteria with the following subgroups: spastic bilateral and unilateral, dyskinetic, ataxic or not further classified. Functional level was classified by the Gross Motor Function Classification System (GMFCS) and Manual Ability Classification System (MACS), which distinguishes five levels (I–V), with level V being the most severe (Eliasson et al. 2006, Novak et al. 2012). The children with CP were noted to have significantly higher problem behavior screening SDQ scores, with two-thirds scoring above the 90th centile on TDS. More than half (57%) of the children met criteria for a DSM-IV-R mental disorder with a sensitivity of 0.85 and a specificity of 0.55. In the study sample, 10% of children had ID/IDD, 9% had epilepsy, and 19% had visual impairments. A population-based study also in Norway gave the rate of co-occurring epilepsy rate of 37% among 11-year-old children (Surén et al. 2012).

Specific mental and neurodevelopmental disorders

An early epidemiological study of hemiplegic CP reported that more than half of the affected children and adolescents had a co-occurring mental disorder (Goodman and Graham 1996). Among the specific mental disorders, anxiety and mood are the most common internalizing mental conditions; ADHD being the most prevalent neurode-velopmental disorder in children and adolescents with CP. In the United States, the associated rate of ASD has been noted to be as high as 1 in 5 children with non-spastic CP (CDC 2012). Despite such an important footprint for challenging problem behaviors and specific mental disorders in individuals with CP, there has been very limited research on this topic worldwide. The mental and neurodevelopmental disorders that ought to be carefully considered in children and adolescents with CP are listed in Tables 13.2 and 13.3, respectively.

Table 13.2 Common mental disorders in children and adolescents with cerebral palsy

- Anxiety disorders predominantly anxiety disorder-unspecified; anxiety disorder, due to another condition, and generalized anxiety disorder

- Sleep–wake disorders, predominantly insomnia and hyper-somnolence disorders

- Feeding and eating disorders, predominantly unspecified and avoidant/restricted food intake disorders

- Elimination disorders, predominantly unspecified with urinary and fecal symptoms

- Mood disorders, predominantly depressive disorder, disruptive mood dysregulation disorder, or mood disorder-unspecified; and

- [a]Neurodevelopmental disorders.

[a]See listing in Table 13.3.

Table 13.3   Common neurodevelopmental disorder in children and adolescents with cerebral palsy

- Attention-deficit–hyperactivity disorder (ADHD)
- Communication disorders, predominantly language and speech sound disorders
- Intellectual disability/intellectual developmental disorders (ID/IDD)
- Specific learning disorders usually not accounted for by the presence of ID/IDD; and
- Motor disorders including stereotyped movement disorder and developmental coordination disorder.
- Autism Spectrum disorder (ASD)

Disruptive mood dysregulation disorder

Disruptive mood dysregulation disorder (DMDD) is a serious mental disorder in children and adolescents with CP and ought to be considered in differential diagnosis if temper outbursts and irritability persist 3–4 times per week for 12 or more weeks. These outbursts may occur in response to frustration and can be verbal or behavioral in the form of aggressive conduct with damage of property, self, or others. The outbursts need to occur in at least two of three settings, ranging from home, school, or with peers (American Psychiatric Association 2013).

Bipolar and other related mood disorders

To meet the full criteria for Bipolar II disorder, a child and adolescent with CP needs to be in a distinct period of persistently elevated and/or irritable mood with heightened levels of activity and energy, lasting for at least 4 consecutive days, most of the day. These episodes cannot be attributable to an underlying physiological/medical condition that is causing chronic pain or physical discomfort that may be triggering the behavior. It is therefore essential to rule out contributory factors, working collaboratively with the primary care and specialist medical team.

Mood disorder, unspecified type, is also associated with persistent mood swings that range from periods of acting silly or being disinhibited with high-level of activity and diminished sleep. These episodes can be associated with distress, labile affect, and even self-injury. In these circumstances, any suggestion of unsafe behavior or increased risk of self-harm needs to be carefully monitored and prevented in a closely supervised environment.

Although DMDD is classified under depressive disorders, both Bipolar II and DMDD are more akin to mood disorders in children and adolescents with CP, and may respond to pharmacotherapy with mood stabilizers with the goal of reducing the acute interfering nature of the mood changes.

Depressive disorders and the question of bereavement exception
Children and adolescents with CP who experience a depressive episode often look sad, and may also complain about somatic symptoms, for example, stomachache, headaches, or any type of bodily pain. They may eat or drink less, sleep fewer hours, and appear exhausted, with diminished interest in enjoyable activities to which they are drawn. Depending on their developmental age and cognitive level, they may talk of death and dying.

Often a limited circle of meaningful relations, i.e. parents, siblings, grandparents, close aunts, uncles, and cousins, characterize the social environment of children and adolescents with CP. They are, therefore, extremely vulnerable to loss and bereavement, for example, death or serious illness and absence of a loved one, as well as separation, for example, an older beloved sibling moving away to college. Any such loss can lead to heightened mourning that may progress to complicated traumatic grief over time (Brickell and Munir 2008). Such states of mourning may be non-distinguishable from melancholic depression and may respond poorly to treatment with even multiple trials of antidepressant medication, unless the psychological factors are addressed at the emotional, cognitive, and family levels through encouragement with an increased level of support and activities. Unfortunately, the elimination of 'bereavement exclusion' in diagnostic criteria for major depressive disorder in the DSM-5 (American Psychiatric Association 2013) may often lead to pharmacological management of complicated grief, that also requires intensive psychotherapeutic interventions.

Attention-deficit–hyperactivity disorder
Attention-deficit–hyperactivity disorder (ADHD) is the most common neurodevelopmental disorder observed in children and adolescents with CP, which manifests by inattention, hyperactivity, and impulsivity, with often all ADHD symptom domains being endorsed. It is also important to be mindful of executive and cognitive function impairments associated with CP that may invariably lead to inattention, distractibility, forgetfulness and switching from one activity to another. Furthermore, interfering performance anxiety, or sensorimotor problems, can also modify a child's ability to stay focused and diminish task performance. A child with CP may appear disinterested in an activity, by seeming tired or bored, and may readily give it up after a few minutes. The assessments need to include an appropriate level of difficulty in focusing attention, organizing and completing a task, or learning new things. Children and adolescents with CP may appear as if they are not listening when spoken to as they take a much longer time to process information and to respond to others. They may have difficulty communicating and articulating words because of deficits in communication abilities. They also may appear as though they are daydreaming or confused and have difficulty in following instructions. The co-occurrence of ADHD therefore needs to be carefully evaluated using good clinical judgment before hurriedly leading to interventions with stimulant medications.

The children and adolescents with CP who have ADHD and especially exhibit symptoms of hyperactivity, which includes fidgeting, squirming in their seats, being constantly in motion, or those who also exhibit a significant degree of impulsive behaviors (e.g. being impatient, acting without regard for consequences, showing difficulty in waiting for things or for their turn, interrupting others' conversations and activities) are better candidates for pharmacotherapy and psychosocial treatments that incorporate academic and organizational skills.

Autism spectrum disorders

Autism Spectrum Disorders (ASD) have been reported to be prevalent in children with quadriplegic, mixed, and hemiplegic CP, and in children with epilepsy and low level of speech (Kilincaslan and Mukaddes 2009). ASD is often part of multiple neurodevelopmental conditions with a considerable overlap of factors, as described in the ESSENCE model (Gillberg 2010). The prevalence of co-occurring ASD per se has been noted to be 6.9% among 8-year-old children with CP in the ADDM Network, and much higher (18.4%) among children with non-spastic CP, particularly hypotonic CP (CDC 2012). The higher frequency of ASD in non-spastic compared to spastic subtypes of CP requires further study, as it has been a consistent finding. The co-occurring seizure disorder frequency was 41% overall and did not differ by ASD status or CP subtype, and was noted to be highest with those who have limited or no walking ability (CDC 2012).

Intellectual disability/Intellectual developmental disorder

The co-occurrence of Intellectual Disability/Intellectual Developmental Disorder (ID/IDD) in children and adolescents with CP has not been carefully assessed. Many registry surveillance studies measure distinct prevalence figures for CP and ID/IDD and, therefore, do not report on overlap across CP and ID/IDD in representative population samples. Maenner et al. (2016) using the 2011–12 National Survey of Children's Health (NSCH), and the 2011–13 National Health Interview Survey (NHIS), determined the unique prevalence figures for CP and ID/IDD based on parent reports among children aged 2–17 years as 2.6–2.9 per 1 000 for CP, and 12.2–12.1 per 1 000 for ID/IDD. Overall, the figures range from 10 to 50% of children with CP having concurrent ID/IDD. Among those, the majority are represented by mild ID/IDD, and 1 in 5 have moderate to severe ID/IDD. Generally, the greater the level of a person's brain impairment, the more likely it is that they will have ID/IDD. Children with CP and ID/IDD frequently have other co-occurring developmental and health conditions (Schieve et al. 2012).

Cerebral palsy as a mental health risk condition across the lifespan

A number of mediating factors may influence the emergence of challenging problem behaviors and specific mental disorders in children and adolescents with CP. Some of these include presence of pain, chronic fatigue, disrupted sleep and nutritional status. In fact, 65% of adolescent girls and 50% of adolescent boys report experiencing pain, mostly in the feet, ankles, knees, and lower back. The pain interferes with everyday activities and limits their ability to focus. For a given child or adolescent with CP, a number of mediating family characteristics are also relevant in predicting resilience and mental well-being. These include lower levels of parental education, parental age, household income, limited access to special education, rural versus urban households, less availability of vocational and recreational services, parental and family supports and higher level of perceived parental stress and associated physical and medical comorbidities.

Insight is often a positive predictor of mental well-being. However, many children and adolescents with CP with greater degree of awareness of their differences compared to neurotypical adolescents may be at greater risk for developing persistent feelings of sadness that may lead to disillusionment and depression if unrecognized and unaddressed in a timely fashion. Such adverse outcomes for children with CP despite positive predictive characteristics, are highly unfortunate and represent nodal points for intervention in later years. It is not surprising therefore that many children and adolescents with CP, who demonstrate higher levels of cognitive and adaptive functioning, require specialized mental health services. These children may channel this disappointment as anger directed toward others or as self-injury directed to themselves. Such behaviors can prevent a child and adolescent with CP from being in an optimal academic placement, which may lead to further adverse consequences.

Since separation and individuation is inevitably delayed in children and adolescents with CP, especially given their dependence on parents/caregivers for day-to-day living, the stage in which these challenging problem behaviors and mental disorders occur depends on the home environment. Encouraging the families to join support groups and to participate actively in developmentally informed counseling is paramount to bolster self-esteem and improve coping mechanisms. The relational and family-oriented support approaches are highly important strategies. In addition, the lack of connection to other families, scarcity of programs designed to support children adolescents with CP, and the discontinuity of services have important adverse effects on maintaining healthy trajectories.

Early interventions promoting mental well-being

Parents of children and adolescents with CP, as in other disabilities, report a larger number of problems during the first year of life (Blackman and Cobb 1989). Early detection, diagnosis and interventions to mitigate the long-term ill effects of challenging problem behaviors and specific mental disorders is likely to significantly reduce the burden of CP measured across multiple sectors of society – family life, education, health and social care. The assessment of psychological well-being of each child and adolescent, at various ages, and with varying adaptive and cognitive skills, ought to be a crucial component of each medical examination. This calls for work within coordinated multidisciplinary teams.

Navigating transitions

Navigating postsecondary education, transition to independent living and vocational training for employment are inherently difficult. The limitations in motor function is a challenging barrier for social participation for children with CP (Donkervoort et al. 2007). The multidisciplinary teams need to play an active role in the formulation and implementation of individualized educational and subsequent individual service plans – these transitions represent important opportunities points for intervention and can also be times when a young people or an adult with CP is referred for specialized mental health services. Adults with CP have lower rates of participation than the overall population in employment, marriage, and independent living. This may result in high levels of loneliness and resultant depression (Liptak 2008). Very few studies have identified interventions that will help physically disabled adults achieve optimal health and well-being, maintain mobility, community interaction, and access to support services.

Supporting families

Apart from the challenges to mental health in individuals with CP, there is also an impact on family dynamics. Parents of children and adolescents with CP face a range of stressors depending on their child's age, development, and functioning. At the time of initial diagnosis, parents typically grieve when confronted with the fact that their child is not developing normally and life will present ongoing struggles for them and their child. In the second phase, parents experience the desire to help their child operate as normally as possible. They seek appropriate support services when the child's needs change, including the transition from home to independent adult-living settings (Rentinckt et al. 2006). The trend toward family-focused, rather than short-term interventions focused on children alone, have improved outcomes and reduced family stress (Raina et al. 2005).

Unfortunately, single parents carrying the sole responsibility to care for a child and adolescent with CP face much higher levels of stress compared to two-parent families (see Case study). Additional factors, such as Adverse Childhood Experiences (ACEs), loss of family income, increased odds of living in housing areas where there is limited access to services, all compound the situation. One of the biggest threats to self-esteem and happiness is bullying. This needs to be assessed as part of a health examination for all age groups. School administrators, program personnel and parents may not be aware of it and the child or adolescent with CP may not be able to express their concerns and fears.

Case study

Carol was a 14-year-old girl with bilateral spastic CP with mild ID/IDD. She was referred for treatment for intermittent episodes of agitation especially exacerbated during daily transitions. She was in an excellent highly structured therapeutic educational program. Six months prior to her referral she had become increasingly difficult to manage at home. She also developed episodes of moodiness with irritability, anger and aggression especially directed toward her mother, who was her sole caregiver in view of earlier parental separation and subsequent divorce. Carol's mother began to find it highly challenging to manage these behaviors. It was particularly disappointing as she had been very comfortable over the years in fostering an excellent relationship with her daughter. Carol underwent multidisciplinary medical team evaluation, which was highly helpful. The team emphasized that the exacerbations of her daughter's mental health functioning needed to be evaluated within a complex framework that took into consideration Carol's increasing emotional and neurocognitive challenges in the areas of her attention, executive functioning, and social understanding (Bottcher 2010). It was explained that children and adolescents with CP often experience physical as well as emotional and environmental stressors that may result in emergence of mental disorders, exacerbated by the transitions in development, as well as possible environmental influences in the home and school contexts. All these factors needed to be considered in evaluating Carol's challenging behaviors. Additionally, potential contributing medical factors, including pain, needed to be ruled out, which the team was able to do.

Carol's specific mental health conditions included a mood disorder and exaggerated generalized anxiety. Carol had a modest response to psychopharmacological interventions in alleviating her anxiety and mood changes. Consideration was even given to admitting her for an acute residential or in-patient program for stabilization. She would engage in intense periods of behavioral outbursts. The situation was alleviated some months later when Carol's mother began a supportive and loving relationship with a partner toward whom Carol developed a unique affinity. The arrival of an additional supportive and loving figure facilitated much greater opportunities for structured activities for Carol at home, in the community, and in helping with the transitions. The emotional tenor in the household changed. Carol's anxiety and moods improved. The additional companionship and support for Carol's mother was also critically important in making her feel more confident, as their interactions had become a great source of stress and self-blame. Over time, Carol's problem behaviors ceased, she was more communicative and interested in a range of fun activities, including a wider network of peers.

Conclusions

There is an important need for funding future studies to better identify and classify children with CP, the causal factors, effects of disability, and improved management as well as implementation of preventive measures (Gladstone 2010). The magnitude of the problems related to mental well-being and isolation of individuals with CP in resource-poor settings and in particular those living in low-income countries is an urgent global public health as well as a human rights concern (Erol et al. 2017). Individuals with CP continue to receive suboptimal care with greater likelihood long-term residential or institutional placements with limited social inclusion and family involvement.

For every individual with CP, the challenges to their well-being can be assessed at each new stage in life. From the very outset, care must be taken in the early identification, assessment and management of children with CP to ensure that psychological problems are not overlooked and potentially preventable risk factors, such as pain, are treated in a timely and effective manner. Comprehensive and coordinated medical services ought to include mental health surveillance and supports that are integrated within traditional medical services. Awareness of these challenges and sensitivity to the signs of emotional and behavioral problems are essential, but can be improved by strengthening the training of mental health professionals. As emphasized in this chapter, one in two children with CP have co-occurring specific mental disorders with two-thirds presenting persistent challenging problem behaviors that interfere in the individual's functioning, which warrant a specialist referral.

Transitions from childhood to adolescence and from adolescence to adulthood represent critical periods that require additional support and guidance for families. Participation in a community and social engagement through relationships with peers, neighbors, friends and relatives provide important benefits. Celebrating birthdays or holidays with loved ones, or participating in events like the Special Olympics, can be a force for good by advocating the strength of people living with CP or disabilities in general.

Key points

- Mental health related conditions in children and adolescents with CP are both substantial and persistent across the lifespan.

- Mental health conditions in CP interfere with the quality of life and social participation of children and adolescents and their families. Multidisciplinary care of persons with CP ought to include mental health services as a high proportion of people with CP will have co-occurring mental disorders across their lifespans.

- Despite the significant burden of mental health conditions in children and adolescents with CP, only a minority receive direct specialized mental health services.

- Greater attention must be paid to development of multidisciplinary programs for early identification, mental health assessment, and early interventions for co-occurring mental health disorders in children and adolescents with CP.

- The co-occurring mental health disorders in children and adolescents with CP are predictive of the restrictions these children face in educational and vocational participation and inclusion in society.

- Transitions from childhood to adolescence, and from adolescence to adulthood, in people with CP, represent critical opportunities that underscore the need for provision of additional support and professional guidance for families.

- Mental well-being of the parents of children and adolescents with CP can be strongly influenced by the severity of their children's co-occurring mental health disorders as much as the severity of their CP.

References

American Psychiatric Association (2013) *Diagnostic and Statistical Manual of Mental Disorders*, fifth edn. (DSM-5). Washington, DC: American Psychiatric Publishing, Inc.

Andersen GL, Irgens LM, Haagaas I, Skranes JS, Meberg AE, Vik T. (2008) Cerebral palsy in Norway: prevalence, subtypes and severity. *Eur J Paediatr Neurol* **12**: 4–13.

Arneson CL, Durkin MS, Benedict RE, Kirby RS, Yeargin-Allsopp M, Van Naarden Braun K, Doernberg NS. (2009) Prevalence of cerebral palsy: Autism and Developmental Disabilities Monitoring Network, three sites, United States, 2004. *Disabil Health J* **2**: 45–8.

Bhasin TK, Brocksen S, Avchen RN, Van Naarden Braun K (2006) Prevalence of four developmental disabilities among children aged 8 years – Metropolitan Atlanta Developmental Disabilities Surveillance Program 1996 and 2000. *MMWR Surveillance Summaries* **55**(1): 1–9.

Bjorgaas HM, Elgen I, Boe T, Hysings M (2013) Mental health in children with cerebral palsy: Does screening capture the complexity? *Scientific World Journal* Article ID **46** 7 pages.

Blackman JA, Cobb LS (1989) A comparison of parents' perceptions of common behavior problems in developmentally at-risk and normal children. *Children's Health Care* **218**(2): 108–13.

Bottcher L (2010) Children with spastic cerebral palsy, their cognitive functioning, and social participation: a review. *Child Neuropsychol* **38**: 457–63.

Brickell C, Munir K (2008) Grief and its complications in individuals with intellectual disability. *Harv Rev Psychiatry* **16**: 1–12.

Brossard-Racine M, Hall N, Majnemer A, et al. (2012) Behavioural problems in school age children with cerebral palsy. *Eur J Paediatr Neurol* **16**: 35–41.

Cans C, Surman G, McManus V, Coghlan D, Hensey O, Johnson A (2004) Cerebral palsy registries. *Semin Pediatr Neurol* **11**: 18–23.

CDC (2012) Prevalence of autism spectrum disorders—Autism and Developmental Disabilities Monitoring Network 14 sites, United States 2008. *MMWR Surveillance Summaries* **61**: 1–19.

Donkervoort M, Roebroeck M, Wiegerink D, et al. (2007) Determinants of functioning of adolescents and young adults with cerebral palsy. *Disabil Rehab* **29**: 453–63.

Downs J, Blackmore AM, Epstein A, et al. (2018) The prevalence of mental health disorders and symptoms in children and adolescents with cerebral palsy: a systematic review and meta-analysis. *Dev Med Child Neurol* **60**: 30–8.

Durkin MS, Benedict RE, Christensen D, et al. (2016) Prevalence of cerebral palsy among 8-year-old children in 2010 and preliminary evidence of trends in its relationship to low birthweight. *Paediatr Perinat Epidemiol* **30**: 496–510.

Einfeld SL, Emerson E (2011) Comorbidity of intellectual disability and mental disorder in children and adolescents: a systematic review. *J Intellect Dev Disabil* **36**: 137–43.

Eliasson AC, Krumlinde-Sundholm L, Rösblad B, et al. (2006) The Manual Ability Classification System (MACS) for children with cerebral palsy: scale development and evidence of validity and reliability. *Dev Med Child Neurol* **48**: 549–54.

Gillberg C (2010) The ESSENCE in child psychiatry: early symptomatic syndromes eliciting neurodevelopmental clinical examinations. *Research Developmental Disabilities* **31**(6): 1543–51.

Gladstone M (2010) A review of the incidence and prevalence, types and aetiology of childhood cerebral palsy in resource-poor settings. *Ann Trop Paediatr* **30**: 181–96.

Goodman R, Ford T, Simmons H, Gatward R, Meltzer H (2000) Using the Strengths and Difficulties Questionnaire (SDQ) to screen for child psychiatric disorders in a community sample. *British Journal of Psychiatry* **177**: 534–9.

Goodman R, Graham P (1996) Psychiatric problems in children with hemiplegia: a cross sectional epidemiological survey. *BMJ* **312**: 1065–9.

Kilincaslan A, Mukaddes NM (2009) Pervasive developmental disorders in individuals with cerebral palsy. *Dev Med Child Neurol* **51**: 289–94.

Liptak GS (2008) Health and well-being of adults with cerebral palsy. *Curr Opin Neurol* **21**: 136–42.

Maenner MJ, Blumberg SJ, Kogan MD, Christensen D, Yeargin-Allsopp M, Schieve LA (2016) Prevalence of cerebral palsy and intellectual disability among children identified in two U.S. National Surveys 2011 –2013. *Ann Epidemiol* **26**: 222–6.

Munir K (2016) The co-occurrence of mental disorders in children and adolescents with intellectual disability/intellectual developmental disorder. *Curr Opin Psychiatry* **29**: 95–102.

Munir K, Friedman SL, Leonard EL (2018) Section III. Psychiatric Disorders in Children and Adolescents: Intellectual Disabilities (Intellectual Developmental Disorders). In: Ebert, M. Leckman J, Petrakis I, (eds). *Current Diagnosis & Treatment in Psychiatry*, 3rd edn. New York: LANGE CURRENT Series, McGraw-Hill Education / Medical, pp. 447–66.

Munir K, Friedman SL, Szymanski LS (2015) Neurodevelopmental Disorders: Intellectual Disability/Intellectual Developmental Disorders. In: Tasman A, Kay J, Lieberman JA, First MB, Riba M (eds.) *Psychiatry*, vol 1. Chichester: John Wiley & Sons, pp. 672–705.

Novak I, Hines M, Goldsmith S, Barclay R (2012) Clinical prognostic messages from a systematic review on cerebral palsy. *Pediatrics* **130**: 1285–312.

Odding M, Roebroeck E, Stam HJ (2006) The epidemiology of cerebral palsy: incidence, impairments and risk factors. *Disabil Rehab* **28**: 183–91.

Paneth N, Hong T, Korzeniewski S (2006) The descriptive epidemiology of cerebral palsy. *Clinics in Perinatology* **33**: 251–67.

Parkes J, White-Koning M, Dickinson HO, et al. (2008) Psychological problems in children with cerebral palsy: A cross-sectional European study. *J Child Psychol Psychiatry* **49**: 405–13.

Parkes J, White-Koning M, McCullough N, Colver A (2009) Psychological problems in children with hemiplegia: a European multicentre survey. *Arch Dis Child* **94**(6): 429–33.

Pies R (2014) The bereavement exclusion and DSM-5: an update and commentary. *Innov Clin Neurosci* **11**(7–8): 19–22.

Raina P, O'Donnell M, Rosenbaum P, et al. (2005) The health and well-being of caregivers of children with cerebral palsy. *Pediatrics* **115**: e626-e636.

Ramstad K, Jahnsen R, Skjeldal OH, Diseth TH (2012) Mental health, health related quality of life and recurrent musculoskeletal pain in children with cerebral palsy 8–18 years old. *Disabil Rehab* **34**: 1589–95.

Reid SM, Meehan E, McIntyre S, Goldsmith S, Badawi N, Reddihough DS (2016) Temporal trends in cerebral palsy by impairment severity and birth gestation. *Dev Med Child Neurol* **58** (Suppl. 2): 25–35.

Rentinck ICM, Ketelaar M, Jongmans MJ, et al. (2006) Parents of children with cerebral palsy: A review of factors related to the process of adaptation. *Child Care Health Dev* **33**: 161–9.

Schieve LA, Gonzalez V, Boulet SL, et al. (2012) Concurrent medical conditions and health care use and needs among children with learning and behavioral developmental disabilities, National Health Interview Survey 2006–2010. *Res Dev Disabil* **33**: 467–76.

Sigurdardottir S, Indredavik MS, Eiriksdottir A, et al. (2012) Behavioural and emotional symptoms of preschool children with cerebral palsy: A population study. *Dev Med Child Neurol* **52**: 1056–61.

Stevens SE, Steele CA, Jutai JW, Kalnins IV, Bortolussi JA, Biggar WD. 1996 Adolescents with physical disabilities: some psychosocial aspects of health. *J Adolesc Health* **19**: 157–64.

Surén P, Bakken IJ, Aase H, Chin R, Gunnes N, Lie KK, et al. (2012) Autism spectrum disorder, ADHD, epilepsy, and cerebral palsy in Norwegian children. Pediatrics **130**: 152–8.

Surveillance of Cerebral Palsy in Europe (2002) Prevalence and characteristics of children with cerebral palsy in Europe. *Dev Med Child Neurol* **44**: 633–40.

Winter S, Autry A, Boyle C, Yeargin-Allsopp M (2002) Trends in the prevalence of cerebral palsy in a population-based study. *Pediatrics* **110**: 1220–5.

Chapter 14

Pain and Irritability

Julie Hauer

Introduction

Irritability is defined as a disorder characterized by an abnormal response to stimuli or physiological arousal that can be in response to pain, medications, an emotional state, an acute illness or medical condition (US Department of Health and Human Services 2010). This chapter will focus on individuals with severe impairment of the central nervous system (CNS) resulting in life-long inability to communicate information about irritability, a group often referred to as individuals with severe neurological impairment (SNI). Pain is a frequent cause of irritability in this group, highest in those with severe to profound intellectual disability and in Gross Motor Function Classification System (GMFCS) level IV and V (Chapter 1), with many identified to have weekly to daily pain (Stallard et al. 2002; Breau et al. 2003; Houlihan et al. 2004; Hunt et al. 2004; Hauer and Houtrow 2017;).

Sources of discomfort to consider in children with complex cerebral palsy (CP) include everyday routine causes of discomfort, such as the need to be repositioned. This chapter will focus on acute and chronic sources of pain when symptoms persist despite attending to these routine needs.

Identifying pain in nonverbal children with cerebral palsy

Pain behaviors refer to the features observed when nonverbal individuals with central nervous system impairment experience pain (Herr et al. 2011). Pain behaviors are changes from a child's typical baseline behavior in the following categories:

- Vocalizations: crying, whimpering, moaning

- Facial expression: grimacing, frowning, furrowed brow, eyes wide open

- Consolability: inability to be made comfortable

- Interaction: withdrawn, seeking comfort

- Sleep: increased or decreased sleep

- Movement: increased baseline movement, restless, startles easily, pulls away when touched

- Tone: stiffening of extremities, clenching of fists, back arching

- Physiological: tachycardia, sweating, shivering, change in color, tears

Intermittent increases in tone, movement, and changes in body position are common pain behaviors in children with SNI. This is described on pain assessment tools as 'stiffens or spasms', 'spastic', 'tense', 'tremors', 'twists or turns', and 'arches back' (Breau et al. 2002a; Breau et al. 2002b; Hunt et al. 2004; Malviya et al. 2006; Solodiuk et al. 2010). Such features were the most common pain behaviors noted in 22 children with SNI and recurrent pain episodes, with 19 of 22 of the children having muscle spasms during episodes. although 20 of 22 children were already on one or more medications for spasticity (Hauer and Solodiuk 2015). Some children with SNI will display less typical pain behaviors, such as laughing, a blunted facial expression, or self-injurious behavior (Hunt et al. 2004; Malviya et al. 2006).

Pain assessment tools have been developed for use in children who are unable to indicate pain due to significant intellectual disability (Breau et al. 2002a; Breau et al. 2002b; Hunt et al. 2004; Malviya et al. 2006; Solodiuk et al. 2010). Parents and caregivers should undergo a detailed review of the use of these tools to determine their child's baseline behaviors and specific features noted when pain occurs. Pain assessment tools include the revised Face, Legs, Activity, Cry, Consolability (r-FLACC; Malviya et al. 2006) scale and the Individualized Numeric Rating Scale (INRS; Solodiuk et al. 2010), tools that can be used to indicate behaviors specific to each child. Other tools include the Paediatric Pain Profile (PPP; Hunt et al. 2004), Non-Communicating Children's Pain Checklist-Postoperative Version (NCCPC-PV), and the Non-Communicating Children's Pain Checklist-Revised (NCCPC-R; Breau et al. 2002a; Breau et al. 2002b;). These tools have been studied in children with intellectual disability, most in the severe to profound range, and typically with associated CP. In children who acquire a developmental age of 3 years or more, age-appropriate pain assessment tools, such as the FACES pain scale, can be used.

Pain assessment tools can assist with pain identification following surgery. For children noted to have intermittent pain episodes over a longer period, it is appropriate not to become overly dependent on such tools. Instead, parents can be asked to rate typical and worst pain episodes as mild, moderate, or severe, along with reviewing the frequency and length of pain episodes. This information can then be used to determine if the frequency, duration, and severity of pain episodes have sufficiently decreased after a medication trial.

In addition to pain assessment following surgery or when a parent notes concerns about pain in a child, other reasons to assess for pain behaviors include:

- When a routine comprehensive assessment is carried out: parents can be asked 'Do you have concerns that your son is uncomfortable or agitated at times, or is he typically calm and easily comforted?'

- When a child is identified to have intermittent muscle spasms and changes in body position: determine whether the child appears calm during such movement or if pain behaviors are noted with intermittent muscle spasms and movement.

- When gastrointestinal symptoms are identified: nociceptive sources include gastroesophageal reflux disease (GERD) and cholecystitis, and CNS sources include central neuropathic pain and autonomic dysfunction.

Sources of acute and chronic pain

The mechanisms that generate pain include (1) nociceptive pain due to tissue injury or inflammation, or (2) neuropathic pain due to abnormal transmission of pain signals as a result of injury, dysfunction, or altered excitability in the peripheral or central nervous system (World Health Organization 2012). It is helpful to assess for pain behaviors that can be due to these mechanisms when descriptive terms such as 'agitation' or 'neuro-irritability' are used. The use of such terms can inadvertently shift focus away from pain and thereby away from treatment directed at the mechanisms of action that result in observable pain behaviors.

Sources of acute pain in children with SNI include everyday routine discomfort, such as muscle spasms or an uncomfortable position, and pain from a new nociceptive source. New-onset pain behaviors may also be observed with any acute illness that can result in distress. When a child with SNI is identified as having recurrent pain behavior episodes, it is important to consider sources attributable to altered function of the CNS (Table 14.1). These sources can be a cause of pain or have features that include pain behaviors.

New onset acute pain
Acute nociceptive sources include common childhood problems, such as otitis media, corneal abrasion, hair tourniquet, testicular or ovarian torsion, or appendicitis. Children

Table 14.1 Chronic sources of pain or pain behaviors due to the altered nervous system

Problem	Features and Comments
Central neuropathic pain	• Symptoms include pain localized to the GI tract, such as pain triggered by distention of the GI tract (suggested by pain associated with tube feedings or intestinal gas, with relief following a bowel movement or flatus) • Pain features can occur spontaneously and with no trigger, described by adults as 'shock-like' • Attributable to impairment of the spinothalamic tract and thalamus
Visceral hyperalgesia	• Altered threshold to pain generation in response to a stimulus in the GI tract • Attributable to the altered enteric nervous system due to sensitization of visceral afferents as well as central sensitization in the CNS
Autonomic dysfunction (dysautonomia)	• Features that suggest dysautonomia: skin flushing, hyperthermia, pain localized to the GI tract, retching, bowel dysmotility, general discomfort, agitation, tachycardia, sweating, arching, stiffening • Dysautonomia can be a source of discomfort, and pain can trigger the features that occur with dysautonomia
Paroxysmal autonomic instability with dystonia (PAID)	• Involves features of both autonomic dysfunction and dystonia • Indicates altered function of the CNS areas that regulate autonomic function and movement • Pain can trigger and worsen the observed features
Spasticity	• Velocity-dependent increase in muscle tone that results in muscles that are resistant to movement • Spasticity is often not painful but can result in musculoskeletal pain over time
Muscle spasms	• Sudden involuntary contraction of a muscle or group of muscles; associated features can include arching, stiffening, tremors, and clonus • Pain behaviors can indicate pain from muscle spasms or indicate pain from another source as the trigger for muscle spasms

GI, gastro-intestinal; CNS, central nervous system

with SNI may also be at increased risk for GERD; constipation, acute pancreatitis (associated with valproic acid and hypothermia); cholecystitis (associated with tube feedings); urinary tract infection (UTI); urinary retention, nephrolithiasis (associated with immobility, topiramate, and the ketogenic diet); hip subluxation, fracture (osteoporosis risk attributable to immobility and certain anti-seizure drugs); and dental pain. Problems such as hip subluxation can be a source of symptoms in some and an incidental finding in others. Features observed with medication withdrawal or toxicity (i.e. serotonin syndrome or neuroleptic syndrome) include pain behaviors.

Evaluation in search of a nociceptive source can be guided by details from the child's history and examination, and factor in how long the symptoms have been occurring (Hauer and Houtrow 2017). A child with no history of intermittent irritability requires a more extensive evaluation if the initial tests are negative. In contrast, a child with a history of intermittent episodes with pain behaviors may benefit from an empirical medication trial directed at central sources of symptoms, following the initial evaluation.

The history can determine if any medications were recently started or stopped, when the last dental assessment occurred, if the child has a ventriculoperitoneal shunt, whether symptoms are associated with movement (fracture or hip subluxation), and other details that are relevant to the potential sources. Older children with moderate intellectual disability may be able to point to the location of pain. Details from the physical examination include determining whether the gastrostomy tube is too tight due to weight gain and whether pain occurs with positioning or palpation of the extremities, along with a general comprehensive examination with the child unclothed.

There is no agreed on standard nociceptive evaluation for children with SNI. The initial tests can be guided by the risk of missing a specific source, such as tests assessing for urinary tract infection and acute pancreatitis. Baseline studies often include the following: blood tests (basic metabolic panel, complete blood cell count, alanine aminotransferase, total bilirubin, alkaline phosphatase, gamma-glutamyl transpeptidase, lipase); urine (urine analysis and culture); and radiography or bone scan if a fracture is suspected. Following this initial assessment of a child with no history of irritability and recurrent pain behaviors, further diagnostic evaluation would be warranted. This work-up may include abdominal ultrasonography or computed tomography (CT), upper gastrointestinal tract series, impedance study, and endoscopy, as directed by the history, examination, and initial tests. In addition to potential medical etiologies, behavioral, mental health and environmental contributors to acute irritability need to be considered, depending on intellectual level and circumstances (see Chapter 13).

Chronic pain

Chronic pain is continuous or recurrent pain that may involve a persistent nociceptive stimulus or persist in the absence of an identifiable cause. When a nonverbal child with CP first presents because symptoms are reaching a threshold for parental concern, history can identify the child with recurrent episodes of irritability that are assessed to include pain behaviors versus the previously comfortable child with new acute pain. Following the initial assessment for a pain source, this history can then guide clinicians when to pursue further testing in search of a new nociceptive source versus when to initiate an empirical trial while considering further testing.

Children with recurrent episodes of irritability may have had multiple tests and interventions for commonly recognized problems, such as treatment directed at GERD and spasticity. Children with SNI are vulnerable to repeated testing over months in the search for a cause. This results in delayed consideration of empirical medication trials directed at CNS sources (Table 14.1) that cannot be identified by diagnostic tests (Hauer 2012). This can delay pain management and expose a child to invasive testing.

Sources of recurrent pain episodes include an impaired nervous system (Table 14.1). Several challenges exist in considering these sources, including the lack of diagnostic tests and the fear of missing a nociceptive cause. It can also be challenging to assess the child with spasticity and associated pain features. Spasticity is typically not painful, although it is often considered a chronic source of pain. Alternatively, the associated intermittent alterations in muscle tone and posture may be pain behaviors indicating an underlying chronic pain source.

In the child with a chronic history of recurrent episodes with pain behaviors, reasons to initiate an empirical trial directed at sources indicated in Table 14.1 include the following (Hauer 2012):

- Chronic irritability that is assessed to include pain behaviors and persists following treatment for possible nociceptive sources

- Muscle spasms or autonomic dysfunction with associated pain behaviors

- Symptoms localized to the gastrointestinal tract that persist despite treatment directed at GERD (i.e. central neuropathic pain and visceral hyperalgesia)

- Symptoms that can occur 'out of the blue' (i.e. central neuropathic pain)

- Surgery weeks to months before the onset of symptoms (i.e. post-surgical neuropathic pain)

It is possible for a child to have an altered CNS resulting in a baseline of recurrent pain as well as a new nociceptive source as a trigger for an acute escalation of symptoms. The section on pain management will provide suggested guidelines, including when to consider an empirical trial and what interventions to consider.

Pain management

Causes of nociceptive pain can typically be identified by a diagnostic test and have a known treatment for the problem. Treatment then results in resolution of presenting pain features. In contrast, sources of chronic intermittent pain episodes due to the impaired CNS typically do not have a diagnostic test. As a result, treatment directed at such sources will be empirical.

The decision to initiate an empirical trial for recurrent pain episodes will be guided by the frequency, duration, and severity of episodes. Children with the greatest impairment of the CNS are also most likely to have a CNS source for recurrent pain behaviors.

In a child with pre-existing pain behavior episodes, the history, physical examination, and blood and urine tests can assess for acute sources that are critical to identify (e.g. UTI, nephrolithiasis, acute pancreatitis, fracture, cholecystitis). Following this initial assessment, it may be reasonable then to initiate an empirical trial while considering further diagnostic testing. Initiating a medication trial while considering invasive tests, such as endoscopy or impedance study, can avoid the need for such tests when symptoms improve.

Medications for chronic pain

Pain treatment for recurrent pain is summarized in Table 14.2. Empirical medication selection for persistent pain behaviors is best guided first by the safety of medications, given the lack of a standard approach, with information on efficacy for chronic sources of pain primarily guided by evidence in adults. A proposed 'neuro-pain' ladder has been developed, factoring in safety of medication trials, such as suggesting a gabapentin trial before using a tricyclic antidepressant or methadone (Hauer 2012).

The literature reports benefits from the use of gabapentin for children with SNI and recurrent pain episodes (Hauer et al. 2007; Haney et al. 2009; Siden et al. 2013; Hauer and Solodiuk 2015). Gabapentin and pregabalin are the most commonly used medications for neuropathic pain in adults. Table 14.3 shows suggested dosing guidelines. Use of other medications is guided by general principles of pain treatment in children and treatment of specific pain syndromes in adults, such as central neuropathic pain (World Health Organization 2012; Moulin et al. 2014).

When pain escalates in a child with chronic pain under reasonable control, considerations include assessment for a new nociceptive pain source. Effective pain treatment does not mask pain from a new pain source, as noted in a case series of children with SNI when, at a time of effective symptom management of recurrent pain behaviors, UTIs were identified in three patients by the onset of new pain behaviors (Hauer and Solodiuk 2015). Other considerations include revisiting non-pharmacologic strategies that lessen triggers, adjusting medications for weight gain, and adding another medication with a different mechanism of action.

Non-pharmacologic strategies

Non-pharmacologic strategies often used by caregivers include cuddling, rocking, tight swaddling, repositioning, and massage. Supportive equipment can minimize positional pain. Other interventions include warm baths, weighted blankets, vibratory mats, and music. Complementary and integrative therapies can include essential oils, Reiki, and

Table 14.2   Medications for acute and chronic pain

Medications	Evidence for Use
Gabapentinoids: Thought to inhibit excitation by binding to the alpha-2-delta subunit of voltage-dependent Ca^{2+} ion channels in the CNS	
Gabapentin Pregabalin	• Neuropathic pain, peripheral, and central • Visceral hyperalgesia • Dysautonomia • Spasticity
Tricyclic antidepressants (TCAs): Reuptake inhibition of serotonin and norepinephrine in the CNS, both inhibitors of pain transmission (also antagonists of 5HT-2, H-1, and Ach)	
Nortriptyline Amitriptyline	• Neuropathic pain, peripheral, and central • Visceral hyperalgesia
Opioids: Opioid receptor agonists, including mu receptors	
Tramadol Morphine Methadone	• Pain • Autonomic storms • Methadone has added benefit for neuropathic pain
Alpha-2 adrenergic receptor agonist	
Clonidine	• Dysautonomia • Spasticity • May enhance pain management
Cannabinoids: Cannabinoid receptor agonist (C-1 and C-2)	
Dronabinol	• Central pain in adults with multiple sclerosis
Benzodiazepines: Increases affinity of GABA for GABA$_A$ receptors	
Clonazepam Lorazepam Midazolam	• Benzodiazepines do not treat pain, can be used as an adjuvant • As needed for autonomic storms

5HT indicates serotonin; Ach, acetylcholine; C, cannabinoid; GABA, gamma-aminobutyric acid; H, histamine

acupuncture. Distention of the gastrointestinal tract is an important consideration, given the lower threshold to symptom generation associated with visceral hyperalgesia and central neuropathic pain. Strategies include gastrostomy tube venting, equipment that allows venting during feedings, and a decrease in the total volume of fluids and nutrition given by feeding tube. This is important given the risk for overestimating metabolism and fluid requirements (Hauer and Houtrow 2017).

Table 14.3   Suggested dosing guidelines for gabapentinoids

Gabapentin

Day 1–3   2 mg/kg (100 mg maximum) enteral three times daily (TID)

Day 4–6   4 mg/kg TID

Day 7–9   6 mg/kg TID

Day 10–12   8 mg/kg TID

Increase every 2–4 days by 5–6 mg/kg/day until

1. Effective analgesia reached (often noted at 35–45 mg/kg/day[10])
2. Side effects experienced (nystagmus, sedation, tremor, ataxia, swelling)
3. Maximum total dose of 50–72 mg/kg/day reached (2400–3600 mg/day)
4. Younger children (<5 years) may require a 30% higher mg/kg/day dosing, such as a total dose of 45–60 mg/kg/day[10]
5. Half of the total daily dose may be given as the evening dose if symptoms occur mostly in the evening and overnight
6. Titrate more rapidly for severe pain or as tolerated

Pregabalin

Day 1–3   1 mg/kg/dose (50 mg maximum) once or twice daily

Day 4–6   1 mg/kg/dose twice daily (or dose increase if started twice daily)

1. Increase every 2–4 days up to 3 mg/kg/dose two or three times daily (maximum 4 mg/kg/dose)
2. Titrate more rapidly for severe pain or as tolerated

Care plans for break-through pain episodes

Break-through symptoms can occur given that scheduled medications modify the symptoms generated by the altered CNS yet do not 'fix' the cause. Care plans can help families manage these break-through symptoms and may include

- presenting pain behavior features;

- initial routine interventions (e.g. check for wet diaper, reposition);

- initial non-pharmacologic strategies (e.g. remove orthotics, massage legs, rocking, headphones with favorite music, place on a vibratory mat);

- interventions for triggers such as excessive stimulation to the nervous system (e.g. hospital environment) and gastrointestinal tract distention (e.g. use as-needed suppository or enema, vent gastrostomy feeding tube, hold feeds and give electrolyte replacement overnight, reduce total feeds/fluids);

- use of as-needed medications (options include as-needed antacid, acetaminophen, ibuprofen, morphine, clonidine, or benzodiazepine) (Hauer and Houtrow 2017.

Working with families and caregivers

Discussing side effects is an important first step when considering an empirical medication trial. When anticipating the side effect of sedation, a discussion with the child's family can determine if it is more important to minimize sedation or to improve symptoms sooner while accepting transient sedation. This information can then guide decisions about initial starting dose and the titration schedule to the initial trial dose.

Potential fears can also be identified and addressed, such as the fear of harm, drug addiction with an opioid, and masking pain caused by a new problem. Fear of respiratory depression is one of the greatest barriers with use of an opioid. The risk of significant respiratory depression is low when following evidence-based dosing guidelines and slow titration, from a starting dose that is individualized to the patient. Knowing the intent of pain treatment can also assist by considering the difference in opioid use following surgery versus when the primary goal is to maintain comfort in a child with a life-limiting condition. The former involves monitoring to identify and manage respiratory depression, meeting the intent to promote comfort safely and avoid any harm. With the latter it is ethically permissible to accept the low risk of respiratory depression and forgo monitoring at such a time. Expert consultation can be helpful at such times to avoid fears interfering with adequate symptom treatment.

Families and caregivers also benefit from being helped to understand that it is not always possible to remove or 'fix' central sources of pain episodes. Medications can modify symptoms by increasing inhibition or decreasing excitation in the CNS. Parents should be informed that many children have a decrease in symptoms, though some do not have the degree of benefit hoped for and symptoms originating from the CNS can return or persist. Framing this information is especially helpful when a second or third trial is initiated, to avoid the assumption that all symptoms can be eliminated. The goal can always remain to lessen symptoms due to the impaired CNS while acknowledging the hoped-for goal may not be achieved in all children. For the occasional child with intractable symptoms, such information can also help families with other goals, such as accepting a greater level of sedation to achieve symptom control and determining when invasive interventions such as intubation will not be used to avoid prolonged suffering (Hauer and Houtrow 2017). Fortunately for most children, adequate symptom management can be achieved.

Finally, it is critical that the person and team providing oversight are clearly identified. This includes determining the team that a family is to contact when questions about symptom management and side effects arise. For complex symptom management, this might involve a specialty pain team or palliative medicine team.

Conclusions

Pain can be a frequent problem in children with significant impairment of the CNS. New onset pain involves assessment for a nociceptive pain source and chronic intermittent pain involves consideration of pain episodes due to the impaired CNS, such as CP. Tests can identify when a nociceptive source exists and indicate the problem to treat. Alterations in the CNS that can result in recurring pain episodes require empirical medication trials given the lack of tests to identify these problems. This framework can significantly improve our ability to improve comfort in this population of children.

Key points:

Pain management in children with impairment of the CNS involves:

• Recognition of pain behaviors

• Obtaining a history that distinguishes the previously comfortable child from the child with a history of irritability and agitation (i.e. pre-existing pain behaviors)

• Assessment for nociceptive sources, factoring in this history

• Knowledge of history, physical examination, and diagnostic tests to consider when assessing for a nociceptive source

• Consideration of alternative sources for irritability, such as mental health and environmental causes, including abuse

• An empirical medication trial in a child with a history of intermittent pain over months, following the initial evaluation for a nociceptive pain source

• Access to experts in pain and symptom management for children with SNI

• Awareness of triggers that can worsen symptoms, including GI tract distention

• Use of non-pharmacologic strategies

References

Breau LM, Camfield CS, McGrath PJ, Finley GA (2003) The incidence of pain in children with severe cognitive impairments. *Arch Pediatr Adolesc Med* **157**: 1219–1226.

Breau LM, Finley GA, McGrath PJ, Camfield CS (2002a) Validation of the non-communicating children's pain checklist-postoperative version. *Anesthesiology* **96**: 528-535.

Breau LM, McGrath PJ, Camfield CS, Finley GA (2002b) Psychometric properties of the non-communicating children's pain checklist-revised. *Pain* **9**: 349–357.

Haney AL, Garner SS, Cox TH (2009) Gabapentin therapy for pain and irritability in a neurologically impaired infant. *Pharmacotherapy* **29**: 997–1001.

Hauer J (2012) Improving comfort in children with severe neurological impairment. *Prog Palliat* **20**: 349–356.

Hauer J, Houtrow AJ (2017) AAP Section on Hospice and Palliative Medicine, Council on Children with Disabilities. Pain Assessment and Treatment in Children with Significant Impairment of the Central Nervous System. Pediatrics. 139, e20171002.

Hauer J, Wical B, Charnas L (2007) Gabapentin successfully manages chronic unexplained irritability in children with severe neurologic impairment. *Pediatrics* **119**: e519–e22.

Hauer JM, Solodiuk JC (2015) Gabapentin for management of recurrent pain in 22 nonverbal children with severe neurological impairment: a retrospective analysis. *J Palliat Med* **18**: 453–456.

Herr K, Coyne PJ, McCaffery M, Manworren R, Merkel S (2011) Pain assessment in the patient unable to self-report: position statement with clinical practice recommendations. *Pain Manag Nurs* **12**: 230–250.

Houlihan CM, O'Donnell M, Conaway M, Stevenson RD (2004) Bodily pain and health-related quality of life in children with cerebral palsy. *Dev Med Child Neurol* **46**: 305–310.

Hunt A, Goldman A, Seers K, et al. (2004) Clinical validation of the paediatric pain profile. *Dev Med Child Neurol* **46**: 9–18.

Malviya S, Voepel-Lewis T, Burke C, et al (2006) The revised FLACC observational pain tool: improved reliability and validity for pain assessment in children with cognitive impairment. *Paediatr Anaesth* **16**: 258–265.

Moulin D, Boulanger A, Clark AJ, et al (2014) Pharmacological management of chronic neuropathic pain: revised consensus statement from the Canadian Pain Society. *Pain Res Manag* **19**: 328–335.

Siden HB, Carleton BC Oberlander TF (2013) Physician variability in treating pain and irritability of unknown origin in children with severe neurological impairment. *Pain Res Manag* **18**: 243–248.

Solodiuk JC, Scott-Sutherland J, Meyers M, et al (2010) Validation of the Individualized Numeric Rating Scale (INRS): a pain assessment tool for nonverbal children with intellectual disability. *Pain* **150**: 231–236.

Stallard P, Williams L, Velleman R, et al (2002) Brief report: behaviors identified by caregivers to detect pain in noncommunicating children. *J Pediatr Psychol* **27**: 209–214.

US Department of Health and Human Services, National Institutes of Health and National Cancer Institute. (2010) *Common Terminology Criteria for Adverse Events (CTCAE) Version 4.03.* [Online] Available from: http://www.hrc.govt.nz/sites/default/files/CTCAE manual - DMCC. pdf [Accessed April 2, 2018].

World Health Organization (2012) WHO guidelines on the pharmacological treatment of persisting pain in children with medical illnesses. Available at: http://www.who.int/medicines/areas/quality_safety/guide_perspainchild/en/. Accessed June 15, 2016.

Chapter 15

Seizures and epilepsy in children with cerebral palsy

John R. Mytinger and Howard P. Goodkin

Introduction

An underlying predisposition for recurrent unprovoked seizures (i.e. epilepsy) occurs in more than a third of children with cerebral palsy (CP) (Ashwal et al. 2004). Children with more severe forms of CP (e.g. spastic quadriplegia) or who are nonambulatory are more likely to have epilepsy (Shevell et al. 2009). Early recognition and appropriate treatment of epilepsy may prevent serious complications (e.g. injury, status epilepticus, sudden death in epilepsy) and can have a significant impact on developmental outcomes and academic performance. In this chapter, we review important aspects of seizures and epilepsy associated with CP.

Terminology

The terminology used to describe seizures and epilepsy syndromes continues to evolve. The International League Against Epilepsy (ILAE) updated seizure terminology in 2010 (Berg et al. 2010). Seizures are organized into three categories: generalized, focal and unknown (Table 15.1). Studies of children with CP and epilepsy that include seizure type often do not differentiate primary generalized seizures from secondarily generalized seizures. It appears, however, that focal seizures are the most common seizure type in children with CP. One study that differentiated focal from primary generalized seizures reported that just over 70% of children with CP and epilepsy experience focal seizures while just less than 30% of children experienced primary generalized seizures (Delgado et al. 1996).

Table 15.1 Seizure organization

Generalized seizures
Tonic-clonic
Absence
Myoclonic
Clonic
Tonic
Atonic
Focal seizures (see text)
Unknown
Epileptic spasms
Infantile spasms

Modified from Berg et al. (2010)

The ILAE allows for the diagnosis of epilepsy in the setting of (1) two or more unprovoked seizures occurring at least 24 hours apart, (2) a single unprovoked seizure with evidence (clinical, electroencephalogram [EEG] or neuroimaging) suggesting a recurrence risk of at least 60%, or (3) an epilepsy syndrome (Fisher et al. 2014).

Focal seizures
Focal seizures can remain localized to a single area of the brain (often causing limited clinical manifestations) or spread to other brain regions (often with more obvious clinical manifestations). Focal seizures that remain localized can occur with and without alteration in consciousness and may present with numerous possible clinical manifestations depending on the brain region involved. Focal seizures can evolve to a bilateral convulsive seizure (i.e. a secondarily generalized seizure). Spread to other brain regions can occur after a delay or occur rapidly. Sometimes, the spread from a focal area to bilateral networks is so rapid that the seizure is confused with a primary generalized seizure (a physiological phenomenon referred to as rapid bisynchrony). The convulsion can include tonic (sustained increase muscle tone), clonic (regularly repetitive) or tonic-clonic (tonic followed by clonic) movements.

Generalized seizures
The current concept of generalized seizures is that they originate at some point within the brain and rapidly engage bilaterally distributed networks (Berg et al. 2010). In other words, even primary generalized seizures start at some area within the brain. Differentiating between primary generalized versus focal seizures is critically important when choosing therapies. For example, only children with focal-onset seizures would be considered for epilepsy surgery and some anti-seizure drugs (e.g. carbamazepine) can exacerbate some types of generalized seizures. As described above, for secondarily

generalized seizures, tonic, clonic and tonic-clonic seizures are common manifestations of primary generalized seizures.

Typical absence seizures (classically with 3Hz spike-and-wave on the EEG, as seen with childhood absence epilepsy) are a type of generalized seizure that do not result from brain injury. In a child with CP and 'staring spells', the diagnosis is almost never child-hood absence epilepsy (unless the child was destined to have it regardless of the CP). Whereas children with focal seizures with an alteration in consciousness often have postictal sedation, children with typical absence seizures do not experience postictal sedation. Other helpful distinctions include the age at onset (childhood absence epi-lepsy beginning most often after 3 years of age and focal seizures starting anytime) as well as the frequency of seizures (many per day for childhood absence epilepsy and few per week or month for focal seizures).

Atypical absence seizures are often of longer duration and are more likely to occur with associated clinical changes such as reduced postural tone or with tonic or myoclonic movements. Atypical absence seizures almost always occur in children with multiple seizure types and cognitive disability. Likewise, atonic seizures ('drop attacks'), charac-terized by a sudden loss of postural tone, almost always occur in children with severe epilepsy and cognitive disability. It is critically important to differentiate these seizures from children who fall because of impairments in coordination or gait. Myoclonus is characterized by sudden and rapid ('shock-like') movements. Myoclonic jerks can be nonepileptic (e.g. sleep myoclonus), or epileptic.

Unknown seizures (seizures difficult to characterize as either focal or generalized)

Within this category are epileptic spasms. An infantile spasm is a type of epileptic spasm that can be caused by brain pathology that is focal or widespread. Infantile spasms are most often seen in infants with West syndrome. A brief discussion of West syndrome and Lennox-Gastaut syndrome (LGS) is imperative because these syndromes often occur in the setting of brain injury with coexisting CP. These syndromes are examples of 'epileptic encephalopathies' – a term that "embodies the notion that the epileptic activity itself may contribute to severe cognitive and behavioral impairments above and beyond what might be expected from the underlying pathology alone (e.g. cortical malformation), and that these can worsen over time" (Berg et al. 2010). West syndrome is characterized by infantile spasms, developmental abnormalities and an abnormal EEG – classically hypsarrhythmia (a chaotic background pattern of high amplitude slow waves and multifocal independent spikes). Overall, about 15% of children with CP will develop West syndrome (Hadjipanayis et al. 1997). More wide-spread brain injury increases the risk of West syndrome. For example, children with spastic quadriplegic CP have a higher incidence of West syndrome – 27% in one series (Hadjipanayis et al. 1997).

It is crucial that infantile spasms be recognized because early recognition and treatment may favorably influence the response to treatment and outcome. The most common pattern of infantile spasms is paroxysmal onset simultaneous symmetrical extension of the arms and flexion of the neck and hips, typically occurring in clusters and often following sleep-wake transitions (in the morning or after naps). However, any combination of mixed flexion-extension is possible. Infantile spasms can be asymmetrical especially with focal brain pathology. Infantile spasms can be subtle and involve small movements of the eyes or face. The occurrence of these 'odd' movements in 'clusters' is often the key to the diagnosis. Half of children with infantile spasms go on to develop an alternative seizure type and roughly a third of children with infantile spasms evolve to LGS. LGS is characterized by cognitive impairment, intractable epilepsy with multiple seizure types and slow spike-and-wave (i.e. less than 3Hz) on EEG. Although any seizure type can be seen in children with LGS, tonic seizures are the most common type. Atypical absence and atonic seizure are also common in LGS. Children with LGS typically have life-long epilepsy that is difficult to control.

Patterns of brain injury affecting the manifestation of epilepsy

Although there appears to be important genetic contributions to the development of epilepsy even in those with a remote symptomatic etiology like brain injury, the development of epilepsy in children with CP most often occurs following damage to cortical neurons. The term 'remote symptomatic' describes a history of a major brain injury (e.g. trauma) or the presence of a condition such as CP, developmental delay or cognitive disability that indicates brain pathology. Seizures arise from cortical neurons that lack an appropriate balance of inhibitory and excitatory electrical connectivity. It is intuitive then that children with more severe CP are more likely to have cortical disease and thus comorbid epilepsy. The pattern of brain injury, and thus the type of CP, has a profound effect on the incidence, age at onset and type of epilepsy. For example, the incidence of epilepsy is highest (Kudrjavcev et al. 1985; Kwong et al. 1998; Carlsson et al. 2003 Kułak and Sobaniec 2003,, Shevell et al. 2009, Zelnik et al. 2010) and the age at onset is earliest (Hadjipanayis et al. 1997, Kwong et al. 1998, Carlsson et al. 2003,) in children with spastic quadriplegic CP given the greater degree of brain injury in these patients. Approximately two out of three of patients with spastic quadriplegic CP will develop epilepsy (Hadjipanayis et al. 1997, Kwong et al. 1998, Kułak and Sobaniec 2003, Zelnik et al. 2010).

Spastic quadriplegic CP is often related to widespread brain injury (e.g. ischemia) or severe brain malformation. The widespread involvement can lead to the development of generalized seizures. In contrast, focal seizures are more common in the other forms of CP where the injury is likely more circumscribed. Epilepsy is commonly seen in children with hemiplegic CP that most often results from an infarct (typically in the middle cerebral artery territory) with associated loss of the perfused brain tissue (porencephaly) including the overlying cortex.

Spastic diplegic CP is less commonly associated with epilepsy (Hadjipanayis et al. 1997, Shevell et al. 2009). Spastic diplegic CP is associated with preterm birth with injury occurring between 26 and 32 weeks' gestational age with the subsequent development of periventricular leukomalacia and damage to the descending corticospinal tracts. Given the anatomical arrangement of the corticospinal fibers, with the leg fibers closer to the area of injury, the spasticity typically involves the legs in isolation or preferentially. However, the cortex is often spared, explaining the lower incidence of epilepsy in children with spastic diplegic CP.

Epilepsy is often absent in patients with extrapyramidal CP due to the damage associated with the deep gray structures (basal ganglia), often with sparing of the cortex. Possible etiologies for injury to the basal ganglia include kernicterus and hypoxic-ischemic encephalopathy. Regardless of the type of CP, epilepsy is far more common in children with CP who are nonambulatory (Gross Motor Function Classification System IV and V, see Chapter 1) when compared to those who are ambulatory (Shevell et al. 2009, Kirby et al. 2011, Sellier et al. 2012,).

Presentation

A thorough history and examination often reveals the diagnosis of epilepsy. The history will aid in the distinction between epileptic and nonepileptic phenomena. The clinician should be aware of seizure mimics. Important examples of nonepileptic spells include childhood syncope (e.g. breath-holding spells) that can lead to reflex anoxic seizures, psychogenic nonepileptic seizures, shuddering, gratification behavior, tics, stereotypies, and others. The history for a patient with spells should include a careful assessment of the clinical changes that occur during an event. For example, psychogenic nonepileptic seizures can be variable in semiology and include features atypical of epileptic seizures such as long duration, preservation of consciousness during an apparent convulsion, head movements in a 'no-no' pattern, eyes closed during the event and hip thrusting (to name a few). Epileptic seizures within a single person are almost always stereotypical from seizure to seizure (unless there are multiple seizure types) and usually relatively brief (less than 2 to 3 minutes). In addition, identification of focal features (e.g. eye deviation, unilateral clonic movements or dystonic posturing) early in the seizure can have diagnostic implications (focal versus generalized seizures) and lateralizing value (left or right hemisphere). Unilateral weakness after a seizure (i.e. Todd paralysis) may also indicate a seizure arising from the contralateral hemisphere. Further history should include the age at onset, the frequency, precipitating factors (e.g. sleep deprivation, illness, fever), risk factors for the development of epilepsy (e.g. brain injury, history of meningitis) and a family history of seizures. A history of neonatal seizures strongly predicts the later development of epilepsy in children with CP (Kwong et al. 1998, Zafeiriou et al. 1999, Carlsson et al. 2003, Kułak and Sobaniec 2003, Zelnik et al. 2010).

As noted above, seizures can range from subtle (e.g. behavioral arrest) to severe convulsions with status epilepticus. The seizure presentation depends on the brain region(s) involved and can take on numerous forms. Of note, seizures should be considered in any child who is confused, lethargic, or falls asleep after the event, regardless of the appearance of the event. While these symptoms can occur after spells unrelated to seizures or epilepsy, these changes are common findings after seizures and are referred to postictal symptoms. These postictal symptoms should gradually improve. In the absence of improvement, it is possible that the seizure is continuing and medical evaluation should be immediately sought.

Evaluation

The examination should include both a general and neurological examination. Within the general examination, the cardiac evaluation is especially important to identify a pathological murmur or an irregular heart rhythm that might suggest a cardiogenic cause of the spell (e.g. cardiogenic syncope). As a supplement to the examination, a 12-lead EKG is an important and inexpensive test in the evaluation of spells. Particularly important to the neurological examination are assessments for asymmetries of tone, strength, and reflexes. The finding of a smaller or shorter limb or digit (e.g. thumbs and first toes) when compared to the other side can be a clue to brain pathology in the contralateral hemisphere. Hyperreflexia and up going toes may also be present in the wake of a seizure and similarly can subsequently resolve (if not present at baseline).

In the evaluation of seizure, an understanding of provoked and unprovoked seizure is necessary. The classic provoked seizure is the febrile seizure. Several additional examples of provoked seizures are those that occur in the setting of significant head trauma immediately preceding the seizure, electrolyte disarray, medication/drug toxicity, or those seizures occurring in the setting of central nervous system infection or tumor. These conditions that lead to provoked seizures must be differentiated from the circumstances or triggers that lower the seizure threshold in patients who possess an enduring predisposition for epileptic seizures (i.e. individuals with epilepsy). Such triggers frequently include sleep deprivation, illness, and fever. Children with epilepsy who present with seizures in the setting of fever *do not* have febrile seizures (although occasionally the two conditions coexist). It is far more likely that these children have epilepsy and have experienced a seizure in the setting of a lowered seizure threshold. Many clinicians withhold anti-seizure drug adjustment in this setting because 'the seizure was provoked by fever'. However, these children typically do require medication adjustment (an increased dose or the addition of/transition to another anti-seizure drug) so that they have a greater degree of protection from seizure in the setting of a future fever. Typical febrile seizures have an age of occurrence of between 6 months and 6 years, clinically involve bilaterally symmetric tremulousness of the upper extremities (often without tonic-clonic movements), are without focal features, such as eye deviation, and have a duration of less than 15 minutes without recurrence. If there is deviance from this typical pattern, especially in the setting of a possible remote symptomatic etiology (e.g. brain injury in a patient with CP), an epileptic seizure should strongly be considered.

An EEG is not indicated in a patient with CP for determining the etiology of CP but is indicated in a patient with findings concerning for unprovoked seizures (Ashwal et al. 2004). Following a first unprovoked seizure, the EEG can provide information regarding seizure type, epilepsy syndrome, the need for neuroimaging and risk of recurrence – all findings that affect management decisions (Hirtz et al. 2000). The EEG need not be obtained acutely and can be obtained as an outpatient. In the acute setting, a laboratory evaluation (for electrolytes such as sodium, glucose, calcium, and magnesium) could be considered in a child presenting with vomiting, diarrhea or dehydration, a child failing to return to baseline alertness, or children less than 6 months of age (Hirtz et al. 2000). In children not returning to baseline, especially in the setting of suspected intracranial space-occupying lesion, neuroimaging and subsequent lumbar puncture should be considered. The clinician should strongly consider brain imaging prior to lumbar puncture if there is any concern for increased intracranial pressure. This is particularly true in the setting of an incomplete neurological examination such as an inability to assess for the presence of papilledema.

If non-urgent neuroimaging is obtained, it should be with an MRI protocol designed by a neuroradiologist experienced in the assessment of children with epilepsy. Children with CP and epilepsy are more likely to have brain imaging abnormalities when compared to children with CP and no epilepsy (Zelnik et al. 2010). Although non-urgent neuroimaging after a first unprovoked seizure is of low yield in terms of its effect on management decisions, it should be considered in patients with unexplained neurological signs and symptoms, focal seizures not due to a benign focal epilepsy of childhood or children less than one year of age (Hirtz et al. 2000). Once the diagnosis of epilepsy is made, a brain MRI should be obtained (if not already performed) to determine the etiology of the epilepsy and aid in prognosis.

Treatment

Whether to initiate treatment for epilepsy depends in part on the risk of seizure recurrence after a first unprovoked seizure. Whereas recurrence occurs in 30–50% of children with an unknown cause of epilepsy, a seizure will recur in greater than 50% of children with a remote symptomatic etiology (Hirtz et al. 2003). Camfield et al. (1985) reported that just over half of all children with a first unprovoked seizure go on to have a second. Of those children that have a second unprovoked seizure, nearly 80% go on to have a third seizure (Camfield et al. 1985). In addition, these authors found three predictors of a second unprovoked seizure: focal seizure type (79% recurred), focal spikes on EEG (68% recurred) and an abnormal neurological examination (73% recurred) (Camfield et al. 1985). Overall, it appears that focal spikes on the EEG and a remote symptomatic etiology or abnormal neurological examination are the strongest predictors of seizure recurrence after a first unprovoked seizure (Berg and Shinnar 1991, Berg 2008).

Anti-seizure drugs

Anti-seizure drugs are used to reduce neuronal excitability with the goal of preventing seizures. Anti-seizure drugs do not change the natural history of the epilepsy. Reducing neuronal excitability (and other less well-known mechanisms) can cause potentially significant cognitive and behavioral adverse effects. The decision to initiate an anti-seizure drug for epilepsy is based on a risk-to-benefit assessment that considers the likelihood of seizure recurrence, the risk of injury from seizures, comorbidities (e.g. migraine), medication side effects and the wishes of the family and patient. While adverse side effects are a concern, clinicians familiar with epilepsy and anti-seizure drugs can often find a balance between tolerability and efficacy. To limit adverse effects, it is optimal to use the least number of medications (e.g. monotherapy) at the lowest effective dose. Given that ongoing seizures (especially convulsions) are an independent risk factor for death in epilepsy, the authors advocate for the aggressive treatment of epilepsy to the point of complete remission, if possible. Unfortunately, about a third of patients continue to have seizures despite adequate trials of anti-seizure drugs.

The initial goal of treatment using anti-seizure drugs is complete seizure control without side effects. Fewer side effects and interactions are seen with monotherapy. When compared to patients with epilepsy without CP, those with epilepsy and CP are more likely to require polytherapy (Gururaj et al. 2003, Hadjipanayis et al. 1997, Zafeiriou et al. 1999). When compared to other forms of CP, those with spastic quadriplegic CP are at greatest risk (one third to two thirds) for needing polytherapy (Hadjipanayis et al. 1997, Gururaj et al. 2003, Kułak and Sobaniec 2003). Intractable epilepsy is more common in those with spastic quadriplegic CP when compared to other forms of CP, (Kułak and Sobaniec 2003).

Several anti-seizure drugs (particularly phenobarbital) are associated with cognitive and behavioral side effects in children. Although phenobarbital is the treatment of choice for neonatal seizures because of its safety profile in this group, it is now common practice to largely restrict the use of phenobarbital to the neonatal and early infantile period with a subsequent transition to an alternative medication, if needed, before 3, 6, or 12 months of age depending on the clinical scenario and country of practice. In general, second generation anti-seizure drugs (e.g. lamotrigine, levetiracetam, oxcarbazepine) are better tolerated and often require less drug level monitoring than first generation anti-seizure drugs (e.g. phenobarbital, phenytoin, carbamazepine). Despite the concern regarding adverse side effects, most children tolerate individual medications without clinically significant side effects. However, trials of several medications are often required before both tolerability and efficacy are achieved.

Prescribers should know that some hepatic enzyme inducing anti-seizure drugs (e.g. phenobarbital) can lower the serum concentration of other drugs that are hepatically metabolized. Hepatic induction also reduces vitamin D levels (potentially reducing bone mineral density) and decreases the effectiveness of oral contraceptive pills by reducing estrogen levels. There are now over 20 anti-seizure medications available for use. Medication management is typically carried out by a specialist who is familiar with the potential adverse effects of anti-seizure drugs as well as their potential drug-drug interactions. Levetiracetam has gained favor as a broad spectrum (i.e. useful with multiple seizures types) anti-seizure medication with a favorable safety profile (aside from the 10–15% of patients who experience irritability) and absence of drug-drug interactions.

Diet therapy

The ketogenic diet is a regimen that is high in fat and low in carbohydrates and protein leading to ketosis. It can be used for both generalized and focal seizures. About half of children treated with the ketogenic diet experience a 50% reduction in seizures. If the ketogenic diet is used, it is typically initiated in the hospital under close observation that includes monitoring of glucose and ketones. Guidance and education by an experienced dietician is critical. Clinician experience with the ketogenic diet is especially important in children with an unknown cause of epilepsy as several inborn errors of metabolism can result in clinical deterioration with initiation of the ketogenic diet. The ketogenic diet is contraindicated in patients with pyruvate carboxylase deficiency, organic acidurias and porphyria. Potential adverse effects include reduced bone mineral density, kidney stones and growth impairment. Children with CP who are nonambulatory are already at risk for low bone mineral density and this added risk is undesirable. Children are supplemented with vitamin D and B vitamins. Some clinicians discontinue topiramate and valproate before starting the diet because of the risk of kidney stones and liver disease respectively. In children taking the diet by mouth, compliance can be challenging. When the diet is discontinued, it should be done gradually as sudden discontinuation can exacerbate seizures or may even cause status epilepticus. Less restrictive diets such as the modified Atkins diet or low glycemic index treatment appear to offer efficacy similar to the ketogenic diet but with improved compliance.

Epilepsy surgery

Children who fail to become seizure free following adequate trials of two anti-seizure drugs are said to have refractory epilepsy. Children with refractory epilepsy with focal-onset seizures should be referred to a specialized epilepsy center for consideration of epilepsy surgery or other specialized treatments and resources. Successful surgical resection of the seizure onset zone is far more likely to lead to seizure freedom when compared to additional trials of anti-seizure drugs. Not all children who undergo an epilepsy surgery evaluation are candidates for resection.

Vagal nerve stimulation

Vagal nerve stimulation (VNS) is a less invasive potential treatment for refractory epilepsy. This device is implanted under the skin of the chest and, via a wire running to the vagus nerve in the neck, delivers intermittent electrical stimulation. It is particularly effective for atonic seizures – a seizure type common in patients with LGS. Both focal and generalized seizures may respond to VNS. About 50% of children will experience a 50% decrease in seizure frequency. The likelihood of seizure freedom with VNS is very low and so VNS should only be considered in those children who are not candidates for resective surgery.

Prognosis

In all children with epilepsy, half will grow out of their epilepsy and discontinue anti-seizure drugs. About half of children with epilepsy who are seizure free for 1 to 2 years can successfully stop medication (Berg and Shinnar 1991, Dooley et al. 1996). Those with an unknown cause of epilepsy and those who achieve early remission have nearly an 80% chance of remission (Berg et al. 2011). However, the presence of a remote symptomatic etiology negatively impacts the likelihood of successful remission following medication withdrawal. Thus, children with CP are less likely to experience prolonged remission after medication withdrawal when compared to children without a remote symptomatic etiology. In addition, children with epilepsy onset at or beyond 10 years of age are less likely to experience remission (Dooley et al. 1996, Berg et al. 2011,).

Although the risk of recurrence is high, some children with CP and epilepsy may successfully discontinue their anti-seizure drugs and experience a prolonged remission (Delgado et al. 1996, Zafeiriou et al. 1999). Delgado and colleagues (1996) reported rates of prolonged seizure remission following medication withdrawal in children with CP after a seizure-free period of at least 2 years. Overall, nearly 60% of these children experienced a prolonged period of seizure remission after medication withdrawal with a relapse occurring in 40% of those with spastic quadriplegia and in only 14% of those with spastic diplegia (Delgado et al. 1996). The decision to withdraw medication should consider whether the anti-seizure drug is causing side effects, the likelihood of a prolonged remission and the potential risk of a recurrent seizure.

Key points

- Epilepsy occurs in more than a third of children with cerebral palsy.

- Focal seizures are the most common seizure type in children with cerebral palsy.

- More severe cerebral palsy increases the risk of epilepsy.

- Patterns of brain pathology often influence the clinical presentation of seizures.

- In addition to medication, treatments such as the vagal nerve stimulator, epilepsy surgery and diet therapy are available.

References

Ashwal S, Russman BS, Blasco PA, et al (2004) Practice parameter: diagnostic assessment of the child with cerebral palsy: report of the Quality Standards Subcommittee of the American Academy of Neurology and the Practice Committee of the Child Neurology Society. *Neurology* 62: 851–863.

Berg AT (2008) Risk of recurrence after a first unprovoked seizure. *Epilepsia* 49 Suppl **1**: 13–18.

Berg AT, Shinnar S (1991) The risk of seizure recurrence following a first unprovoked seizure: a quantitative review. *Neurology* **41**: 965–972.

Berg AT, Berkovic SF, Brodie MJ, et al (2010) Revised terminology and concepts for organization of seizures and epilepsies: report of the ILAE Commission on Classification and Terminology, 2005–2009. *Epilepsia* **51**: 676–685.

Berg AT, Testa FM, Levy SR (2011) Complete remission in nonsyndromic childhood-onset epilepsy. *Ann Neurol* **70**: 566–673.

Camfield PR, Camfield CS, Dooley JM, et al (1985) Epilepsy after a first unprovoked seizure in childhood. *Neurology* **35**: 1657–1660.

Carlsson M, Hagberg G, Olsson I (2003) Clinical and aetiological aspects of epilepsy in children with cerebral palsy. *Dev Med Child Neurol* **45**: 371–376.

Delgado MR, Riela AR, Mills J, Pitt A, Browne R (1996) Discontinuation of antiepileptic drug treatment after two seizure-free years in children with cerebral palsy. *Pediatrics*. Feb; **97**: 192–197.

Dooley J, Gordon K, Camfield P, et al (1996) Discontinuation of anticonvulsant therapy in children free of seizures for 1 year: a prospective study. *Neurology* **46**: 969–974.

Fisher RS, Acevedo C, Arzimanoglou A, et al (2014) ILAE official report: a practical clinical definition of epilepsy. *Epilepsia*. Apr; **55**(4): 475–482.

Gururaj AK, Sztriha L, Bener A, Dawodu A, Eapen V (2003) Epilepsy in children with cerebral palsy. *Seizure*. Mar; **12**(2): 110–114.

Hadjipanayis A, Hadjichristodoulou C, Youroukos S (1997) Epilepsy in patients with cerebral palsy. *Dev Med Child Neurol* **39**: 659–663.

Hirtz D, Ashwal S, Berg A, et al (2000) Practice parameter: evaluating a first nonfebrile seizure in children: report of the quality standards subcommittee of the American Academy of Neurology, The Child Neurology Society, and The American Epilepsy Society. *Neurology* **55**(5): 616–623.

Hirtz D, Berg A, Bettis D, et al (2003) Practice parameter: treatment of the child with a first unprovoked seizure: Report of the Quality Standards Subcommittee of the American Academy of Neurology and the Practice Committee of the Child Neurology Society. *Neurology* **60**: 166–175.

Kirby RS, Wingate MS, Van Naarden Braun K, et al (2011) Prevalence and functioning of children with cerebral palsy in four areas of the United States in **2006**: a report from the Autism and Developmental Disabilities Monitoring Network. *Res Dev Disabil* **32**: 462–469.

Kudrjavcev T, Schoenberg BS, Kurland LT, Groover RV (1985) Cerebral palsy: survival rates, associated handicaps, and distribution by clinical subtype (Rochester, MN, 1950–1976). Neurology 35: 900–903.

Kułak W, Sobaniec W (2003) Risk factors and prognosis of epilepsy in children with cerebral palsy in north-eastern Poland. *Brain Dev*. Oct; **25**(7): 499–506.

Kwong KL, Wong SN, So KT (1998) Epilepsy in children with cerebral palsy. *Pediatr Neurol* **19**: 31–36,

Sellier E, Uldall P, Calado E, et al *(2012)* Epilepsy and cerebral palsy: characteristics and trends in children born in 1976–1998. *Eur J Paediatr Neurol* **16**: 48–55.

Shevell MI, Dagenais L, Hall N; REPACQ Consortium (2009) Comorbidities in cerebral palsy and their relationship to neurologic subtype and GMFCS level. *Neurology* **72**: 2090–2096.

Zafeiriou DI, Kontopoulos EE, Tsikoulas I (1999) Characteristics and prognosis of epilepsy in children with cerebral palsy. *J Child Neurol* **14**: 289–294.

Zelnik N, Konopnicki M, Bennett-Back O, et al. (2010) Risk factors for epilepsy in children with cerebral palsy. *Eur J Paediatr Neurol* **14**: 67–72.

Chapter 16

Urologic issues in children with complex cerebral palsy

Stuart Bauer

Introduction

Cerebral Palsy (CP) is the most common physical disability in childhood, affecting approximately 2.1 per 1 000 8-year-old children in the United States with variable degrees of disability (Oskoui et al. 2013). Despite this, cerebral palsy is one of the lesser causes of urinary incontinence in children, probably accounting for fewer than 1% of all etiologies affecting lower urinary tract (LUT) function (Bauer et al. 2012). Part of the reason for this is likely related to the fact that little attention has been paid to its presence and there has been under-reporting of its prevalence in the literature. Investigating LUT function in older children with cerebral palsy has revealed that specific areas of the cerebral cortex and brainstem that control urinary function are less affected by the insults causing cerebral palsy than other locations along the central nervous system (CNS) (Fowler et al. 2008). Urinary and fecal incontinence gradually begin to play a major role in social acceptability as children with complex cerebral palsy age (Samijn et al. 2016). As primary care and consulting physicians develop a greater understanding of the urologic issues important to children with cerebral palsy and their families, they can provide improved quality of care and help affected individuals achieve their best possible outcomes. Thus, the aim of this chapter is to promote a better working knowledge of the LUT so early signs of dysfunction may be identified and targeted therapy instituted.

Physiology of the lower urinary tract

Lower urinary tract function is under the influence of multiple areas of the CNS. The sacral spinal cord (S2–4) provides the parasympathetic reflex arcs that allow for sensory input when the bladder is full and needs to empty and for stimulating a detrusor contraction to empty it. At the same time, Onuf's nucleus in the sacral cord is responsible for modulating the striated muscle component of the external urethral sphincter function, tightening the muscle with bladder filling and during increases in abdominal pressure as well as relaxing the muscle completely during normal voiding to insure emptying takes place efficiently and at low pressure.

The thoraco-lumbar portion of the spinal cord (T10 – L1) provides sympathetic innervation to the bladder and bladder neck that allows the detrusor (bladder muscle) to expand at low pressure while providing increasing resistance at the bladder neck (a sort of second sphincter mechanism) in order to maintain continence during filling. Spinal thalamic tracts and the posterior and lateral columns of the spinal cord carry messages to and from these centers of control to the base of the brain stem in the pontine mesencephalic center. It is this latter critical nexus that coordinates the function of the two lower spinal cord centers to ensure normal function of the lower urinary tract unit.

From the pontine mesencephalic center, impulses traverse to several locations higher in the brain including the peri-aqueductal gray matter, the right insula, the prefrontal cortex and the anterior cingulate gyrus that allow the individual to both sense the need to void and either allow it to happen if appropriate, or prevent micturition if not (Tadic et al. 2010). It has been clearly shown, using measurements of blood flow during functional magnetic resonance imaging (MRI) of the brain that these areas are active when a person senses the need to void (urgency) and either prevents it or allows it to happen (depending on the physical and social circumstances of the individual) (Tadic et al. 2010). As will be discussed later, oftentimes, these portions of the brain do not seem to be or are only minimally affected by the cerebral insults associated with cerebral palsy (Fowler et al. 2008, Richards and Malouin 2013). Rather, it is the limitations of physical and/or cognitive abilities that often lead to episodes of urinary incontinence (Wang et al. 2008, Kaerts et al. 2012, Murphy et al. 2012).

Causative factors for incontinence

Children with cerebral palsy will often achieve urinary continence, albeit at a later age than their typically developing peers (Richards and Malouin 2013, Roijen et al. 2001, Ozturk et al. 2006). Not infrequently, daytime continence is achieved first, followed by nighttime continence within the next year, but this is clearly dependent on either the ability to get to a bathroom facility quickly enough independently or the ability to signal for assistance that there is a need to empty the bladder. Overall, 14% (Silva et al. 2009) to 34% (Richardson and Palmer 2009) of all children with cerebral palsy are continent of urine before 5 years of age. The median age for achieving continence in those with high intellectual capacity and diplegia or hemiplegia varies from

3.6 to 4.1 years. For those with low intellectual capacity and quadiplegia, those children with complex cerebral palsy, this milestone is achieved much later (10.1 to 13.2 years) (Roijen et al. 2001). Most studies do not evaluate the correlation of mobility (or Gross Motor Function Classification System (GMFCS) level; see Chapter 1) with achievement of continence (Murphy et al. 2012, Silva et al. 2009, Ersoz et al. 2009). In 97 children with cerebral palsy evaluated via a standardized dysfunction voiding symptom survey, investigators found 25% of those who were able to walk had LUT dysfunction compared with 75% in those who were unable to do so ($P < 0.001$) (Silva et al. 2009). LUT symptoms became more prevalent as children aged, from 11% in children under age 5 to 30% in those over 30 years (Murphy et al. 2012, Silva et al. 2009).

Symptomatology

The reported incidence of urinary symptoms in children with cerebral palsy varies by the specifics of the investigation, namely the breadth and numbers of patients evaluated and in what settings – an outpatient clinic versus a school for children with complex medical conditions. Thus, the range of symptomatology is quite varied – 16% (Murphy et al. 2012) to 94% (Gündoğdu et al. 2013). Part of this may be due to a child's communication skills, including their ability to relate their needs to parents or caregivers (Murphy et al. 2012). Despite the fact that males are slightly more likely to have cerebral palsy, girls are more prone than boys to have LUT symptoms (Silva et al. 2009, Ersoz et al. 2009). Daytime urinary incontinence is the most common symptom, occurring in 23% to 94% of affected youths with cerebral palsy with an overall prevalence of 35% to 45% (Murphy et al. 2012, Roijen et al. 2001, Richardson and Palmer 2009, Gündoğdu et al. 2013, Reid and Borzyskowski 1993, Karaman et al. 2005). Urgency and frequency are also part of this constellation of symptoms (Murphy et al. 2012, Karaman et al. 2005). Monosymptomatic enuresis (nighttime wetting without daytime symptoms) is seen in as little as 3% (Richards and Malouin 2013) but it has been reported in up to 13% (Silva et al. 2009, Karaman et al. 2005), again depending on age of the patient. The occurrence of urinary tract infection (UTI) is also variable, being noted in 5% to 57% (Silva et al. 2009, Ersoz et al. 2009, Gündoğdu et al. 2013, Silva et al. 2010). When using Rome III criteria (≤ 2 defecations per week; ≥ 1 episode of fecal incontinence per week; history of retentive posturing or excessive volitional stool retention; history of painful or hard bowel movements; presence of a large fecal mass in the rectum; and history of large diameter stools that obstruct the toilet (Rasquin, Di Lorenzo et al. 2006)), constipation can be detected in 33% to 66% of affected children with cerebral palsy (Silva et al. 2009, Gündoğdu et al. 2013, Karaman et al. 2005). Upper urinary tract deterioration, primarily hydronephrosis, is uncommon, appearing in less than 5%, but with a range of 0.5% to 12% (Murphy et al. 2012, Silva et al. 2009, Gündoğdu et al. 2013, Silva et al. 2010). Other parameters of 'deterioration' being reported include, asymmetric renal size, vesicoureteral reflux and renal calculi (Murphy et al. 2012, Silva et al. 2009, Gündoğdu et al. 2013). Factors that raise the risk of upper urinary tract deterioration include

Table 16.1 Summary: International children's continence society recommendations for the diagnostic evaluation and follow-up of congenital neuropathic bladder dysfunction in children

Condition	Type of investigation	Indications
Cerebral palsy	Renal/bladder ultrasound	Lower urinary tract symptoms persisting beyond the expected time for toilet training
	Uroflowmetry/postvoid residual	Wetting despite timed voiding, adequate fluid intake, effective bowel regimen & double voiding
	KUB	Wetting despite timed voiding, adequate fluid intake, effective bowel regimen & double voiding
	Voiding cystourethrography	Upper urinary tract abnormalities, (thick-walled bladder)
		Febrile UTI
		Recurrent afebrile urinary infection
	Urodynamic studies:	
	Cystometrogram/sphincter EMG	Signs suggesting dyssynergy: • Thick-walled bladder on ultrasound; • Persistent incontinence despite appropriate oral intake & an effective bladder / bowel regimen
		Incomplete emptying on uroflowmetry;
		Evidence of a structural abnormality, unexplainable by X-ray imaging

increasing age, clinical symptoms of detrusor sphincter dyssynergia (urinary retention, interrupted uroflow patterns, hesitancy), and recurrent UTI (Gündoğdu et al. 2013).

Pathogenesis

The majority of children with cerebral palsy have normal LUT function. When symptoms are present they seem to be related less to abnormal bladder function than to decreased mobility or an inability to communicate. The type of dysfunction involving the LUT, when it does occur, is related to specific areas of the CNS affected by the insult causing the cerebral palsy (Fowler et al. 2008): cerebral cortical involvement can lead to detrusor overactivity; lesions at or below the pontine mesencephalic center may produce detrusor sphincter dyssynergy. When the sacral spinal cord is affected, which may arise in the setting of tethering, this can cause detrusor areflexia and incontinence from paralysis of the pelvic nerves (Wang et al. 2008). When urodynamic testing has been undertaken in those with symptoms, normal LUT function has been found in only one third (Silva et al. 2009). Detrusor overactivity is noted in approximately 30% (Murphy et al. 2012, Gündoğdu et al. 2013, Decter et al. 1987), whereas detrusor underactivity is documented in 6% (Murphy et al. 2012). Smaller than expected bladder capacity for age has been detected in 42% to 93% (Silva et al. 2009, Ersoz et al. 2009, Gündoğdu et al. 2013), most likely related to the presence of an overactive detrusor contraction leading to urgency and urgency incontinence from an earlier than expected evacuation of urine (Karaman et al. 2005). Sphincter incoordination (dyssynergy) between the bladder and external urethral sphincter during voiding is found in approximately 12% (Silva et al. 2009, Karaman et al. 2005, Decter et al. 1987). It should be noted the incidence of these abnormal urodynamic parameters is related to the selection bias involved when only investigating patients with symptoms of unresolved incontinence or recurrent UTI. The true population prevalence of abnormal urodynamic LUT function is unknown but probably much less than what has been quoted, as a considerable number of individuals with cerebral palsy, across the complexity spectrum, have normal continence and no UTIs. However, some investigators have noted abnormal urodynamics in the absence of clinical LUT symptoms and recommend such testing in everyone (Houle et al. 1998, Bross et al. 2007).

Elevated residual urine volume (greater than 25ml) has been found to occur in 13% of children with cerebral palsy (Silva et al. 2009). Uroflow patterns may vary from normal (a bell-shaped curve) in 63%, to staccato in 17%, to interrupted in 13%, to a flat (plateau-shape) curve in 3%, and a high peaked (tower-shape) pattern in 3% (Murphy et al. 2012). Obviously, this variability is related to many factors such as the degree of spasticity noted in each individual and its effect on the external urethral sphincter, the presence of detrusor over- or under- activity and how extensively each person may strain to empty. No one has correlated upper urinary tract deterioration with the type of LUT function these patients exhibit on urodynamic evaluation nor with uroflow patterns and/or the amount of residual urine volume they may have. Frequency and urge incontinence often persist into adulthood (Mayo.1992, Yokoyama et al. 1989).

Management

Management of the urinary tract in affected individuals varies depending on the presentation, the severity of symptoms and the clinician's proclivity for full evaluation. In infancy, urinary tract imaging is probably not necessary unless there is a suspicion that an anatomic abnormality is likely, based on family history or prenatal ultrasonography. Most often babies have normal voiding and bowel habits. It is only after toilet training is attempted that symptoms of incontinence or subtle signs of dysfunction may surface. It is important at this stage to reassure parents or caregivers who may become frustrated with the slow pace of achieving continence, as this depends on many factors including cognitive and language development and mobility. Ensuring that the child is well hydrated and on an appropriate bowel regimen are the first measures to institute

Table 16.2   Approach to the child with cerebral palsy based on symptomatology

Asymptomatic ambulatory child:

- Observation

Symptomatic non-ambulatory child:

- Regular (periodic) toileting

- Adequate fluid intake based on age and weight

- Avoidance of caffeinated beverages and foods as they may lead to detrusor overactivity

- Effective bowel management with ample high fiber foods & periodic stimulant laxatives

- Determine if baclofen therapy is responsible for urinary retention (bladder scan residual).

Symptomatic non-ambulatory child (persistent incontinence):

- Bladder scan for post-voided volume measure after a reasonable void

- KUB to determine colonic distension and fecal burden

- Renal ultrasound to assess bladder wall thickness and possible rectal stool burden

- Determine if baclofen therapy is responsible for urinary retention (bladder scan residual).

Symptomatic non-ambulatory child (recurrent non-febrile UTI):

- Bladder scan for post-voided volume measure after a reasonable void

- KUB to determine colonic distension and fecal burden

- Renal ultrasound to determine presence of bladder and/or renal calculi, degree of hydronephrosis, bladder wall thickness and possible rectal stool burden

- Determine if baclofen therapy is responsible for urinary retention (bladder scan residual).

Symptomatic child with febrile UTI:

- Same as for afebrile UTI

- Voiding cystography to rule out vesicoureteral reflux or another structural bladder abnormality

(Van Laecke et al. 2001, Van Laecke et al. 2009, Wyman et al. 2009). This cannot be emphasized enough as it has been shown that urgency decreases with increased fluid intake (Van Laecke et al. 2009). As the child matures, setting a defined and regular toileting schedule and encouraging him/her to void should eventually lead to a successful outcome for many, particularly those with sufficient cognitive capacity. In addition, an appropriate diet, minimizing caffeine intake, providing adequate fluids throughout the day and having a proper amount of fiber in the diet should help to encourage regular and timely bowel movements.

Regardless of the degree of success in toilet training, urinary tract imaging or residual urine measurements are not generally needed. It is only when medical intervention is being considered that obtaining a KUB, or pelvic ultrasound, to determine the degree of constipation (or assessment of rectal fullness) and residual urine measurements are necessary, to ensure medical therapy has not altered the ability to empty.

Management of urinary tract pathology such as stones, vesicoureteral reflux, and/or hydronephrosis is based on the same principals employed for treating those conditions in children without cerebral palsy. Children with complex cerebral palsy often take medications, particularly anti-convulsants, which may predispose them to kidney stones and may warrant routine monitoring. The key for the clinician is to considering this possibility when relatively non-specific symptoms arise (e.g. see Chapter 14: Pain and Irritability).

No specific surveillance measures are needed in this population, especially since the neurologic condition is not dynamic. If the individual is able to remain continent and empty the bladder at regular intervals without the onset of new incontinence, they can be followed expectantly, especially if there has been no deterioration in upper or LUT function. However, when assessing affected adults it often comes to light that they have suffered from frequency and urge incontinence for many years without anyone investigating why (Mayo.1992, Yokoyama et al. 1989). The key point here for clinicians is to ask patients and their caregivers about urinary symptoms.

Specific recommendations

Given the fact that affected children often have LUT symptoms, upper urinary tract deterioration is rare. Therefore, recommendations for evaluation must be cautiously promoted. Most patients can be managed initially with minimal investigation and conservative treatment, as outlined in the Management section. In those with frequency, urgency, and/or incontinence, initial investigation should include a urinalysis and culture to rule out UTI and if possible, a minimally invasive uroflow and/or a bladder ultrasound scan to measure residual urine volume. It is important to determine if the incontinence is the result of delayed signaling or awareness by the child, or an inability to get to a bathroom facility once the urge to void is experienced. Conservative measures, such as adequate hydration, closely adhered to timed voiding (or toileting), making sure the individual has regular and complete bowel movements and is not suffering from constipation, have been shown to reduce symptoms substantially (Van Laecke et al. 2009, Wyman et al. 2009). Baclofen treatment is a common treatment for spasticity but it can lead to urinary retention as it paralyzes detrusor muscle function (Vignes et al. 2007). If this is the cause for urinary retention, there is a fine balance between titrating the baclofen dose to reduce spasticity and emptying ability (Ordia et al. 2002, White. 1985).

Once considered an initial mainstay of treatment, antimuscarinic (e.g. Ditropan (oxybutynin HCl)) therapy is now only employed following implementation of an effective bowel management program that routinely empties the colon and rectum. Residual urines should be measured after this class of drugs is instituted. This is due to their potential adverse effect of slowing down colonic and rectal muscle function as well as detrusor muscle function, as antimuscarinics affect M3 receptors in the bowel just as they do in the bladder. Obtaining a KUB can corroborate the suspected stool burden as well as provide a visual image that enjoins the patient and his/her caregivers to consider other measures (i.e., stimulant laxatives taken at specific intervals to ensure the gastro-intestinal tract does not retain excessive amounts of fecal matter). If these routine standards of care have been initiated and if the judicious addition of anticholinergic medication has not resulted in resolution of urologic symptoms, referral to Urology for further investigation with urodynamic studies should be considered.

Recurrent, non-febrile urinary tract infection may be further investigated with renal and bladder ultrasonography, looking for the presence of hydronephrosis, renal parenchymal thinning, nephrolithiasis, discrepancy in size between the two kidneys, distal ureteral dilation and residual urine volume after a purposeful void. If any of these findings are noted or the individual has a febrile urinary infection then urologic referral for LUT imaging (voiding or nuclear cystography) is undertaken to rule out vesico-ureteral reflux, or bladder outlet obstruction. Increased bladder wall thickness (greater than 6mm in a bladder that is filled to at least 60% of its expected capacity) on ultrasound imaging may signify detrusor overactivity or detrusor sphincter dyssynergy that then warrants urodynamic investigation. In addition, children with other factors known to be associated with the potential for upper urinary tract deterioration (urinary retention, interrupted urinary stream, hesitancy) should also undergo urodynamic testing.

Conclusions

Although cerebral palsy is a non-progressive CNS disorder, urologic symptoms often only come to light as affected children along with their caregivers attempt toilet training. The evaluation of the urinary tract depends on the extent and type of symptoms these children exhibit. Management is based on a stepwise program that initially insures adequate hydration, appropriate diet, proper bowel evacuation regimens and realistic timed voiding schedules. Initial investigations should be non-invasive, with only more involved studies undertaken when minimally intrusive tests suggest a significant abnormality. Referral to Urology is necessary when non-invasive tests and simple measures as outlined in this chapter do not adequately manage symptoms or in the presence of additional confounding factors such as recurrent urinary tract infections, urinary retention or nephrolithiasis.

Summary points

- Most children with cerebral palsy develop awareness of the need to urinate at a reasonably young age as areas of the brain affecting urinary function are less likely to be affected by the cerebral insult that caused their cerebral palsy.

- It is usually the limitations of physical abilities or cognitive co-morbidities that lead to urinary incontinence; between 14% and 34% of children with cerebral palsy are continent by 5 years of age. The medical literature does not clearly provide guidance regarding severity of functional status and continence.

- Most children with cerebral palsy have normal lower urinary tract function; when an abnormality exists, detrusor overactivity is the most likely finding.

- Because the condition is nonprogressive, most children who achieve continence rarely develop problems at a later age. When they do occur, minimal investigations and conservative treatment are the primary approaches.

- Noninvasive studies include: residual urine after a purposeful void (to measure residual urine), renal ultrasonography (to assess upper and lower urinary tract appearance) and a KUB (to evaluate stool burden).

- Baclofen, a commonly used muscle relaxant, can inadvertently cause urinary retention.

- Oxybutynin (Ditropan) or other antimuscarinics should only be considered after adequate fluid intake, avoidance of caffeinated foods and an effective bowel regimen have been instituted.

- All children and young people with complex cerebral palsy, and/or their caregivers, should be questioned about urinary symptoms, particularly urgency and incontinence.

- Invasive urologic evaluation is only undertaken after conservative measures fail to achieve continence, recurrent UTIs take place or a febrile urinary infection has occurred.

References

Bauer SB, Austin PF, Rawashdeh YF, de Jong TP, Franco I, Siggard C, Jorgensen TM, Society ICC (2012) International Children's Continence Society's recommendations for initial diagnostic evaluation and follow-up in congenital neuropathic bladder and bowel dysfunction in children. *Neurourol Urodyn* **31**: 610–614.

Bross S, Honeck P, Kwon ST, Badawi JK, Trojan L, Alken P (2007) Correlation between motor function and lower urinary tract dysfunction in patients with infantile cerebral palsy. *Neurourol Urodyn* **26**: 222–227.

Decter RM, Bauer SB, Khoshbin S, Dyro FM, Krarup C, Colodny AH, Retik AB (1987) Urodynamic assessment of children with cerebral palsy. *J Urol* **138**: 1110–1112.

Ersoz M, Kaya K, Erol SK, Kulakli F, Akyuz M, Ozel S (2009) Noninvasive evaluation of lower urinary tract function in children with cerebral palsy. *Am J Phys Med Rehabil* **88**: 735–741.

Fowler CJ, Griffiths D, de Groat WC (2008) The neural control of micturition. *Nat Rev Neurosci* **9**: 453–466.

Gündoğdu G, Kömür M, Avlan D, Sarı FB, Delibaş, A, Taşdelen B, Naycı A, Okuyaz C (2013) Relationship of bladder dysfunction with upper urinary tract deterioration in cerebral palsy. *J Pediatr Urol* **9**: 659–664.

Houle AM, Vernet O, Jednak R, Pippi Salle JL, Farmer JP (1998) Bladder function before and after selective dorsal rhizotomy in children with cerebral palsy. *J Urol* **160**: 1088–1091.

Kaerts N, Van Hal G, Vermandel A, Wyndaele JJ (2012) Readiness signs used to define the proper moment to start toilet training: a review of the literature. *Neurourol Urodyn* **31**: 437–440.

Karaman MI, Kaya C, Caskurlu T, Guney S, Ergenekon E (2005) Urodynamic findings in children with cerebral palsy. *Int J Urol* **12**: 717–720.

Mayo ME (1992) Lower urinary tract dysfunction in cerebral palsy. *J Urol* **147**: 419–420.

Murphy KP, Boutin SA, Ide KR (2012) Cerebral palsy, neurogenic bladder, and outcomes of life-time care. *Dev Med Child Neurol* **54**: 945–950.

Ordia JI, Fischer E, Adamski E, Chagnon KG, Spatz EL (2002) Continuous intrathecal baclofen infusion by a programmable pump in 131 consecutive patients with severe spasticity of spinal origin. *Neuromodulation* **5**: 16–24.

Oskoui M, Coutinho F, Dykeman J, Jetté N, Pringsheim T (2013) An update on the prevalence of cerebral palsy: a systematic review and meta-analysis. *Dev Med Child Neurol* **55**: 509–519.

Ozturk M, Oktem F, Kisioglu N, Demirci M, Altuntas I, Kutluhan S, Dogan M (2006) Bladder and bowel control in children with cerebral palsy: case-control study. *Croat Med J* **47**: 264–270.

Rasquin A, Di Lorenzo C, Forbes D, Guiraldes E, Hyams JS, Staiano A, Walker LS (2006) Child-hood functional gastrointestinal disorders: child/adolescent. *Gastroenterology* **130**: 1527–1537.

Reid CJD, Borzyskowski M (1993) Lower urinary tract dysfunction in cerebral palsy. *Arch Dis Child* **68**: 739–742.

Richards CL, Malouin F (2013) Cerebral palsy: definition, assessment and rehabilitation. *Handb Clin Neurol* **111**: 183–195.

Richardson I, Palmer LS (2009) Clinical and urodynamic spectrum of bladder function in cerebral palsy. *J Urol* **182**: 1945–1948.

Roijen LE, Postema K, Limbeek VJ, Kuppevelt VH (2001) Development of bladder control in children and adolescents with cerebral palsy. *Dev Med Child Neurol* **43**: 103–107.

Samijn B, Van Laecke E, Renson C (2016) *Neurourol Urodynam*.

Silva JAF, Alvares RA, Barboza AL, Monteiro RTM (2009) Lower urinary tract dysfunction in children with Cerebral Palsy. *Neururol Urodyn* **28**: 959–963.

Silva JAF, Gonsalves MC, Saverio AP, Oliveira IC, Carrerette FB, Damião R (2010) Lower urinary tract dysfunction and ultrasound assessment of bladder wall thickness in children with cerebral palsy. *Urology* **76**: 942–945.

Tadic SD, Griffiths D, Schaefer W, Cheng CI, Resnick NM (2010) Brain activity measured by functional magnetic resonance imaging is related to patient reported urgency urinary incontinence severity. *J Urol* **183**: 221–228.

Van Laecke E, Golinveaux L, Goossens L, Raes A, Hoebeke P, Vande Walle J (2001) Voiding disorders in severely mentally and motor disabled children. *J Urol* **166**: 2404–2406.

Van Laecke E, Raes A, Vande Walle J, Hoebeke P (2009) Adequate fluid intake, urinary incontinence, and physical and/or intellectual disability. *J Urol* **182**: 2079–2084.

Vignes J-R, Deloire MSA, Petry KG, Nagy F (2007) Characterization and restoration of altered inhibitory and excitatory control of micturition reflex in experimental autoimmune encephalomyelitis in rats. *J Physiol* **578**: 439–450.

Wang M-H, Harvey J, Baskin L (2008). Management of neurogenic bladder in patients with cerebral palsy. *J Pediatr Rehabil Med* **1**(2): 123–125.

White WB (1985) Aggravated CNS depression with urinary retention secondary to baclofen administration. *Arch Intern Med* **145**: 1717–1718.

Wyman JF, Burgio KL, Newman DK (2009) Practical aspects of lifestyle modifications and behavioural interventions in the treatment of overactive bladder and urgency urinary incontinence. *Int J Clin Pract* **63**: 1177–1191.

Yokoyama O, Nagano K, Hirata A, Hisazumi H, Izumida S (1989) [Clinical evaluation for voiding dysfunction in patients with cerebral palsy]. *Nippon Hinyokika Gakkai Zasshi* **80**: 591–595.

Chapter 17

Adolescence and sexuality

Susan Hayden Gray and Laurie J. Glader

Introduction

Increasingly the topic of sexual health for adolescents with disabilities is being approached as a human rights issue. The World Health Organization defines sexual health as 'a state of physical, mental and social well-being in relation to sexuality…[that] requires a positive and respectful approach to sexuality and sexual relationships, as well as the possibility of having pleasurable and safe sexual experiences, free of coercion, discrimination and violence' (World Health Organization 2010). The American Academy of Pediatrics describes sexual development as a 'multidimensional process, intimately linked to the basic human needs of being liked and accepted, displaying and receiving affection, feeling valued and attractive, and sharing thoughts and feelings' (Murphy et al. 2006). This human rights approach lies in stark contrast to the anxiety and even panic experienced by many parents when considering the onset of puberty in their children with cerebral palsy (CP). Health care providers can provide a great service to families by making pubertal development and sexual health education a routine part of anticipatory guidance starting at an early age, prior even to the physical changes of puberty (Quint and O'Brien 2016).

Puberty, growth and physical maturation

It is important for practitioners to have an idea of what is normal in pubertal development to be able to advise families about abnormal development. Studies about the timing of puberty in young people with CP are limited in number and limited in the diversity of participants. Puberty appears to start at an earlier age in white children with CP compared to age-matched controls in the National Health And Nutrition Examination

Survey (NHANES) and Pediatric Research in Office Setting (PROS) studies, but is prolonged in duration (Worley et al. 2002). For white girls with CP, Tanner stage 2 pubic hair development started at mean age of 8.2 years (95% confidence intervals [CI] 6.7–9.2) and Tanner stage 2 breast development started at mean age of 10.1 years (95% CI 8.8–11.2). For white boys with CP, Tanner stage 2 testicular development occurred at mean age of 10.0 years (95% CI 9.0–11.3) and Tanner stage 2 pubic hair 10.7 years (95% CI 9.6–11.6). Menarche occurs later in white girls with CP (median age of 14, vs 12 years 10 months in general population) (Worley et al. 2002). Girls are considered skeletally mature and reach final adult height approximately 2 years after menarche; this milestone may be an important consideration in terms of timing of orthopedic interventions.

Children with neurodevelopmental disabilities, such as complex CP, may be at increased risk of precocious puberty,compared to the general population.(Siddiqi et al. 1999) The development of pubic hair, often accompanied by axillary hair development, body odor and/or acne, is common in children with CP, and may represent premature adrenarche of benign type. The literature is sparse regarding the indications for further evaluation of these symptoms, but if there is rapid tempo progression, or for girls who have additional signs of precocious development before age 8 or boys who have testicular enlargement before age 9, further evaluation is warranted.

Growth attenuation to maintain a small body habitus is an intervention that may be raised by caregivers. Generally, the interest in this type of intervention stems from recognition that caring for an adult who is entirely dependent on others for all aspects of daily living such as dressing, diapering, bathing and transfers, can be challenging for the caregiver. Quite often caregivers seeking growth attenuation are doing so out of a desire to continue being able to easily physically care for their child into adulthood. However, this type of intervention is controversial, is not supported by organizations such as the American Association on Intellectual and Developmental Disabilities, and is generally not pursued. Any decisions regarding growth attenuation merit consultation with an ethicist.

Menarche and menstrual management

In one survey of families of young women with CP, more than half sought medical guidance about managing menses before menarche in their children. The amount of parental anxiety generated was directly proportional to the severity of disability of the child (Zacharin et al. 2010). Our recommendation is that health care providers address the issue proactively before menarche occurs. Parents may dread the onset of menarche because it is a reminder of the possibility of sexuality or even the risk of sexual abuse of their daughters, or because hormonal changes may bring mood fluctuations, worsened spasticity, or catamenial (peri-menstrual) seizure patterns. For many, the added hygiene and personal caretaking responsibilities compound their anxiety, and may be amplified when caregivers are male.

1. Ensure all girls and their parents receive anticipatory guidance prior to menarche.

2. At time of menses: discuss hygiene, menses as a 'vital sign' (should occur about every 21–40 days and for 3–7 days at a time), anticipate plan for dysmenorrhea.

3. Assess regularity (consider using phone apps for family to keep track), hygiene, and impact on quality of life.

4. For primary dysmenorrhea: initiate trial of nonsteroidal anti-inflammatory drugs (NSAIDs) starting on first day of recognized menstrual period: ibuprofen 10mg/kg/dose up to 600mg every 6 hours or naproxen sodium 275mg to 550mg twice a day, with food, for first 2 days of menses.

5. For dysmenorrhea not responding to NSAIDs, desire to shorten or eliminate menses, or need for contraception: consider hormonal management. Reassess possibility of sexual activity at least annually and send urine gonorrhea and chlamydia Nucleic Acid Amplification Test (NAAT) if suspected or confirmed sexual contact.

Figure 17.1   Stepwise approach to menstrual concerns in young women with severe cerebral palsy

The presence of menstruation should be considered a 'vital sign' in young women. A normal menstrual period lasts from 3 to 7 days and occurs every 21–45 days in adolescents. There is slightly more variability in adolescents, especially in the first year or two after menarche, but amenorrhea lasting longer than 3 months should be investigated, regardless of gynecologic age (American College of Obstetricians and Gynecologists (ACOG) Committee Opinion No. 349 2006). Although menarche may occur at a later age in young women with CP, amenorrhea past the age of 15 years should also be investigated. A thorough workup of primary amenorrhea includes genital exam to confirm patency of introitus in addition to hormonal testing, and so referral may be indicated. Dysmenorrhea is common in most young women, especially after menstruation has been present for several years and ovulatory cycles are established. Patients whose pain fails to respond to standard doses of nonsteroidal anti-inflammatory drugs (NSAIDs) (e.g. ibuprofen 10 mg/kg/dose up to 600 mg every 6 hours or naproxen sodium 275 mg to 550 mg twice a day) should receive further evaluation and be considered for hormonal management (see Figure 17.1).

Many young women with disabilities and their families desire greater control of their menstrual cycles and request hormonal treatment (see Figure 17.2). As noted in the recent American Academy of Pediatrics (AAP) guidelines about menstrual management for those with disabilities, amenorrhea is often desired but is difficult to achieve and should not be promised. Sometimes regular periods at less frequent but predictable intervals are a more realistic goal, and health care providers should be open with families in setting and prioritizing goals of hormonal treatment (Quint and O'Brien 2016). Obtaining a medical history and a blood pressure reading are the only prerequisites for prescription of hormonal methods; pelvic examination should not be a requirement

Clinical situation	Consider using:	Notes
Patients desiring less frequent menses	Extended cycle (e.g. 42/7, 63/7, 84/7) or continuous use of monophasic COCs, the contraceptive vaginal ring, or contraceptive patch[a]	This dosing is considered off-label unless using an 84/7 pill, but can often provide predictable but less frequent menses.
Catamenial symptoms	Combined oral contraceptives, the contraceptive vaginal ring, or contraceptive patch (consider extended cycle or continuous use) or depot medroxyprogesterone	Catamenial symptoms such as increased seizure frequency are best treated with a method that provides consistent suppression of ovulation.
Patients taking high doses of anticonvulsants	Depot medroxyprogesterone or an IUD	High doses of anticonvulsants may lower effective hormone dose (see CDC Medical Eligibility Criteria, https://www.cdc.gov/ reproductivehealth/contraception/mmwr/ mec/summary.html)
Patients who have limited mobility	IUD, contraceptive implant, or progestin-only oral contraceptive	Patients with limited mobility may be at higher risk of thrombosis with estrogen containing contraceptives. Patients with limited mobility may also be at higher risk of loss of bone density with prolonged use of depot medroxyprogesterone.

Figure 17.2 Special clinical situations for hormonal management in young women with severe cerebral palsy

[a]Extended cycle or continuous use of contraceptive patch may deliver a higher dose of estrogen and should be used with caution, families should be counseled about the possibility of blood clot.

COC, combined oral contraceptive

as this can set up an unnecessary barrier to receiving medication. The medical history should focus on potential contra-indications to the use of estrogen, such as migraine with aura or personal history of deep venous thrombosis or other clotting problems. For other medical conditions which are contra-indications to estrogen use, clinicians should familiarize themselves with the WHO and Centers for Disease Control (CDC) Medical Eligibility Criteria (MEC) for contraceptive use criteria available at https://www.cdc.gov/ reproductivehealth/contraception/mmwr/mec/ and the CDC MEC 2016 app in which risks and benefits of contraceptive methods are outlined (World Health Organization 2015, Curtis et al. 2016). There are no guidelines specific to CP, although the CDC guidelines (CDC 2016) do include recommendations for women with multiple sclerosis with and without prolonged immobility. More research about hormones and clotting risk in women with CP, and specifically about the interaction of mobility and clotting risk, is needed.

Estrogen containing methods (combined hormonal contraceptives)
Estrogen containing combined hormonal contraceptives offer the possibility of predictable withdrawal bleeding and menstrual control. Oral contraceptive pills are the most familiar birth control method for many young women and their parents, although the intravaginal ring and transdermal patch offer the advantage of less frequent dosing (monthly and weekly, respectively). The intravaginal ring provides the equivalent of 15mcg of ethinyl estradiol in addition to progestin – a benefit for those looking for the smallest amount of hormone necessary to control cycles – but it requires a certain amount of manual dexterity or a willing partner to insert. The transdermal patch provides the equivalent of 35mcg daily of ethinyl estradiol in addition to progestin and can be placed on the upper arm, lower abdomen, buttocks, or medial to the scapula – a position that may be useful in girls with intellectual disability who display tactile hypersensitivity or chronic picking behaviors. In patients with severe CP, interactions with other medications may require changing doses or may limit the use of estrogen. In particular the use of antiepileptic drugs (such as carbamazepine, topiramate, and oxcarbazepine) that induce hepatic enzymes may lower the contraceptive effectiveness of combined oral contraceptives, progestin-only pills, and the progestin implant and may produce more irregular bleeding. Lamotrigine is known to lower the effectiveness of combined hormonal contraceptives, and combined hormonal contraceptives also (conversely) lower the effectiveness of lamotrigine; dose adjustment or elimination of the pill-free interval may be required to avoid fluctuations in bioavailability (World Health Organization 2015, Curtis et al. 2016). Extended cycle (e.g. 84/7) combined oral contraceptives may provide less frequent menses in selected patients who are able to adhere to an extremely regular pill-taking schedule. Continuous use of combined oral contraceptives, the transdermal patch, or occasionally intravaginal ring are considered off-label but is frequently tried to reduce frequency of bleeding even further (see Figure 17.2).

Progestin-only contraceptives
Progestin-only methods include progestin-only pills, depot injections, implantable devices, and hormone eluting intrauterine devices (IUDs). The implantable device and the IUD offer maximum contraceptive efficacy and long-term use, but irregular suppression of ovulation and unpredictable bleeding patterns. There is limited data about long-term use of progestin-only methods and bone health for adolescents. The depot formulation of medroxyprogesterone acetate (DMPA) offers convenient dosing and excellent suppression of ovulation, which may be important in preventing catamenial syndromes, but its downsides are weight gain and bone loss in some adolescents during use (Cromer et al. 1996, Bonny et al. 2006) (see Figure 17.2). While most bone loss is thought to be potentially reversible, in a wheelchair-using patient with some degree of immobility this is an additive risk to bone health, and caution should be urged with DMPA use, and regular monitoring of bone density using DEXA (with

age-matched controls) considered. Use of another progestin, norethindrone acetate 5 mg daily, continuously for menstrual suppression is another option in those with a contraindication to estrogen. This use is considered off-label. This medication has been also used as 'add-back' therapy to decrease bone loss in young women taking puberty-suppressing GnRH analogs and has been associated with stable bone mass (Hornstein et al. 1998).

Hormone-free contraceptive methods
The copper IUD provides up to 10 years of contraception and offers the advantage of no medication interactions, but may increase menstrual flow and menstrual cramping.

Pregnancy prevention

Many patients initially requesting help with menstrual management may also want to use hormonal therapies for contraception, and they should be asked routinely and confidentially if they are having sex so that they can be screened appropriately for sexually transmitted infections. Despite having conversations about menstrual management and birth control, many young women with CP report that they have never been asked by pediatric providers about future childbearing plans. (Gray et al. 2016). In addition to discussion about sexual practices, sexual identity, and sexual orientation, we recommend adopting a reproductive life plan approach, as recommended by Centers for Disease Control and Prevention. The typical recommendation is to ask, the following questions regularly of all female patients: 'Do you have any children now? Do you want to have (more) children? How many (more) children do you want to have and when?' (Gavin et al. 2014). These questions are a simple way to open the door to preconception counseling or contraceptive counseling. For younger patients, the simple question, 'Have you ever thought about having children?' is broad and can similarly open the door to further discussion about fertility.

The potential for childbearing in intellectually disabled girls is an anxiety-provoking topic for many families, and discussion requires sensitivity and knowledge of therapeutic options. Some families of young women with profound intellectual disabilities request sterilization for their daughters. In general, this an option which, in addition to raising ethical questions, is less utilized due to the availability of long acting and reversible contraceptive methods. Implants or IUDs can be placed under anesthesia if necessary and have greater effectiveness than methods such as endometrial ablation, much lower risk of complication to the patient than surgical procedures such as hysterectomy or salpingectomy, and no need for a court order if the parent requesting the procedure has medical guardianship. It is important to recognize that all of these approaches only address pregnancy prevention. They do not address risk for sexually transmitted diseases, carry with them concerns about side effects, and do not address the deeper, sometimes unstated, concern of vulnerability to abuse. In general, when the issue of preventing pregnancy in a severely intellectually impaired woman is raised, it is important to address the ethical questions underlying the request, oftentimes through team discussion or even with ethicists.

Voluntary sexual activity and sexual history taking

Adolescents with physical disabilities alone are just as sexually active as their peers (Cheng and Udry 2002) (although the data on women with CP who function at a Gross Motor Function Classification System level IV or V is less specifically delineated), and they deserve access to the same services for their reproductive health. The importance of having access to confidential services is paramount, because adolescents may choose to forgo care if not assured of confidentiality (Ford et al. 1997). It is vital that practitioners separate the physically disabled adolescent from his/her parent to ask questions about sexual history, a habit that may not come easily when parents are used to being involved in many more aspects of daily care. When taking a sexual history, the CDC's recommendation is to ask about the 'Five Ps': partners, practices, protection from sexually transmitted infections (STI), past history of STIs, prevention of pregnancy (Workowski and Berman 2010) (See Figure 17.3). There is some evidence that physically disabled adolescents have higher rates of same sex attraction than peers, so asking specifically about gender identity ('do you think of yourself as a man, woman or neither?') and sexual orientation ('are you attracted to men, women, or both?') is important (Cheng and Udry 2002).

For certain patients with intellectual disabilities, fully confidential care may not be possible or ethical. For patients with mild intellectual disability who function independently in the community, having a confidential discussion about sex with a health care provider may be very appropriate. Patients with mild intellectual disability are likely to be as sexually active as their peers, and there is some evidence that they are less likely to use birth control or condoms, so it is important that they receive sexual health education and individualized health counseling (Servais 2006). In an ideal world, health care providers can involve parents in discussions about sexuality and contraception. If the parent does leave the room, it is vital that the health care provider is transparent with both the patient and with parents about what can and cannot remain confidential. Health care providers need to be vigilant in screening for coercion in this particularly vulnerable population.

Condom use is crucial to discuss because condoms are the only contraceptive method that also provides protection against STIs. For patients with latex allergy, polyurethane condoms are an acceptable alternative, although patients should always be encouraged to use two forms of birth control. For those with dexterity/coordination issues, the female condom is larger (and made of polyurethane) and may be an acceptable alternative.

1. Partners

- 'Do you have sex with men, women, or both?'

- 'In the past 2 months, how many partners have you had sex with?'

- 'In the past 12 months, how many partners have you had sex with?'

- 'Is it possible that any of your sex partners in the past 12 months had sex with someone else while they were still in a sexual relationship with you?'

2. Practices

- 'To understand your risks for STIs, I need to understand the kind of sex you have had recently.'

  o 'Have you had vaginal sex, meaning "penis in vagina sex"?' If yes, 'Do you use condoms: never, sometimes, or always?'

  o 'Have you had anal sex, meaning "penis in rectum/anus sex"?' If yes, 'Do you use condoms: never, sometimes, or always?'

  o 'Have you had oral sex, meaning "mouth on penis/vagina"?'

- For condom answers:

  o If 'never': 'Why don't you use condoms?'

  o If 'sometimes': 'In what situations (or with whom) do you use condoms?'

3. Prevention of pregnancy

- 'What are you doing to prevent pregnancy?'

4. Protection from STIs

- 'What do you do to protect yourself from STIs and HIV?'

5. Past history of STIs

- 'Have you ever had an STI?'

- 'Have any of your partners had an STI?'

- Additional questions to identify HIV and viral hepatitis risk include:

  o 'Have you or any of your partners ever injected drugs?'

  o 'Have you or any of your partners exchanged drugs for sex?'

  o 'Is there anything else about your sexual practices that I need to know about?'

Figure 17.3   STI/HIV risk assessment with the five Ps: Partners, Practices, Prevention of pregnancy, Protection from sexually transmitted infections (STIs), and past history of STIs[a]
[a]Workowski and Berman 2010.

Screening for chlamydia and gonorrhea is now easily accomplished by nucleic acid amplification testing (NAAT) of urine, vaginal self-swab, or vaginal swab obtained by a provider for those who do not have the motor control to obtain one independently, so full pelvic examination with a speculum may only be necessary in symptomatic patients if sexually active (e.g. vaginal discharge with itching) and for Pap screening starting at the age of 21. HIV testing is recommended for all patients at age 13, and after that based on risk behaviors. Other sexually transmitted infection screening is also based on risk assessment (Workowski and Bolan 2015).

Sexual abuse

The exact prevalence of sexual violence and sexual abuse in young people with CP is unknown. It is known, however, that both physical and developmental disabilities are associated with higher lifetime risk of sexual abuse, with estimates ranging from 2- to 10-fold increased odds of sexual abuse in children with disabilities compared to children without disabilities (Baladerian 1991, Sullivan, and Knutson 2000, Hibbard et al. 2007, Murphy 2011). Presenting symptoms in cases of sexual abuse can be nonspecific, e.g. problems with eating, abdominal pain, sleep disturbance, increased or newly identified masturbation, and mood changes. In most cases of sexual abuse there are no physical findings, so the health care provider must maintain a high level of suspicion. Perpetrators of sexual abuse are most likely to be male and to be known to the young person, including family members, friends, personal care attendants, teachers, and transportation providers. For adolescent patients who have the intellectual capacity to participate in a one-on-one discussion, it is vital for the health care provider to separate the patient from all care providers routinely in order to screen for sexual abuse and violence, and to create an open and supportive relationship with the patient to facilitate disclosure (the screening recommended by ACOG (2012) for adult women with disabilities available at https:// www.acog.org/Clinical-Guidance-and-Publications/Committee-Opinions/Committee-on-Health-Care-for-Underserved-Women/Intimate-Partner-Violence for screening questions recommended by ACOG for women with disabilities).If a patient discloses that sexual violence or abuse is ongoing, the first priority is safety. Consultation with social workers domestic violence services, and/or legal services may be indicated to intervene in such a way that the patient can be protected from an abuser who may be in close proximity during his/her daily life. Health care providers are mandated reporters of child sexual abuse, but may also be mandated reporters of adult sexual abuse in case of intellectual disability in adult victims depending on state law.

Prevention of sexual violence and abuse starts with patient education. It is vital that young people with CP receive medically accurate and comprehensive sexual education at home, at school, and in the clinic. Sexual education must acknowledge that sexuality itself is not inherently wrong, that it is natural for young people with CP to have sexual feelings, but then draw a distinction between sexuality and sexual exploitation. Physicians can also support prevention of abuse by advocating for Americans with Disabilities Act (ADA) accessibility of shelters for victims of sexual violence, increased education of teachers and care providers about abuse, increased availability of respite services for families under stress, and greater public awareness of sexual abuse of persons with disabilities (Marge 2003).

Problematic sexual behaviors

Inappropriate sexual behavior is sometimes raised as a concern by caregivers of youth with intellectual disability and complex forms of CP. This occurs most commonly among young men and includes behaviors such as touching of private parts or masturbating in public, or touching others inappropriately. These behaviors can create difficulties in an individual's daily life at school or in the community. In general, behavioral interventions should be recommended as first-line therapies. This can include strategies such as re-direction, reminding the individual of an appropriate time and place for the behavior, and providing opportunities for masturbation in private. Individualized behavioral plans working one-on-one with a therapist over time can have a positive impact. Parental or caregiver education about the normal nature of masturbation is an important element in addressing this concern. While pharmacologic interventions are often mentioned (and read about on the internet by caregivers) the quality of the literature to support their use is not robust enough at this time to support their routine use in clinical practice (Sajith et al. 2008, Coshway et al. 2016). In general, the goal should be not to eliminate masturbation entirely but rather to limit it to a safe and appropriate behavior.

Human papillomavirus vaccination and Papanicolaou testing

Human papillomavirus (HPV) is the most common sexually transmitted infection in the United States. HPV vaccination is recommended universally for boys and girls starting at age 9. We have found some parents question the need for HPV vaccination in children with CP because they assume their child may not become sexually active. There is limited data about the sexual behavior of adolescents with complex physical disabilities. Because predicting onset of sexual activity in any given individual is difficult, because many adolescents with physical disabilities are sexually active at the same rates as peers, and because there is increased vulnerability to abuse in this population, it is critical not to make assumptions, and therefore we recommend adherence to American Academy of Pediatrics (AAP) and Advisory Committee on Immunization Practices (ACIP) guidelines for universal vaccination, especially because if pelvic examination and Papanicolaou (Pap) testing are physically challenging, HPV vaccination may prevent the need for more frequent screening and intervention later in life.

Pap testing for cervical cancer screening is now recommended to start at the age of 21, and many pediatric providers prefer to refer patients to an adolescent specialist or gynecologist experienced with examining those with mobility limitations at this juncture. Strategies for making pelvic examination more comfortable in young women with CP include verbal preparation and description of examination procedures, allowing the patient to bring a person of her choice to help her position herself, breathing techniques, premedication with NSAIDs or with a benzodiazepine such as diazepam, use of a motorized examiniation table to facilitate transfer, use of alternate examination positions (such as knee-chest, diamond-shape, M-shape, or V-shape), use of a smaller

Huffman Pederson speculum, warming the speculum, use of anesthetic jelly for speculum insertion, or use of blind swab for Pap smear or HPV DNA testing (Cox, Signore, nd; Simpson 2001).

Where to find further information about sexual health

Parents often ask for health care providers' recommendations about where to seek further information online about sexual health. Depending on the question, the most personalized information may come from seeking consultation with an experienced urologist, adolescent specialist, or gynecologist. If a sexual education curriculum is offered at a student's school, an analogous program at a developmentally appropriate level should be offered to the individual with disability. For online information searches, we recommend that parents start at the National Library of Medicine website (MedlinePlus).

Key points

- Menses should be considered a 'vital sign' and a marker of health. Amenorrhea lasting longer than 3 months should be investigated, regardless of gynecologic age.

- Amenorrhea past the age of 15 years should be investigated.

- Obtaining a medical history and a blood pressure reading are the only prerequisites for prescription of hormonal interventions for menstrual management or contraception; pelvic examination should not be a requirement.

- Masturbation is common and may become problematic if it occurs in inappropriate settings. In general, it can be managed with behavioral interventions; the goal should be not to eliminate masturbation entirely but rather to limit it to a safe and appropriate behavior.

- Adherence to AAP and ACIP guidelines for universal HPV vaccination is recommended.

References

ACOG Committee Opinion No. 349 (2006) Menstruation in girls and adolescents: using the menstrual cycle as a vital sign. *Obstet Gynecol* **118** : 1323–8.

ACOG (2012) 'Intimate partner violence: Committee opinion no. 518', *Obstetrics & Gynecology*, 119, pp. 412–417. doi: 10.1097/AOG.0b013e318249ff74.

Baladerian NJ (1991) Sexual abuse of people with developmental disabilities. *Sexuality and Disability* **9** : 323–35.

Bonny AE, Ziegler J, Harvey R, Debanne SM, Secic M, Cromer B (2006) Weight gain in obese and nonobese adolescent girls initiating depot medroxyprogesterone, oral contraceptive pills, or no hormonal contraceptive method. *Arch Pediatr Adolesc Med* **160**: 40–5.

CDC (2016) US Medical Eligibility Criteria (US MEC) for Contraceptive Use, 2016. Available at www.cdc.gov/reproductivehealth/contraception/mmwr/mec/ and the CDC MEC 2016 app.

Cheng MM, Udry JR (2002) Sexual behaviors of physically disabled adolescents in the United States. *J Adolesc Health* **31** (1): 48–58.

Coshway L, Broussard J, Acharya K, Fried K, Msall ME, Lantos JD, Nahata L (2016) Medical therapy for inappropriate sexual behaviors in a teen with autism spectrum disorder. *Pediatrics* **137**: e20154366-e20154366.

Cox RL, Signore C, Q. E. (nd) *Reproductive Health Care for Women with Disabilities, ACOG.* Available at: http://www.acog.org/About-ACOG/ACOG-Departments/Women-with-Disabilities/Interactive-site-for-clinicians-serving-women-with-disabilities (Accessed: 27 September 2016).

Cromer BA, Blair JMA, Mahan JD, Zibners L, Naumovski Z (1996) A prospective comparison of bone density in adolescent girls receiving depot medroxyprogesterone acetate (Depo-Provera), levonorgestrel (Norplant), or oral contraceptives. *J Pediatrics* **129** : 671–6.

Curtis KM, Tepper NK, Jatlaoui TC, Berry-Bibee E, Horton LG, Zapata LB, et al. (2016) U.S. Medical Eligibility Criteria for Contraceptive Use 2016. MMWR Recomm Rep **65** (3): 1–103.

Ford CA, Millstein SG, Halpern-Felsher BL, Irwin CE (1997) Influence of physician confidentiality assurances on adolescents willingness to disclose information and seek future health care. A randomized controlled trial. *JAMA* **278** : 1029–34.

Gavin L, Moskosky S, Carter M, Curtis K, Glass E, Godfrey E, et al. (2014) Providing quality family planning. *MMWR Recomm Rep* **63** : 1–60.

Gray SH, Wylie M, Bloom Z, Byrne R, Glader, L (2016) Reproductive health education received by young women with cerebral palsy. Poster presented at Pediatric Academic Societies, Baltimore, MD.

Hibbard RA, Desch LW, American Academy of Pediatrics Committee on Child Abuse Neglect and American Academy of Pediatrics Council on Children With Disabilities (2007) Maltreatment of children with disabilities. *Pediatrics* **119** : 1018–25.

Hornstein MD, Surrey ES, Weisberg GW, Casino LA (1998) Leuprolide acetate depot and hormonal add-back in endometriosis: a 12-month study. Lupron Add-Back Study Group. *Obstet Gynecol* **91** : 16–24.

Marge DK (2003) A Call to Action: Ending Crimes of Violence against Children and Adults with Disabilities: A report to the Nation 2003. Syracuse, NY: SUNY Upstate Medical University Duplicating and Printing Services.

Murphy N (2011) Maltreatment of children with disabilities: the breaking point. *J Child Neurology* **26** : 1054–1056.

Murphy NA, Elias ER (2006) Sexuality of children and adolescents with developmental disabilities. *Pediatrics* **118** : 398–403.

Quint EH, O'Brien RF (2016) Menstrual management for adolescents with disabilities. *Pediatrics* **137**:e20160295.

Sajith SG, Morgan C, Clarke D (2008) Pharmacological management of inappropriate sexual behaviours: A review of its evidence, rationale and scope in relation to men with intellectual disabilities. *J Intellect Disabli Res* **52**(12) 1078–90.

Servais L (2006) Sexual health care in persons with intellectual disabilities. *Ment Retard Dev Disabil Res Rev* **12** : 48–56.

Siddiqi SU, Van Dyke DC, Donohoue P, McBrien DM (1999) 'Premature sexual development in individuals with neurodevelopmental disabilities', *Dev Med d Child Neurol* 41:, 392–95. doi: 10.1017/S0012162299000857.

Simpson KM (2001) Table Manners and Beyond The Gynecological Exam for Women with Developmental Disabilities. Available at http://lurie.brandeis.edu/pdfs/TableMannersandBeyond.pdf

Sullivan PM, Knutson JF (2000) Maltreatment and disabilities: a population-based epidemiological study. *Child Abuse Neg* 24 : 1257–1273.

Workowski KA, Berman S (2010) Sexually transmitted diseases treatment guidelines. *MMWR Recomm Rep* : 1–110.

Workowski KA, Bolan G. (2015) Sexually transmitted diseases treatment guidelines. *MMWR Recomm Rep* 64: 1–137.

World Health Organization (2010) *Developing Sexual Health Programmes. A Framework for Action.* Geneva: World Health Organization.

World Health Organization (2010) 'Developing sexual health programmes. A framework for action', Geneva: World Health Organization, p. 55.

World Health Organization (2015) *Medical Eligibility for Contraceptive Use*. Geneva: World Health Organization.

Worley G, Houlihan CM, Herman-Giddens ME, O'Donnell ME, Conaway M, Stallings VA, et al. (2002) Secondary sexual characteristics in children with cerebral palsy and moderate to severe motor impairment: a cross-sectional survey. *Pediatrics* 110 : 897–902.

Zacharin M, Savasi I, Grover S (2010) The impact of menstruation in adolescents with disabilities related to cerebral palsy. *Arch Dis Child* 95 : 526–31.

Further resources

For sites specific to reproductive and sexual health, we include several suggestions. Boston Children's Hospital adolescent health websites http://youngwomenshealth.org and http://youngmenshealthsite.org include medically accurate, curated posts about puberty and a wide variety of sexual health topics. The state of Massachusetts has developed an excellent detailed guide with condition-specific resources – www.mass.gov/eohhs/docs/dph/com-health/prevention/hrhs-sexuality-and-disability-resource-guide.pdf . The Center for Parent Information and Resources – www.parentcenterhub.org/repository/sexed/ – and the Sexuality Information and Education Council of the United States – http://www.sexedlibrary.org/ – both also have excellent materials on sexuality education. One website – https://vkc.mc.vanderbilt.edu/healthybodies/ – includes a free online packet 'Healthy Bodies for Boys: A parent's guide for boys with disabilities.'

Chapter 18

Transition to adulthood

Claudio M. de Gusmao and Kitty O'Hare

Introduction

As with most childhood-onset chronic illness, youth with cerebral palsy (CP) are more and more likely to attain adulthood. In the United States, approximately 750 000 youth with special healthcare needs transition into adult health care every year, with a survival rate exceeding 90% (McManus et al. 2013, McPheeters et al 2014). However, improved survival is not always equated with improved quality of life. The transition is often unplanned or poorly executed: fewer than 50% of transitioning youth report receiving adequate support to enter a healthy adult life (McManus et al. 2013). Often, entry to the adult care system for patients with neurologic concerns occurs at a time of crisis and with significant gaps in care (Davies et al. 2013). Even in patients with complex chronic conditions, this interval can be for more than one year (Wisk et al. 2015). In addition, transition to adult care may be delayed or never happen: neurologic conditions are common reasons for adult visits to pediatric emergency rooms (Little and Hirsh 2014). Often these patients are admitted. Resource utilization and length of admission in pediatric hospitals are particularly high for young adults with neurological conditions, such as CP (Goodman et al. 2011).

Many barriers have been identified that preclude a smooth and comprehensive transition. Health care providers may recognize the importance of transition planning but lack the time, support staff and/or appropriate reimbursement. Even when mindful about the relevance of transition, providers may not routinely encourage youth to take charge of their own health care and inconsistently discuss the practical financial considerations of obtaining medical care as an adult. Patients, caregivers and health care staff often express hesitancy and resistance to concluding a long-standing relationship, with difficulty in finding knowledgeable and accepting providers at the time of transfer. Poor communication in the medical system and a gamut of legal, financial and institutional hurdles further complicates the process (Oskoui and Wolfson 2012, Lariviere-Bastien et al. 2013, Borlot et al. 2014, Cheak-Zamora et al. 2014, Brown et al. 2016). Not surprisingly, patients with CP, as well as their caregivers, describe the current state of transition care as being inadequate (DiFazio et al. 2014).

More and more, various medical societies and governmental programs are recognizing that adequate preparation for adult life is a key component of adolescent health. In 2011, the American Academy of Pediatrics, American Academy of Family Physicians and the American College of Physicians issued a joint clinical report on the importance of transition care (Cooley and Sagerman 2011). This report led directly to the creation of the Got Transition program within the US federal government's Maternal Child Health Bureau (The National Alliance to Advance Adolescent Health, no date). In the UK, the Care Act of 2014 called for more routine assessment of children's day-to-day needs as they age into adulthood, and general guidance in supporting youth transition has recently been published (Legislation 2014, Singh et al. 2016).

Unfortunately, the impact on caring for patients with neurologic conditions such as CP has been minimal. To address the issue, the Child Neurology Foundation in North America developed common principles to be considered when transitioning the pediatric neurologic patient to adult services, leading to a consensus statement published in 2016 with endorsement by the American Academy of Neurology (Brown et al. 2016).

Transition of care is a complex intervention that bridges several domains, including pediatric and adult medical care, psychosocial and educational issues, and health care-delivery systems. A comprehensive review is outside the scope of this chapter. As such, we will focus on the medical aspects of transition.

Definitions

'Transition' and 'transfer' are often used interchangeably, yet they have distinct meanings. The Society for Adolescent Medicine defines *transition* to adulthood as 'the purposeful, planned movement of adolescents and young adults with chronic physical and medical conditions from child-centered to adult-oriented health care systems.' (Rosen et al. 2003). The emphasis here is on a *purposeful* and *planned* movement; transition is a gradual change over time. Transfer to adult care, meanwhile, is the actual moment of handover from a pediatric provider to an adult provider. Transferring care is often a source of stress for patients and families, as well as for their health care teams.

Adult medical care

There are substantial differences between the pediatric and adult care delivery models. Pediatric providers have been described as comprehensive and family-oriented, whereas adult colleagues may be disease-centered and focused on the individual (Reiss et al. 2005, Camfield and Camfield 2011). These differences may be particularly striking when caring for patients with CP, due to the multisystem and interdisciplinary nature of the condition. In adult medicine, there is an expectation that knowledge and management of disorders should be imputed to the patient, but these skills are not necessarily fostered during pediatric care.

Transitioning to adult care

With adequate attention to intentional planning over time, the transition to adulthood can be accomplished more smoothly. Several groups recommend that transition planning begin between the ages of 12 to 14 years. This age range is generally recommended as it allows incremental engagement by the adolescent in self-management as well as sufficient time for preparation before attaining the age of legal adulthood (American Academy of Pediatrics et al. 2002, Cooley and Sagerman 2011, Brown et al. 2016, Singh et al. 2016). Further, this is a good time to begin to assess the individual's potential capacity for self-management and the anticipated supports. Individuals who are likely to present with challenges in communication or cognitive impairments may be identified early and measures taken to maximize their potential (see Supported Decision Making section). Both general practitioners and specialists play a role in guiding patients into adulthood.

Primary care providers

Primary care providers (PCPs), also known as general practitioners, play an important role in the transition to adult care. Many families perceive their relationship with their PCP to be their strongest tie to the health care system, whether the PCP is a pediatric-only practitioner or a family medicine specialist. In multisystem diseases such as CP, transition care may be driven by specialists, but nevertheless the PCP is the central hub for ensuring that all transition needs are met.

Even when the primary care provider is comfortable in following patients through adulthood, there should be an effort to adapt to the adult model of care. This includes maximizing self-management and independence (to the extent possible) and ensuring appropriate standard adult care. Often adults with childhood-onset chronic conditions are less likely to receive routine care, such as vaccines or cancer screenings (Christman et al. 2013). Youth who are sexually active, or who are at risk of unwanted sexual conduct, should be routinely screened for sexually transmitted infections, including HIV. Cardiovascular health should be considered, with annual blood pressure measures and periodic cholesterol screening per guidelines. Women should be offered cervical smears and mammograms at appropriate intervals, as well as counseling on reproductive options. All adults should be offered colon cancer screening. Additionally, PCPs should screen adults with CP for mental health concerns, including substance abuse, depression, and anxiety.

Specialists

Specialists are more likely than PCPs to be based in a pediatric system and so to require a formal care transfer to an adult system. Within pediatric institutions, specialists who treat CP often work together as part of a structured multidisciplinary program; there are few such programs in the adult world. A survey of pediatric CP programs in the United States found that the majority of programs described a multidisciplinary adult program as the ideal end-point of transition for adults with CP (Bolger et al. 2017). Perhaps because of the discrepancy between the ideal state and the actual state of adult resources, only one pediatric program reported being at least moderately satisfied with its transfer processes.

For youth with CP, there may be some differences in specialist care needs when attaining adulthood. For example, most young children with CP are closely connected to an orthopedic surgeon. As the child ages, the need for surgery becomes less, while the need for habilitation and rehabilitation becomes more pronounced. By adulthood, patients with CP are less likely to require an orthopedic surgeon and more likely to require regular access to a physiatrist or other physical medicine specialist.

Practical steps to assist patients in the transition process

As previously stated, transition is a planned, purposeful process in the preparation of youth from a child-centered to an adult-centered care model. As such, a variety of flowcharts, algorithms and checklists exist to guide clinicians during the process. An example is illustrated in Figure 18.1.

Developing a practice policy

For primary care and specialty practices that set up an age limit or age range upon which transfer to adult care is expected, a clear written policy should be available. Rather than being a prescriptive document, this statement should ideally reflect the practice's philosophy of care toward youth with chronic health care needs. Essentially, it should outline the expectation of attaining adulthood and the steps that will be taken to assist in preparation for the adult model of care prior to the transfer.

Often, awareness of the transition policy is the first step in transition planning. As such, the document should be posted in a place easily accessible by patients, such as the practice website, posters or brochures. Starting at ages 12–14 years, it should be reviewed annually with patients and families until the handover to adult care is accomplished (Fig. 18.2).

Age 12–14 years

[ ] The patient/family are reminded of the practice transition policy

[ ] The patient is enrolled in the practice transition registry

[ ] Annual skills assessment is initiated

[ ] The patient/family begin to work with the medical team on a Care Summary

[ ] The patient is encouraged to spend time alone with the healthcare provider at each visit

Age 15–17 years

[ ] Annual skills assessment continues

[ ] A care plan can be developed based on the young person's skills assessments and personal goals

[ ] The patient is encouraged to perform more medical tasks, such as refilling prescriptions and scheduling appointments, insofar as abilities allow

[ ] The patient is encouraged to spend more time alone with the healthcare provider at each visit

[ ] Potential adult specialists are identified

[ ] The care summary is updated at least annually, or with any critical change in status

[ ] Adult vocational planning is underway at school

[ ] Plans are being made for adult home life including recreation, social activities, transportation, self-care

[ ] Planning for limited or full guardianship begins

[ ] Financial planning begins, including assessment of adult insurance needs

Age 18–21 years

[ ] Care transfers from pediatric specialists to adult specialists; adult model of care is initiated

[ ] The care summary is updated at least annually, or with any critical change in status

[ ] The patient is encouraged to perform most medical tasks, in so far as abilities allow

Figure 18.1   Transition checklist

We at the Children's Hospital Cerebral Palsy Program are proud to serve children from birth to age 21 years. Starting at age 14 years, we will ask to spend a few minutes alone with your child at each visit, so that your child becomes more comfortable with the medical team. During this time, we will try to encourage you to take responsibility for their care and support them on their road to independence.

By age 16 years, we will assess your child's long-term care needs. This may involve different members of the care team and will assist in determining what services your child will need. If your child has a condition that prevents him/her making health care decisions, we will help you to consider options for supported decision making.

At age 18, children legally become adults. We respect and encourage a family-centered approach, but at this point we will need the young adult's consent to involve families in health care decisions – unless the need for supported decision making has been legally established.

We suggest that most patients should be considered for transferring to adult care between the ages of 18-21. We will assist with this transfer process, including helping to find adult providers, sending medical records to the new adult providers, and communicating with adult providers about the unique needs of your child.

Figure 18.2   Sample adult transition policy

Setting up a registry

Though all youth require some preparation for adulthood, youth with chronic conditions such as CP require more care and attention over time. PCPs and specialists should have a system in place for identifying the youth with chronic conditions in their practice. Many electronic health records have a registry development feature; a spreadsheet or simple list also has utility. Once youth with chronic conditions are identified, starting at ages 12–14 years there should be an annual review of their progress in transition care.

Progress in transition – skills assessment

Youth with CP have a range of abilities, both intellectual and physical. As the patient matures, their self-care abilities and level of independence may also evolve. Each patient's unique needs must be considered in navigating the road to adulthood. Many validated tools are available to health care providers to assist them to better understand how prepared youth are to manage their medical care as adults (Sawicki et al. 2011, Bolger et al. 2017). An example can be seen in Figure 18.3. Readiness assessments evaluate the young person's strengths in the domains of medication management, ability to schedule appointments, confidence in speaking directly with health care providers (rather than through a guardian), strategies for tracking health care tasks, and ability to manage activities of daily living.

Self-assessment for youth should be done on a periodic basis, perhaps once or twice per year, to set goals for a transition action plan. The questions on the readiness assessment can serve as a prompt for families to continue the preparation for adult life within the home. For example, if the youth indicates that they do not know how to schedule a doctor's appointment, then the family can coach the youth on this process. If the youth is unfamiliar with how to fill a prescription, the family can then invite him or her to participate in the next prescription refill.

One challenge with the available self-assessment tools is that they are designed to be completed by youth themselves. Individuals with intellectual disabilities should not be excluded from this process. Many may be able to develop limited self-management skills. In particular, patients with mild intellectual disability may be able to exert some decision-making capacity and often can become responsible for knowing their diagnosis, taking medication independently, and participating in their care (Wong et al. 2000, Suto et al. 2005). For youth with severe intellectual disabilities, the parent or guardian will be likely to continue as the main activator of care into adulthood. It is critical to identify this lack of capacity for long-term planning (see Supported decision making section). In addition, it is still helpful to assess caregivers' confidence in their caregiving role. For example, caregivers can be asked about their skill and confidence in scheduling appointments with adult specialists, or in finding an appropriate day habilitation program.

Patient Name: _____ Date of Birth: __/__/__ Today's Date __/__/__ (MRN# _____)

Transition Readiness Assessment Questionnaire (TRAQ)

Directions to Youth and Young Adults: Please check the box that best describes your skill level in the following areas that are important for transition to adult health care. There is no right or wrong answer and your answers will remain confidential and private.

Directions to Caregivers/Parents: If your youth or young adult is unable to complete the tasks below on their own, please check the box that best describes ***your*** skill level.   **Check here** If you are a parent/caregiver completing this form. [ ]

	No, I do not know how	No, but I want to learn	No, but I am learning to do this	Yes, I have started doing this	Yes, I always do this when I need to
Managing Medications					
1. Do you fill a prescription if you need to?					
2. Do you know what to do if you are having a bad reaction to your medications?					
3. Do you take medications correctly and on your own?					
4. Do you re-order medications before they run out?					
Appointment Keeping					
5. Do you call the doctor's office to make an appointment?					
6. Do you follow-up on any referral for tests, checks-ups or labs?					
7. Do you arrange for your ride to medical appointments?					
8. Do you call the doctor about unusual changes in your health (For example: Allergic reactions)?					
9. Do you apply for health insurance if you lose your current coverage?					
10. Do you know what your health insurance covers?					
11. Do you manage your money & budget household expenses (For example: use checking/debit card)?					
Tracking Health Issues					
12. Do you fill out the medical history form, including a list of your allergies?					
13. Do you keep a calendar or list of medical and other appointments?					
14. Do you make a list of questions before the doctor's visit?					
15. Do you get financial help with school or work?					
Talking with Providers					
16. Do you tell the doctor or nurse what you are feeling?					
17. Do you answer questions that are asked by the doctor, nurse, or clinic staff?					
Managing Daily Activities					
18. Do you help plan or prepare meals/food?					
19. Do you keep home/room clean or clean-up after meals?					
20. Do you use neighborhood stores and services (For example: Grocery stores and pharmacy stores)?					

© Wood, Sawicki, Reiss, Livingood & Kraemer, 2014

[a]Sawicki et al. 2011, Wood et al. 2014.

Figure 18.3   Sample transition readiness questionnaire[a]

Information from the transition readiness assessment can guide the development of health goals. When these goals are integrated with personal goals, a plan of care can be developed. This document can be helpful to empower youth to attain specific goals within a determined period. An example of a plan of care can be seen in Appendix 1.

Supported decision making

In the United States, if there is no process determining otherwise, competency is automatically assumed upon attaining the age of majority (18 years in most states). At this point, youth legally assume all the rights and responsibilities for making decisions, as well as a right to privacy. This occurs regardless of the degree of the individual's disability, and directly impacts the young adult and those providing care. While many youth eagerly anticipate the rights of adulthood, for families their decreased role in a young person's health care decision can be a source of stress.

Hospitals and clinics should have standardized systems for advising families of the legal changes to communication and decision making at the age of majority. For example, in most areas the legal adult has a right to privacy. Many parents are surprised to learn that they do not have an automatic right to information about their adult child. Providers should ask their adult patients if they wish to designate a proxy for communicating health information, then document that proxy clearly within the medical record. It is also important to document the patient's wishes for addressing emergency situations through a formal advance directive.

For patients known or suspected to have intellectual disability, special consideration must be given to ensure adequate support prior to attaining legal adulthood. Legal guardianship can have many hues, from full to limited – for example, to medical decisions or financial conservatorship. The age of majority and details of the legal process often vary from region to region, and some courts may require report evaluations from different providers as supporting evidence to determine guardianship needs. Reports may need to be performed within a certain time by diverse professionals, such as physicians, social workers and licensed psychologists. Practitioners should become aware of this potentially lengthy process and the laws and standards pertaining to legal adulthood in the locality where they practice. Advance preparation is key.

Therefore, if the need for legal guardianship is anticipated, starting the discussion when the youth are 15–17 years allows adequate planning prior to their 18th birthday. This allows time for arrangements such as consultation with a social worker, formal evaluations by a psychologist and/or neuropsychologist and legal counsel. Neuropsychological testing (when available) can be particularly helpful to illuminate patients' strengths in decision making as well as the areas in which they need support, and may support transition preparation in many ways.

Developing a care summary

The care summary is a written document that summarizes the most salient parts of the patient's medical care. PCPs can coordinate the development with contributions from different appropriate specialists. This is a critical task in assisting patients as they transition. This document can be invaluable whenever patients utilize a new source of care, be it an emergency room, a university health service, or an adult specialist's office. Some electronic health records can generate a care summary; there are also simple templates available online. Essentially, the care summary is a communication tool. With the summary, youth can more easily share the key components of their health history, as well as valuable personal information, such as communication style. See Figure 18.4 for a short sample version and a more comprehensive form in Appendix 2.

Transfer of care

The timing of transfer varies from practice to practice. A survey of CP multidisciplinary clinics in the United States indicated that age is the most common criterion to initiate transfer. Although an age range from 18–22 years old is typical for transfer consideration, a substantial number of pediatric practices continue to care for patients with CP over age 22. Other criteria used to complete the transition process include high school/college graduation, marriage and obtainment of independent living. Less commonly, some practices use pregnancy, substance abuse, nonadherence to treatment and payor source changes as transfer precipitating factors (Bolger et al. 2017).

A major barrier in providing an effective transfer is finding an adult practice that is prepared to accept the patient and provide the full range of care and care coordination. To the extent possible, practices should develop a referral network for patients with CP. This may include adult providers in the specialties of physical medicine and rehabilitation, neurology, orthopedic surgery and primary care.

Training exposure to youth with chronic illness, office systems to coordinate care with subspecialty resources and financial incentives may all potentially increase acceptance of youth with chronic health care needs into adult practices. Although adult providers have the role of assuming the care and management of these patients, they should not be expected to do so without supports that may be more readily available to pediatric providers (Okumura et al. 2010, Cooley and Sagerman 2011).

Once an accepting adult practice is identified, a 'transfer package' can help. These documents ideally include a transfer letter, care summary, previous assessment questionnaires, legal documents (if needed), a condition fact sheet (if needed) and additional provider records (if needed). A sample transfer checklist and transfer letter can be seen in Appendices 3 and 4.

Name	Date of Birth	Emergency Contact
Cell phone	Email	Home address
Communication preference [] Verbal [] Written [] Computer/device [] Gestures [] Other	Language	Insurance
Allergies 1. 2.	Medications 1. 2. 3.	Pharmacy
DME 1. Wheelchair 2. AFOs 3. Stander	DME Supplier	
Surgeries 1. 2.		
Current Medical Conditions 1. Cerebral Palsy 2. 3.		
Care Team 1. GP – 2. Physiatrist – 3. Orthopedic surgeon – 4. Physical therapist – 5. Dentist – 6. Ophthalmologist – 7. Gynecologist – 8. Neurologist – 9. Psychologist –	Address	Phone/fax
Additional Special Needs	Immunization Record Attached	

DME, Durable Medical Equipment; AFO, ankle foot orthosis; GP, general practitioner.

Figure 18.4   Example of a care summary

Ideally, pediatric specialists should become familiar with their colleagues in the adult world who treat patients with CP. Communicating directly with these providers ensures minimal disruption to the patient's health status. The pediatric specialist should remain available to the adult team if questions arise about the patient's history or potential course. Pediatric specialists are also encouraged to follow up with patients, to obtain feedback on the transfer process.

Conclusion

Transition is a planned, purposeful and staged approach to prepare patients to adult-centered care. Inappropriate or ineffective transition of patients with CP may lead to gaps in care and potentially worse health outcomes. We have proposed several tools to assist in the process. Limited evidence suggests that an organized approach to transition improves patients' knowledge of their condition, self-efficacy and confidence (Campbell et al. 2016). Nevertheless, several different models exist in the literature and there is much debate as to what approach is most efficacious. Much like other areas in medicine, quite possibly different approaches will work with different patients in diverse scenarios. Improving transition is an active area of research. Providers are therefore invited to review the tools here described and adapt to their practice according to their needs.

Key points

- The number of children with special care needs surviving into adulthood has dramatically increased in the last decades, but many barriers exist when transitioning to adult care.

- Various publications and guidelines have been published in recent years to assist clinicians in this process.

- Both general practitioners and specialists play a role in guiding patients into adulthood.

- Transition is best viewed as a process that should start early with a series of planned, purposeful steps in the preparation of youth from a child-centered to an adult-centered care.

- Evaluation of competency and the potential need for legal guardianship is an important element of transition. Legal guardianship can have many gradations, from full to limited.

- Six steps can be contemplated: developing a policy, establishing a registry, skills assessments, supported decision making, developing care summary and transferring care.

Further reading

1. Got Transition, a program of the US Maternal Child Health Bureau. Available at www.gottransition.org

2. Child Neurology Foundation Transitions (provider and family resources). Available at www.childneurologyfoundation.org/transitions

3. Pil-pil M, DeLaet D, Kuo AA, Peacock C, Sharma N. (eds) (2016) *Care of Adults with Chronic Childhood Conditions*. Springer.

4. Hergenroeder AC and Wiemann CM (eds) (2018) *Health Care Transition: Building a Program for Adolescents and Young Adults with Chronic Disease and Disability.* Springer

Appendix 1   Care Plan

Young Adults with Neurologic Disorders

Instructions: This plan of care is a written document developed jointly with the transitioning youth to establish priorities and a course of action that integrates health and personal goals. Information from the transition readiness assessment can be used to guide the development of health goals. The plan of care should be updated regularly and sent to the new adult provider as part of the transfer package.

Adapted from www.gottransition.org

Patient Name: Date of Birth:

Primary Diagnosis: Secondary Diagnosis:

WHAT MATTERS MOST TO YOU AS YOU BECOME AN ADULT?

Prioritized Goals	Issues of Concerns	Actions	Person Responsible	Target Date	Completed Date

Initial Date of Plan: _____   Last Updated on: _____

Parent/Caregiver Signature: _____

Clinician Signature: _____

Care Staff Name and Contact Information: _____
_____

Tool developed by the Child Neurology Foundation as part of the ACP HVC Pediatric to Adult Care Transition Project. Available at: www.childneurologyfoundation.org/transitions © 2017 CNF

Appendix 2   Medical Summary: Transitioning Patient

Young Adults with Neurologic Disorders
Instructions: This document should be completed by medical providers, in collaboration with youth and their caregivers.   Intent: This document should be shared with the transitioning patient's new medical providers, as well as the patient himself/herself and his/her caregivers, as appropriate.

Patient Name:	
Date Completed:	Date Revised:
Form Completed by:	

Principal Transition Medical Provider's Contact Information	
Name:	
Address:	
Work number:	Best Time to Reach:
E-Mail:	Best Way to Reach: Phone Email

Transitioning Patient Contact and Insurance Information	
Name:	Nickname:
DOB:	Preferred Language:
Address:	
Cell #: Home #:	Best Time to Reach:
E-Mail:	Best Way to Reach: Text Phone Email
Parent (Caregiver):	Relationship:
Address:	
Cell #: Home #:	Best Time to Reach:
E-Mail:	Best Way to Reach: Text Phone Email
Health Insurance Plan:	Group and ID
Limited Legal Status? (Y/N)	Tutorship (Y/N) Guardianship (Y/N)
Legal documents to be provided by parents of primary caregivers Please attach.	

Appendix 2 (Continued)

Health Care Providers			
	Name	Phone/Fax	e-mail
Primary Care Provider			
	Specialty & Name	Phone/Fax	e-mail
Specialty Provider			
Specialty Provider			
Specialty Provider			
Specialty Provider			
Specialty Provider			
	Name	Phone/Fax	e-mail
Occupational Therapist			
Physical Therapist			
Speech Therapist			
Behavioral Health			
Other			
Other			
Other			

School and Community Information			
Agency/School	Contact Person	Phone/Fax	e-mail

Emergency Care Plan			
Name		Relationship to Patient	
Phone (Cell)	Phone (Home/ Other)		e-mail
Preferred Emergency Care Location			
Special precautions (eg, seizure action plan)			

Appendix 2 (Continued)

Etiology (Check all that apply; describe)		
☐ Genetic/Chromosomal	☐ Prenatal Substance Exposure	☐ Prenatal Viral Exposure
☐ Preterm Birth	☐ Infection	☐ Acquired (eg, TBI, Submersion injury)
☐ Metabolic	☐ Other (specify)	☐ Other (specify)
☐ Unknown (specify)		

Diagnoses and Current Problem	
Primary Neurological Diseases	
Problem List	Details and Recommendations
Secondary Diagnoses	
Problem List	Details and Recommendations
Associated Behavioral Issues	
Please specify:	

Allergies; Medications and Procedures to be Avoided	
Allergies	Reactions
Avoid	Why?
Medications (List)	
Medical Procedures (List)	

Appendix 2 (Continued)

Current Medications (For prior medications, please complete final page)					
Medications	Dose	Frequency	Medications (continued)	Dose	Frequency
1.			7.		
2.			8.		
3.			9.		
4.			10		
5.			11.		
6.			12.		

Prior Surgeries, Procedures and Hospitalizations
Date:
Date:
Date:
Date:
Date:
Date:
Date:
Date:

Adaptive Functioning Domains (current activities)				
Communication	Verbal?	NonVerbal?		
Social				
Nutritional Issues				
Sleep Issues				
Mobility	Independent?	Aides?		Wheelchair?
	Other? Describe			
Functional Academics	Functional Grade Level:		Date Tested:	
	Full scale intelligence quotient: (if available)		Date Tested:	
Self-care				
Leisure				

Appendix 2   (Continued)

Work	
Community Activities	
Safety Issues	
Additional Information	

Equipment, Appliances, and Assistive Technology (note all that apply)						
☐	Gastrostomy	☐	Communication Device	<u>Monitors</u>	☐	Other, Describe:
☐	Tracheostomy	☐	Wheelchair	☐ Apnea		
☐	Suctions	☐	Orthotics	☐ Cardiac		
☐	Nebulizer	☐	Crutches	☐ Oxygen		
☐	Adaptive Seating	☐	Walker	☐ Glucose		

Additional Notes or Information Not Covered Above

Signatures	
Parent/Guardian Name (Printed)	
Parent/Guardian Name (Signature)	
Phone Number	Date

Primary Care Provider Name (Printed)	
Primary Care Provider Name (Signature)	
Phone Number	Date

Appendix 2 (Continued)

Neurology Provider Name (Printed)	
Neurology Provider Name (Signature)	
Phone Number	Date

Prior Medications for Complex Medication Histories (eg, epilepsy)		
Medication	Duration	Reason Discontinued & Comments

Tool developed by the child neurology foundation as part of the acp hvc pediatric to adult care transition project. Available at: www.Childneurologyfoundation.Org/transitions © 2017 CNF

Appendix 3   Transfer Letter Sample

Young Adults with Neurologic Disorders

[ADULT PROVIDER NAME]

[ADDRESS]

[ADDRESS]

[CITY, STATE, ZIP]

Dear *Adult Provider,*

Name is an *age* year-old patient of our practice who will be transferring to your care on date. The patient's primary chronic condition is *condition*, and secondary conditions include *conditions*. The following are included in the *Transfer Package*:

1. Medical summary and emergency care plan
2. Medications
3. Specialists
4. Transition readiness assessment.
5. Legal status: The patient *acts/cannot act* as their own guardian.

I am very familiar with this patient's health condition. I would be happy to provide any consultation assistance to you during the initial phases of transition to adult health care. Please do not hesitate to contact me by phone or email if you have further questions.

Thank you very much for your willingness to assume the care.

Sincerely,

[PEDIATRIC PROVIDER NAME]

Tool developed by the child neurology foundation as part of the acp hvc pediatric to adult care transition project. Available at: www.Childneurologyfoundation.Org/transitions © 2017 CNF

Appendix 4   Transitions Package

Young Adults with Neurologic Disorders

Patient Name: Date of Birth:

Primary Diagnosis:

Transfer of care

☐   Comprehensive transfer package, includes:

    ☐   Transfer letter, including effective of date of transfer of care to adult provider

    ☐   Self-care assessment, completed by patient or caregiver, as appropriate.

    ☐   Plan of care, including goals and actions.

    ☐   Updated medical summary and emergency care plan.

Appendix 4 (Continued)

□ Legal documents, if needed.

□ Condition fact sheet, if needed.

□ Additional provider records, if needed.

□ □ Sent on Date: _____

□ Communicated with adult provider about transfer. Date: _____

Elicited feedback from young adult after transfer from pediatric care. Date: _____

Additional comments/notes: _____

_____

_____

_____

Tool developed by the child neurology foundation as part of the acp hvc pediatric to adult care transition project. Available at: www.Childneurologyfoundation.Org/transitions © 2017 CNF

References

American Academy of Pediatrics, American Academy of Family Physicians and American College of Physicians, American Society of Internal Medicine (2002) A consensus statement on health care transitions for young adults with special health care needs. *Pediatrics* **110**: 1304–1306.

Bolger A, Vargus-Adams J, McMahon M (2017) Transition of care in adolescents with cerebral palsy: a survey of current practices, PM&R. *Amer Acad Physic Med Rehab* 9: 258–264.

Borlot F, Tellez-Zenteno JF, Allen A, Ali A, Snead OC, Andrade DM (2014) Epilepsy transition: Challenges of caring for adults with childhood-onset seizures. *Epilepsia* 55: 1659–1666.

Brown LW, Camfield P, Capers M, et al (2016) The neurologists role in supporting transition to adult health care: A consensus statement. *Neurology* 87: 835–840.

Camfield P, Camfield C (2011) Transition to adult care for children with chronic neurological disorders. *Ann Neurol* 69: 437–444.

Campbell F, Biggs K, Aldiss SK, et al (2016) Transition of care for adolescents from paediatric services to adult health services. *Cochrane Database Syst Rev.* CD009794.

Cheak-Zamora NC, Farmer JE, Mayfield WAet al (2014) Health care transition services for youth with autism spectrum disorders. *Rehab Psychology* 59(3): 340–348.

Christman MP, Castro-Zarraga M, Yeh DD, Liberthson RR, Bhatt AB (2013) Adequacy of cancer screening in adult women with congenital heart disease. *ISRN Cardiol* 1: 1–6.

Cooley WC, Sagerman PJ (2011) Supporting the health care transition from adolescence to adulthood in the medical home. *Pediatrics* 128: 182–200.

Davies H, Rennick J, Majnemer A (2011) Transition from pediatric to adult health care for young adults with neurological disorders: parental perspectives. *Can J Neurosci Nurs* **33**(2): 32–39.

DiFazio RL, Harris M, Vessey JAJA, Glader L, Shanske S (2014) Opportunities lost and found: Experiences of patients with cerebral palsy and their parents transitioning from pediatric to adult healthcare. *J Pediatr Rehab Med* **1**: 17–31.

Goodman DM, Hall M, Levin A, et al (2011) Adults with chronic health conditions originating in childhood: inpatient experience in children's hospitals. *Pediatrics* **128**(1): 5–13.

Lariviere-Bastien D, Bell E, Majnemer A, Shevell M, Racine E (2013) Perspectives of young adults with cerebral palsy on transitioning from pediatric to adult healthcare systems. *Sem Pediatr Neurol* **20**: 154–159.

Legislation Care Act (2014) Queens Printer of Acts of Parliament. Available at: http://www.legislation.gov.uk/ukpga/2014/23/contents/enacted.

Little WK, Hirsh DA (2014) Adult patients in the pediatric emergency department: presentation and disposition. *Pediatr Emer Care* **30**: 808–811.

McManus MA, Pollack LR, Cooley WCet al (2013) Current status of transition preparation among youth with special needs in the United States. *Pediatrics* **131**: 1090–1097.

McPheeters M, Davis A, Taylor J (2014) *Transition Care for Children with Special Health Needs, in Agency for Healthcare Research and Quality*. Rockville, MD: Agency for Healthcare Research and Quality (US).

Okumura MJ, Heisler M, Davis MM, Cabana MD, Demonner S, Kerr EA (2008) Comfort of general internists and general pediatricians in providing care for young adults with chronic illnesses of childhood. *J Gen Int Med* **23**: 1621–1627.

Okumura MJ, Kerr EA, Cabana MD, Davis MM, Demonner S, Heisler M (2010) Physician views on barriers to primary care for young adults with childhood-onset chronic disease. *Pediatrics* **125**: e748–e754.

Oskoui M, Wolfson C (2012) Treatment comfort of adult neurologists in childhood onset conditions. *Can J Neuro Sci* **39**: 202–205.

Reiss JG, Gibson RW, Walker LR (2005) Health care transition: youth, family, and provider perspectives. *Pediatrics* **115**: 112–120.

Rosen DS, Blum RW, Britto M, Sawyer SM, Siegel DM (2003) Transition to adult health care for adolescents and young adults with chronic conditions. *J Adolesc Health* **33**: 309–311.

Sawicki GS, Lukens-Bull K, Yin X, Demars N, Huang IC, Livingood W, Reiss J, Wood D (2011) Measuring the transition readiness of youth with special healthcare needs: Validation of the TRAQ – Transition readiness assessment questionnaire. *J Pediatr Psychol* **36**: 160–171.

Schultz RJ (2013) Parental experiences transitioning their adolescent with epilepsy and cognitive impairments to adult health care. *J Pediatr Health Care* **27**: 359–366.

Singh SP, Anderson B, Liabo K, Ganeshamoorthy T, Committee G (2016) Supporting young people in their transition to adult services: summary of NICE guidance. *BMJ* **353**: i2225.

Suto WMI, Clare ICH, Holland AJ, Watson PC (2005) Capacity to make financial decisions among people with mild intellectual disabilities. *J Intellect Disabil Res* **49**: 199–209.

The National Alliance to Advance Adolescent Health (no date) GotTransition.org. Available at: http://gottransition.org/.

Wisk LE, Finkelstein JA, Sawicki GS, , et al (2015) Predictors of timing of transfer from pediatric-to adult-focused primary care. *JAMA Pediatr* **169**e150951.

Wong JGG, Clare CH, Holland AJJ, Gunn M (2000) The capacity of people with a 'mental disability' to make a health care decision. *Psychol Med* **30**: 295–306.

Wood DL, Sawicki GS, Miller MD, , et al (2014) The Transition Readiness Assessment Questionnaire (TRAQ): its factor structure, reliability, and validity. *Acad Pediatr* **14**: 415–422.

Chapter 19

Evidence-based care: a tool chest for helping families navigate treatment options

Lisa Samson-Fang

Using the research to inform decision making

In a family-centered model of care, the clinician helps a family establish goals and choose from an array of management options realizing that their choice will be influenced by many factors including culture, economics, and the broader context of their lives. For the healthy child with a high prevalence acute or chronic condition (e.g. otitis media, attention-deficit–hyperactivity disorder), the clinician can readily stay up to date on treatment guidelines, side effects, treatment costs and alternatives and present the options to a family efficiently. However, primary care clinicians also care for patients with complex conditions of relatively low prevalence. For example, the typical primary care pediatrician might have within their practice three children with cerebral palsy (CP), two with Down syndrome, and one with congenital hypothyroidism, among many other low prevalence conditions. Staying abreast of the evidence and options for treatment for all these low prevalence conditions is not feasible. For these patients, the clinician relies upon consultants to maintain an up to date knowledge base and present families with treatment options. However, the primary care clinician may still play a pivotal role given the trust and long-term relationship many families have with their medical home and the fact that the medical home oversees the entire clinical landscape. The primary care clinician can fulfill this pivotal role efficiently for families who have children with complex CP if he/she builds a small but robust tool chest of skills.

Skill 1 Define the question or goal

The first step in any evidence-based practice is to define the question. Families often arrive in the clinical setting with concerns which they have yet to formulate into a specific question. A family may desire to explore evaluation or treatment without clearly defining what they hope to learn or improve. Much like the toddler who asks, 'Where do babies come from?' responding with, 'Why do you ask the question?' will result in a more fruitful discussion than reflexively answering the question at face value. A defined question will lead to a more specific discussion about how the evaluation or intervention desired will lead to a clearer pathway forward.

Example
The parents of a child with severe CP bring in a list of nutritional formulas they wish to try. Questioning reveals that their child is sleeping poorly and they feel the high sugar content in the formula is what is keeping their child awake. The questions become:

- Is the high sugar content in commercial formulas a problem?

- What is the role of the night feedings in disrupting the child's sleep?

- What evaluations or interventions can be considered to improve the child's sleep?

While there may be limited evidence to answer all these questions, the path forward including potential consultations, evaluations and interventions is clearer and more likely to result in the desired outcomes than simply responding to the possibility of endorsing or not endorsing a specific formula.

Skill 2 Help families understand why evidence-based care is important

Families don't necessarily understand that, as clinicians, we choose from an array of treatment options weighing evidence of effectiveness in the context of the clinical scenario, patient, and family. For example, we might recommend a therapy where evidence of effectiveness is less robust if we think compliance or tolerance of the most effective therapy is not going to be feasible. The extent that clinicians need to get into the details of this thought process when the condition is straight forward (e.g.. otitis media, urinary tract infection) is less than when a child's condition is chronic or complex (e.g. CP) where choices are often less evident and the need for families to be active participants more critical. If a family is guided to understand that interventions with a higher level of evidence are more likely to have the desired impact, they are better able to make informed choices. Choices must also factor in the subtleties of their child's condition, the treatment alternatives, the context of their family's needs and their belief systems. In the case of a rare condition, where evidence is limited for many therapies, approaching care in an evidence-based model may seem impossible. However, evidence-based practice should be viewed as being aware of the strength of evidence for desired outcomes (which includes the fact that in some cases there is no evidence) and making choices within that context. If families are able to understand that a lack of evidence of effectiveness of a therapy does not necessarily mean that it can never be used, caregivers may feel less overwhelmed when faced with such choices.

Skill 3 Help families get the information they need to make evidence-based choices

The challenges that clinicians face in evaluating a body of evidence for any given intervention are daunting. A primary care clinician is often going to rely on consultants, who treat such conditions much more frequently, to delve into the details. However, the primary care clinician plays an important role in helping families understand the information given to them by consultants, along with information they may have sought out on their own, and putting it in the context of the bigger picture of their child and family.

Families must understand that all research is not equal. Often families will have been exposed to 'research' that has influenced their thought processes without having the skill to process the quality of the information with regards to their child specifically. A common example is an alternative therapy website which cites 'research' that has proven the effectiveness of a particular intervention. Such 'research' is often a few case reports, testimonials, or a small descriptive case series. Even in the context of an academic study, families do not understand that initial studies are designed to be low cost and efficient with the purpose of laying the ground work for more definitive studies. Families may have been exposed to information through the lay press that outlines some observed clinical associations and may misinterpret this information as implying causation. Families may have learned that the randomized controlled trial is the 'criterion standard' but may not understand that there can still be threats to the validity of the study; that the study's characteristics may not apply to their child's situation, or that the impacts of the intervention were statistically but not clinically significant. In these situations, the primary care clinician can help the family put the 'research' they have been exposed to into a proper framework.

Ultimately, there is no perfect research and there are many interventions or outcomes for which no or only preliminary evidence exists. This should not prevent decision making or the use of treatments that show promise. Novak et al. (2013) reviewed the extensive research base for interventions in children with CP. The information was presented using the Evidence Alert Traffic Light System, which is a knowledge translation tool designed to assist clinicians to obtain evidence-based useful information efficiently (Novak and McIntyre 2010). A bottom line summary is provided to the health professional on a specific health condition paired with an 'Algorithm' outlining a logical path from assessment to treatment. The 'Algorithm' is color-coded with the level of treatment evidence highlighted as: effective, recommended by clinical expert opinion, probably/possibly effective, and not effective.

The American Academy of Cerebral Palsy and Developmental Medicine (AACPDM) has used this methodology to publish rapidly accessible and digestible care pathways for the clinician (available at https://www.aacpdm.org/publications/care-pathways). These care pathways are going to be most helpful for the specialty clinician who can put the specific treatments in context, but the primary care clinician who has developed a focus in the care of children with medical complexity will likely find them a useful resource as well. An example of one of the care pathways is presented in Figure 19.1 (Glader et al. 2016). Additional care pathways can be found at the AACPDM website (www.aacpdm.org).

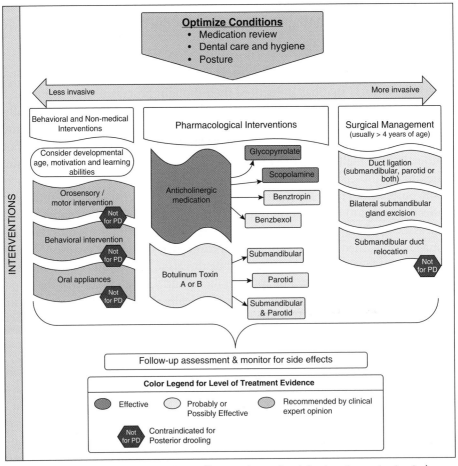

Figure 19.1 Example of a care pathway (Care pathway for sialorrhea in cerebral palsy)
Adapted from https://www.aacpdm.org/publications/care-pathways

Example

A 5-year-old with hemiplegic CP desires treatment for spasticity in the arm and leg to enhance function. Review of the care pathway on the AACPDM website shows diazepam, selective dorsal rhizotomy, and botulinum toxin to be green light therapies for spasticity in children with CP. However, in the context of hemiplegia, only botulinum toxin would be a likely consideration.

Skill 4 Support families in their decision making

For children with complex medical conditions, such as complex CP, families will make treatment decisions frequently and repeatedly throughout their child's life. There are some key tools (see Adams et al. 2017) the primary care provider can implement to support families and children through the following processes.

(1) Provide a framework for considering an intervention. Table 19.1 presents such a framework of decision making that clinicians can share with families to aid them for a wide variety of treatment options (Nickel 1996).

Table 19.1 Framework for family decision making for therapeutic options

What characteristic symptoms am I trying to target and does the treatment that I am considering target these symptoms?
What specific positive effects of treatment would I hope to see?
What short-term and long-term effects might I see with this treatment and how quickly should these effects occur?
What is the evidence that this treatment will result in the desired benefit for my child? If there is no evidence, does the theory behind the treatment fit with what is known and understood about my child's condition?
What are the potential side effects, including medical, emotional and behavioral?
Can this treatment be integrated into my child's current program including integrating with other treatments, other priorities for my child and family, costs and time limitations? Does my child have any contraindications for this therapy?
Do I need additional information from professionals or other families to make this decision?
Are there any red flags I should consider before proceeding (e.g. works for many conditions, improves a vast array of symptoms, no side effects, large profit margin with limited evidence)?
If I proceed, what should be assessed before, during, and after implementing the therapy to track progress? Who will help me with this process? How long will I use this therapy before deciding to continue or discontinue?

Adapted from Nickel (1996)

(2) Help families process the information they have collected from their own research and from meetings with specialists. This is particularly important when they receive conflicting recommendations. Often these mixed messages reflect different clinicians approaching a concern from their particular background and interpretation of the literature and may not necessarily represent disagreement between specialists. In other cases, it may reflect the fact that one of the clinicians misinterpreted the patient or family's concern, was not aware of a treatment option, or was not aware of the broader context of that patient's situation.

(3) Alert families to 'red flags' that should make them pause when a treatment is offered. These include treatments that claim to treat just about any condition or, within a specific condition, to address a vast array of symptoms; treatments that are reported to have major impacts but no side effects; treatments that are being presented with obvious bias; and treatments with significant cost but limited evidence of efficacy.

(4) Encourage families to share information. Families are often reluctant to disclose that they are using an alternative therapy or that they chose not to use a treatment or medication recommended by a clinician. Families may hesitate to go back to the consultant whose advice they didn't follow or hesitate to seek a second opinion, afraid the initial clinician will be offended. The primary care clinician can encourage them to be straight forward with this information and reassure them that, in general, they will not be judged or abandoned by their clinical providers. In the rare case a consultant is not able to continue to provide care for a patient, help them find a new resource.

(5) Be willing to support a trial of some controversial therapies in select situations but suggest clear treatment objectives and pre/post evaluation of symptoms.

(6) Remain actively involved even if you do not agree with the parents' decision. If you feel that their choice is too risky, such as pursuing a controversial therapy with real potential for negative effect or denying therapeutic approaches with clear benefits (e.g.. refusing an anticonvulsant in favor of a vitamin supplement in a child with frequent seizures), explain this clearly to the family.

Skill 5 Empower families to participate in research

The parents of children with conditions such as CP are often strong advocates for their child who want to contribute to the enhancement of care for all children with their child's condition. While there are many forums for advocacy, one forum is the participation in clinical studies. The primary care clinician can help families understand the process of participating in a research study, the pros and cons for their child, the role clinical trials play in informing the care for all children, and the measures in place to insure safety and confidentiality when participating in a study. The clinician can refer families to the clinical trials website (www.clinicaltrials.gov) to find relevant studies or provide input when a family has been offered study participation locally and desire guidance in their decision making.

Conclusion

Given the complexity of care in children with CP, the numerous intervention options, and the extensive and growing literature base, the primary care clinician is not in a position to advise a family of the evidence for most of interventions and outcomes. However, the medical home provider plays a key role in helping families define their questions, connecting them to consultants who can provide them with the needed information, facilitating their thought processes, and guiding their decisions within the broad context of their child's situation.

Key points

- Primary care providers can help families define the question or goal for treatment

- Primary care providers can help families understand the principles of evidence based care and why it is important.

- Families need assistance in getting the information they need to make evidence based choices.

- Navigating decision making can be challenging and families benefit from the trusting relationship they have built with their primary care provider.

- Opportunities to participate in research are often welcomed by families and should be explored when appropriate.

References

Adams, R., Levy, S. and the Council on children with Disabilities. (2017) Shared decision-making and children with disabilities: Pathways to consensus. Pediatrics, 139: e20170956. (doi https:\\doi.org\10.1542\peds.2017-0956)

Glader L, Delsing C, Hughes A, et al. (2016) Sialorrhea: Bottom line 'evidence-informed' recommendations for children/youth with cerebral palsy who have sialorrhea. AACPDM Care Pathways. Available at: www.aacpdm.org/publications/care-pathways.

Nickel R (1996) Controversial therapies for young children with developmental disabilities. *Infants and Young Children* **8**(4): 29–40.

Novak I, McIntyre S (2010) The effect of education with workplace supports on practitioners' evidence-base practice knowledge and implementation behaviors. *Aust Occup Ther J* **57**: 386–393

Novak I, McIntyre S, Morgan C, et al. (2013) A systemic review of interventions for children with cerebral palsy: state of the evidence. *Dev Med Child Neurol* **55**(): 885–910.

Chapter 20

Difficult topics and decision making

Jim Plews-Ogan and Richard I. Grossberg

Children with complex cerebral palsy (CP) and their families face challenging decisions across the lifespan especially when the child is totally dependent on care, non-ambulatory, or coping with multiple, complex medical conditions. Despite such challenges, families of children with medical complexity find meaning and purpose through their experiences and manage to integrate the many medical needs into their daily lives. Over time, though, these families inevitably have to cope with repeated hospitalizations and may need to grapple with decisions regarding out of home placement, in-home services, gastrostomy tube (g-tube) feeding, tracheostomy and mechanical ventilation, major surgeries, and end of life care. Finding adequate information and germane counsel to make these life-altering decisions can be its own task. What follows is a general guide to assist clinicians and families in approaching these tough decisions.

Starting the conversation

Clear, compassionate communication is the bedrock of every clinical interaction and the hallmark of a trusted, therapeutic relationship. Expert communication is never as essential as when we approach families in crisis or at a major life transition. Connecting with a family in the midst of a major transition requires skill and sensitivity that is continuously refined over the course of a career. It also means beginning with a clear-eyed view of our own implicit bias for what we think might be the 'best' decision.

Understanding our own biases helps us to avoid imposing our opinion before it is solicited, or perhaps responding with judgment, instead of compassion and curiosity.

Beginning with open-ended questions and using reflective listening will create trust. Acknowledging the strengths of the family will build a tone of respect. When we allow the patient to take the lead, and move from the concrete and ordinary to the less-defined and emotionally charged, we often end up with a family-centered agenda. Remembering to refer to the child and the parents by name and personalizing the conversation with shared reflections of the child's attributes helps to build connection between the family and provider. Another useful approach is to anticipate potential long-term decision-making and to mention possible issues as soon as the complexity of the child's status becomes clear but before decisions are required. For example, mentioning that 'sometimes children with complex CP need a gastrostomy' opens the door for dialogue before the urgency of a decision is required and may be more comfortable for both the parent and the clinician. These anticipatory, and often brief, discussions lay the groundwork for more difficult conversations later.

Approaching a charged topic

Approaching what we sense is a charged topic, we might begin with a simple question expressing empathy and openness. 'I'm curious. How do you imagine your child with a g-tube?' Or, 'How do you feel when you imagine your child with a g-tube?' An open-ended question such as this, followed by reflective listening, might easily lead to the family's fear that a g-tube heralds a major decline and a failure of sorts. Following this concern with more reflective listening and open-ended questions, we may well uncover fears about mortality, or relief that there is the possibility of sleeping through the night for the first time. It would not be unusual to hear a parent express a sense of guilt for 'giving up' on their child's potential. Or they may feel guilt for taking 'the easy way out' if safe oral feeding is extremely time consuming. Regardless, the process of reflective, non-judgmental, empathic listening gives control to the family, builds trust for the expression of emotional content, and allows us the opportunity to hear what is at the core of the decision for each family at any given moment.

There will be times when the family is not ready to begin a difficult conversation. Sensing or hearing resistance directly from the family, the clinician may need to become more directive. Beginning with our concerns and reflecting on the fear or confusion expressed we can help open up the conversation simply by noting the resistance. Removing physical barriers between the family and the clinician and moving a bit closer or being seated at the level of the child and near the family can create a more engaged environment. The clinician might gently express concerns to focus the conversation such as: 'What will we do the next time the child chokes or aspirates?', 'How will we come to terms with the weight loss?', 'Will we be able to control pain without surgical options?', 'What will be the stress on the family as care givers?', or 'What would you like our emergency plan to be in the next crisis?' Allowing a space of silence after the offering of concern, and reading the family's body language and facial expressions together with their verbal responses will help guide the clinician through the conversation. As the conversation opens up, the opportunity for more reflective listening and the expression and clarification of deeper emotions can herald the needed decisions.

Approaching conflict

Conflict can be frightening and complicated to manage. Avoidance of conflict may lead to a delay in having difficult conversations and result in continued aggressive medical care in the face of perceived futility or alternatively a delay in intervention when the team is fearful of addressing malnutrition or declining oral motor function. Some physicians are more comfortable than others in addressing conflict. Enlisting the help of others or mental health professionals may be useful when situations are particularly charged. Not all conflict is bad and conflict can also lead to growth and resolution when resolved in a suitable fashion. In fact, most stages of development involve the negotiation of a particular conflict that when adequately worked through leads to maturation. While not easy, working through conflict can lead to improvements in care and quality of life. Conflict, in and of itself, may be cathartic and lead to enhanced understanding and transformation. When managing conflict, the physician can help facilitate resolution by clearly restating opposing positions and then with the best interests of the child in mind attempt to create a compromise that all stakeholders can accept. As the situation evolves and changes, continued conversations with trusted stakeholders should continue as one navigates care across the lifespan. Even the most thoughtful plans may change as the child experiences illnesses and crises throughout their lifetime. Healthcare providers should be prepared to accept and work through shifts in care directives, even when parental choices are not what the clinician would recommend. In these cases, the clinician should be explicit about how and if the child and family will continue to be supported by the team.

It's complicated

Children with complex CP face countless interactions with the health care system. They and their families form relationships with a large array of providers, each communicating critical information and offering advice and opinions on optimal health care for the child. It is not unusual to receive conflicting advice or to be confronted with decisions that must be staged and prioritized. In fact, there may be no single, clear path. Families often face the perplexing challenge of sorting through the pros and cons of a decision that has the potential to help and to harm. In cases like this, the primary care clinician can be a trusted sounding board, and can help to sort through facts and offer perspective. We can identify resources and interpret findings. We can offer reassurance and raise further questions. We can help to clarify conflicting opinions, and offer reassurance that the patient and family will not be abandoned, even if the outcome is not what might be hoped for. Often, we support the family as they live with uncertainty. Being open to sharing their uncertainty can be a welcomed comfort. 'I'm not sure,' or, 'I don't know, but we will do our best to figure this out together,' can build trust and deepen the relationship. In many ways, learning to tolerate an enormous uncertainty is the best we can do to assist the family.

When a family hears from a sub-specialist that it's time for a tracheostomy, there may be concerns about how this will change what happens at school, or if school will continue to be an option. There may be real concerns and fears about suctioning, or responding to emergencies that may arise due to the tracheostomy. Families may need an opportunity to reflect on the long-term consequences of any such major decision, and may want to use it as a chance to explore the topic of survival and quality of life. Providing an intentional opportunity for the family to talk through all the components of a decision will allow for an outcome that is more authentic. Facilitating peer to peer support with other families who have gone through the procedure may be helpful too.

By clarifying goals and expectations for quality of life with the family the physician may be able to bring clarity when there is conflicting advice or conflict among family members regarding medical decisions. While studies or standards of care may favor certain interventions, each child is unique and their family circumstances, values, beliefs, and dynamics must be considered when making decisions on medical interventions. Respect for cultural and religious backgrounds must also be considered. Decisions may also be fluid and change over time depending on circumstances and experiences as the child ages. Likewise, taking time to sit with risks and benefits, 'doing nothing' while considering options, can lead to the 'best fit' decision in the end (Mack and Joffe 2014)

Take the time. Create the "space".

It is essential to remember that many complicated decisions evolve over time. Unless there is an emergency, the family and the team have time to engage in the process of considering all the options while carefully planning for the transition. The clinician will often need to be patient with the family through multiple appointments before a decision is made. Focusing on the process rather than the outcome helps everyone to allow for the space it takes to arrive at difficult decisions.

From time to time it is essential to set aside more time, or to clarify that the clinic visit is being set aside to talk through a new plan. This might mean that there are a series of visits to discuss a major transition, or that an hour is set aside for a longer, more detailed conversation. Understanding the limitations and challenges of reimbursement in a fee-for-service setting often needs to be factored into the planning for longer counseling visits. Likewise, selecting a time when parents are free from the distractions of child care so they can enhance the focus and efficiency of the conversation

Organizing a space and time for the intentional consideration of a major decision or life transition is the first step in being prepared for complex decision making. It also gives the clinician the chance to prepare and plan before entering into emotionally charged topics. After all, clinicians and families need the opportunity to consider the options, opinions, biases, data, trends, feelings, impact on family, available resources, finances, training, and readiness for change. Achieving all of this during a routine clinic appointment is rarely feasible, and it is often best to defer the conversation to a later appointment when everyone can be prepared and have adequate time.

Decisions about medical interventions may also evolve more gradually over time as families become more familiar with the healthcare system and the effects of interventions and treatments on their child's quality of life. While families may choose options that are not aligned with the biases of members of the healthcare team, what is essential is that team members explain options and choices and be clear about potential adverse effects as the family weighs the risks and benefits. Team members should be respectful of the family's wishes and remain active participants throughout the lifespan of the patient. By participating on this journey, we remain available to the family as their approach to treatments evolves over time. Decisions exist on a continuum from highly aggressive and interventional to more palliative, and may change rapidly during times of crises.

Who needs to be at the meeting

Deciding who should be at the meeting is part of every major decision-making process. Orchestrating the conversation involves skill, experience, planning and forethought, especially when we move into the realms of placement and palliative care. Managing competing agendas, fears, uncertainty, statistics and hope is all part of the process. At times, a pre-meeting will be helpful for the team to develop a plan for the family meeting. One comment or poorly worded statement can easily disengage an already overwhelmed family.

If a meeting is called, guests should be invited. It is important to include all key decision-makers. Thinking this through with the family in advance of the meeting is essential. If key decision-makers are not available or do not arrive, it may be best to reschedule the meeting. Limiting the numbers of attendees, particularly if there is sensitive information to be shared so as not to overwhelm the family, should be considered. Managing the flow of information needs to be balanced against the dynamics of the room. Planning ahead will contribute to the efficiency and ease of decision making. Stepping in to manage controversy or draw out silent parties is the role of the person coordinating the gathering. Often, it is best to run a family meeting with a team member who is skilled at group dynamics and managing strong emotion. Sometimes, it best to have several meetings over time, rather than try to get it all done in one fell swoop. Often, the family can only hear and digest opinions and options in small doses.

Come to the meeting with a pre-arranged, circulated agenda that allows the family to reflect on their concerns and questions beforehand. The agenda can be broad, 'We are going to consider the options for feeding,' or quite specific, 'We will review the details for out of home placement.' Assigning someone to take notes and assemble them afterward (or recording the discussion) can be exceedingly helpful and welcomed by the family.

Shared goal setting sets the stage

When shared goal setting (see also Chapter 2) is part of the routine care planning for the child and family, the most difficult conversations have roots and history within the relationship over time. Taking account of what is best in the day-to-day, provides the opportunity to plant seeds and raise questions that have future impact. When it is the norm to re-evaluate a plan from many points of view, we have the chance to forecast possibilities and listen for feedback. With some planning and experience, we can test the waters and provide resources in advance of a major decision.

As mobility becomes limited and the child grows, we can initiate conversations about help in the home along with the discussions regarding a motorized chair or other assistive devices as they are relevant. As we address limitations of expressive language and augmented communication, we can raise the issues of safety and autonomy. As we review the notes and recommendations of sub-specialty providers, we can explore readiness for change, and listen for points of conflict, confusion, or ambivalence.

The primary care or complex care provider can have a pivotal role in helping families to negotiate the process of moving through major transitions and decisions, by orchestrating the conversations, providing information, pacing the process, and facilitating the coordination of everyone involved. When a provider has a longitudinal relationship with the family, they can be especially poised to anticipate and manage conflict, and respond to common defenses.

Managing defenses

Defenses are employed when the mind is overwhelmed or in conflict and anxiety is heightened. Defenses generally exist on a continuum from more primitive and less healthy to more mature and helpful, and one's personality and temperament may influence the use of a particular set of defenses.

The defenses we employ occur largely outside of our consciousness. Appreciating when one is encountering a defense can aid in managing discussions and when done tactfully can expose what may be lying beneath in the service of expanding awareness and deepening the conversation. (Grossberg 2008). Less mature defenses may serve to provoke the health care team to become reactive and an awareness of this dynamic may enable members of the health care team to remain more reflective and empathic and avoid making matters worse. When feeling provoked, angry, or frustrated it may be helpful to take a moment to reflect. This more reflective stance will maintain open dialogue and preserve empathy and allow the physician to more appreciate the vulnerability that likely lies beneath.

A list of typically observed defenses, with definitions and examples, are included in Table 20.1. When encountering defenses, the physician may want to address the anxiety that is leading to the defensive posture. This can be difficult and physicians not comfortable with managing conflict and anxiety may want to include social workers or

Table 20.1   Common emotional defenses

Defense	Description	Example
Denial	Distortion or not perceiving a reality as it is too painful	Parent sees feeding as pleasurable when child is showing signs of refusal, pushing for aggressive interventions with little chance for recovery
Intellectualization	Overvaluing thinking and undervaluing feeling	Father insists upon use of hyperbaric oxygen due to claims on internet and shows little if any emotion regarding child's condition
Splitting	Seeing things as 'all good or all bad'; black and white thinking	Parent insists on seeing only one particular physician or only certain staff can care for patient
Projection	Placing one's feeling onto another	Child with near drowning - the family often make caregivers feel guilty about perceived lapses in care at home
Reaction formation	Turning a feeling into its opposite; love turns into hate	Rather than experience more ambivalent emotions about having a child with disability a mother becomes overly devoted and selfless while neglecting self needs, spouse and sibling
Sublimation	Creating less hostile ways to manage negative emotions	Redirection of emotion into positive advocacy through participation in disability rights organizations

psychologists if available to aid in the process. In general, members of the healthcare team most familiar with the patient and family should lead the conversation. When encountering denials over feeding ability or malnutrition, it is helpful for the physician to sensitively state the reality before them. For example, when a patient has significant oral motor dysfunction which is not appreciated by the family, a clinician might say, 'I notice when you are feeding your child by mouth that they are clenching their jaw and turning their head. This made me feel they may be frightened by feeding orally. Did you notice that?' Often the family may not be recognizing these behaviors in their desire to continue oral feeds. Similarly, using growth charts to visually demonstrate the degree of malnutrition may increase awareness of the level of malnutrition. Feeding may be a significant part of the attachment between parent and child, and fears of losing that interaction may fuel denials around feeding abilities and degree of malnutrition. Educational interventions about gastrostomy feedings and particularly focusing on the opportunity to continue oral feeding may relieve anxieties. 'You will still be feeding your child – just differently.'

For parents who are highly intellectualized, it is helpful for the physician to speak to the feelings that may not be apparent by directly asking. 'This must be hard for you, how are you feeling about the frequent pneumonias? I wonder if you're frightened or scared.' By simply labeling the feelings for them you may open up emotion and lessen the focus on medical interventions. When encountering a parent who may be neglecting their own self-care needs, a spouse or sibling in the service of what appears to be a selfless devotion to their disabled child, it may be helpful to bring this dynamic to their attention by asking what they do for themselves or if they can spend time with their partner or siblings. Providing opportunities for respite and encouraging the need for the caregiver to engage in self care can be helpful. Often family members may feel this dynamic but are afraid to address it within the family. An astute physician can recognize this and open up dialogue. Support groups and family therapy may also be helpful.

For parents with more externalizing defenses such as projections or splitting, particularly when there may be comorbid mental illness or a personality disorder, it is helpful to encourage psychotherapy or involvement with mental health professionals. Even when the physician may not be able to change the behavior of the parent it remains helpful to recognize the defensive process so one does not take the behavior personally or respond reactively. As stated earlier, it is helpful when one notes a break in one's own empathy to try to appreciate the underlying dynamic and presence of a defense at play. Educating staff about this dynamic may be helpful so they too do not become reactive. Families who may feel guilty or responsible for their child's impairment from a near drowning or shaken baby syndrome may project their guilt onto healthcare providers and find ways to make those involved in their care to feel guilty. This can present as constant complaints about care issues or making the physician feel as if they are missing a diagnosis. Again, while it may be difficult to stop this dynamic, encouraging the healthcare team to not personalize the accusations may go a long way to disarm the potential for escalating conflict.

Major transitions and challenges in care

Families caring for children with complex CP require a variety of resources in the home. Locating and managing the resources can become a full-time job. The types and intensity of resources can vary over a lifespan, and generally includes community and government sponsored services. Having a clear working knowledge of the necessary and available resources is essential to the comprehensive team management of children with complex CP. Helping families to navigate the options is also an on-going role for the team, while guiding the major transitions in care may fall to the primary clinician.

Obtaining the needed services and entitlements can be overwhelming and confusing. Families may not be prepared to adequately advocate for their child, and may benefit from voluntary or professional assistance. Creating a stepwise plan helps to break down the complexity of the process. Role playing a conversation allows the parent a chance to practice what they might say when advocating for services. Linking families with mentors and peers can prove extremely effective.

Parents often describe the stress of having hired help in the home often feels like having a stranger living with you. They describe the crisis that ensues when in-home providers quit or move away. Not only is there a gap in services, but the child often suffers the loss of a trusted individual who has been providing highly personalized and trusted care. As their primary clinician, we can help to facilitate the process, advocate for services, troubleshoot dilemmas and provide a sounding board for families as they negotiate the in-home care for their child with complex needs.

Out of home care

For any number of reasons, families may elect full or part-time care out of the home. This is always a major life transition for the child and the family, and generally develops over time. Families benefit from the opportunity to talk through the pros and cons, speaking frankly about what they perceive would be best for the child and the entire family.

Some families may be unable to care for their child or may be separated from their child due to abuse/neglect or other legal constraints, necessitating out of home options. Options for out of home care range from foster or adoptive care to group homes and larger congregate care facilities. (Friedman and Norwood 2016) Availability and funding will vary by country and state. Shared parenting is another arrangement that allows the child to remain with trusted friends or family rather than be placed in a facility. In general, group homes and larger facilities within the US are licensed as either Intermediate Care Facilities for the Developmentally Disabled (ICF/DD) or Skilled Nursing Facility (SNF) with varying levels of care. Regardless, most include access to nursing, direct care staff, allied therapy and educational services. Residential care facilities exist in a range of settings, from a small four bed group home with a job coach and community based medical care, to a larger facility with 50–100 beds providing a full nursing and medical staff and on-site access to educational, vocational, recreational and allied therapy services. More specialized centers have access to services akin to those found in a rehabilitation facility and include ventilator care. Residents of congregate care facilities are at greater risk of exposure to infections. Many of these specialized facilities in the US are members of an organization known as the Pediatric Complex Care Organization. Their website contains a directory of facilities (www.pediatriccomplexcare.org).

In addition to medical and nursing services, many facilities also have in-house schools and vocational programs, recreational programs including arts, camps, and allied therapy. Transitional long-term acute care varies by location and may be provided in specialty hospitals or within designated units in acute care settings and are used as a bridge to home when there are substantial technology needs such as the need for ventilator weaning. In more rural settings, this care may be provided in an adult facility with a unit dedicated to pediatric care.

Consideration for non-oral feeding

Children with complex CP are at high risk for oral motor dysfunction that may worsen as the child ages, even when it is not present early on. Alternative options for feeding may need to be considered due to malnutrition, worsening oral motor dysfunction, recurrent aspiration pneumonia, disorders of the esophagus, gastric or intestinal dysmotility, and gastroesophageal reflux (see also Chapters 7, 8, and 9). Decisions regarding alternative feeding are complex and one of the most emotionally charged topics for families. Feeding is a major source of attachment between the child and the family. Disruption of this experience with its concurrent pleasures is troubling for families to consider. For this reason, it is not uncommon for families to be in denial regarding the child's nutritional status or feeding difficulties and for decisions around placing the tube to be among the most challenging for providers and families to navigate. However, most experienced clinicians who care for these children will note many families find the tube helpful and wish they would have placed the tube sooner.

The care team often needs steady patience and repeated educational attempts to have families recognize the benefits of gastrostomy feeds. Often maximizing nutrition and involvement in allied therapies are the mainstays of reaching maximum developmental potential, and families may need to be made aware of these facts. Various educational materials and websites promoting g-tube feedings (e.g. http://www.feedingtubeawareness.org) are available and families may benefit from conversations with families that already have had tubes placed. Gently addressing the underlying concerns or conflicts of attachment may prove useful. Reviewing the options for feeding blended food, prepared by the family, can be helpful. Addressing the potential for on-going oral feeding with a g-tube can also be helpful. Combining the decision for g-tube placement with planning for a major surgery, which will require nutritional support for healing, can be another tactic.

Consideration for tracheostomy

Indications for tracheostomy vary from congenital lesions causing airway obstruction or central apnea to acquired lesions from prolonged intubation. Often as children with CP age and develop worsening spasticity and contractures they may develop upper airway obstruction that contributes to poor oxygenation and ventilation and poor sleep. Prolonged intubation along with the need for frequent suctioning during respiratory illnesses may also raise the need for tracheostomy. As children with complex CP age they have multifactorial contributors to chronic lung disease and failure. Major contributors are neuromuscular weakness and poor cough, aspiration of saliva and gastric contents, scoliosis and possibly underlying reactive airway disease (see also Chapter 9). All these factors over time may contribute to the need for supplemental oxygen, frequent suctioning, Continuous Positive Airway Pressure (CPAP)/BiLevel Positive Airway Pressure (BiPAP) or long-term ventilation. While tracheostomy placement generally leads to improvement for fixed or dynamic upper airway obstructions, there is considerable debate if tracheostomy is beneficial for patients with frequent pneumonia without upper airway obstruction. Often providers may feel a tracheostomy in this situation will aid in suctioning for airway clearance. This may be offset by potential for infection introduced by the presence of an artificial airway and loss of humidification and filtration provided by the upper airway.

As decisions regarding tracheostomy placement are often made in the acute care setting during periods of crises, it is advisable to discuss the potential need for intubation and possible tracheostomy during periods of wellness when the family has time to contemplate and consider the impact of this technology on the child and family. These decisions are complex and often dependent on clinical circumstances at the time of presentation but consideration in advance can often make conversations during a crisis more manageable. In situations where there is definite upper airway obstruction the tracheostomy will likely greatly improve respiratory function and quality of life. In circumstances where tracheostomy is considered for frequent pneumonia and respiratory failure the tracheostomy may necessitate the need for ventilation and increased in-home nursing and equipment. Family members will also have to be trained to manage the tracheostomy to manage changes, suctioning and troubleshooting obstructions and dislodgements. This may be frightening for parents and caregivers and depending on geography there may be difficulty finding qualified in-home caregivers.

Ideally, a physician who has a long-term relationship with the family and is experienced in the management of respiratory complications in CP is the ideal person to have these conversations with families. It may be helpful to have families connect with other families with children with tracheostomies or ventilators. Exploring fully the family's questions and concerns and hopes and expectations will aid in the decision-making process. Discussions regarding more palliative approaches are important for families that do not wish to pursue more aggressive interventions or feel that further medical interventions may prolong their child's suffering.

Consideration for orthopedic procedures and surgery

Orthopedic problems are common in children with complex CP. Surgical interventions are directed at the correction and prevention of deformity, maximizing function, and alleviating pain (see also Chapter 4). Hip dislocation and subluxation, for example, occur with spastic CP, and may lead to pain with joint degeneration. Spasticity can lead to pain and limited movement, with surgical tendon release presented as a way to increase mobility and alleviate symptoms. Spinal surgery for scoliosis is a major surgical intervention that involves complex, peri-operative decision making. Pre-operative preparation includes nutritional, respiratory, and functional status. Post-operative care is may be extensive, painful, and prolonged, often requiring time in the Pediatric Intensive Care Unit (PICU), and followed by completely new seating and functional accommodations.

Since the need for orthopedic interventions evolves over time, the family has an opportunity to discuss options and to prepare. No surgical procedure is without risk, or has a guaranteed outcome. Parents want time to review options and to participate in the decision making and timing of interventions. They may need multiple opinions, requesting recommendations for referrals. In the case of major spinal surgery there can be ethical considerations to consider, given the potentially limited improvement in functional status for the extensive recuperation and cost. While there is an assumption that straightening the spine will improve or prevent respiratory complications, high level evidence to support this is limited and families should be encouraged to obtain consultation with multiple trusted providers in weighing options.

Although the decision for a surgical intervention ultimately lies between the family and the surgeon, primary care and complex care clinicians can be quite helpful in clarifying concerns, reviewing readiness for surgery, planning for post-operative medical management, reviewing the big picture of functional changes and accommodations, overall team management, and being a sounding board throughout the process.

Addressing the needs of the whole family

A child with severe CP and medical complexity affects the life of the entire family (see Chapter 21). Special considerations are made for multiple appointments and hospitalizations. There may be extra people in the home to help; crises may erupt at all the wrong times, displacing planned activities. There are financial concerns, transportation concerns, and unexpected dilemmas. Siblings are asked to delay or limit their desired activities due to time, expense and energy. Marriages suffer from the extra stress and strain of managing all the details and emotional challenges on top of daily life.

Checking in with families on a regular basis about how they are coping is critical to comprehensive care. Yet, it may be difficult to open the topic for fear of generating guilt or creating one more thing for the family to do or think about. Responding to the family's defenses is also a challenge as discussed in the *Managing Defenses* section.

A primary care clinician who cares for all children in the family is in an ideal position to monitor or notice the impact on the family. Noticing that a sibling is having trouble at school, expressing more anger at home, not sleeping well, or having new or increased separation anxiety can be the first step. Inquiring about the sibling's relationship with the patient or affirming the positive aspects you have come to know is a gentle way to approach the possible effects of stress manifesting with the sibling. Asking for the parent's point of view on what might be going on is also key. Having resources and suggestions for how to respond to the sibling's needs via peer support, dedicated time with a parent, engaging extended family and coaches, or professional counseling can also be useful. Similarly, encouraged respite for the parents and activities outside of caregiving will be essential to maintaining balance and enduring caregiving burden. Individual or family therapy and support groups may be helpful as well.

Palliative care

Local resources vary greatly for pediatric palliative care. Many children's hospitals and hospices have a palliative care service that will provide consultation on symptom management, communication, goal setting, and end of life care. An initial visit with a palliative care team member can be arranged during a hospitalization or clinic visit. Often the palliative provider is introduced as an extra layer of care with the time and expertise to assist with symptom control, comfort, and goal setting. When introduced to the family prior to a major crisis, the palliative provider can create trust and build relationship with the family that benefits the entire team (Feudtner 2007). Most palliative providers are skilled at providing telephone consultation to primary and tertiary providers facing challenges about how to address difficult conversations, or provide comfort and symptom relief without feeling like they are giving up on the patient.

Pediatric hospice care is not uniform across the United States as it is throughout the United Kingdom. Many hospice organizations will provide supportive services to the family, even if they are ill-equipped to care for the pediatric patient near the end of life.

Introducing palliative care early is generally helpful to everyone. Even if the family declines services, they know they are available. A palliative care provider checking in with the family once a month or once a quarter has the opportunity to build a relationship. It can be important to clarify for families that palliative care is not limited to end of life care, nor is it hospice care. Palliative care can benefit the family in tandem with on-going medical intervention.

Resuscitation

Palliative providers can assist with discussions regarding resuscitation, but these discussions can be introduced during any goals of care conversation and at many points along the care continuum. The specifics of the conversation change, of course, depending on the age, clinical situation, and context. In general, parents of children with complex CP are acutely aware of or worried about their child's complex and fragile condition and may not be surprised when the topic is addressed directly.

In addition to the goals of care planning, a conversation regarding resuscitation can begin in the context of hospital follow-up, or a requirement for school placement, in-home care, or center-based therapy. The context may create an opportunity to begin the conversation. Consider these opening lines:

- 'Often during a hospitalization, there are questions regarding resuscitation, in the event of an emergency. Did this come up while you were in the hospital? How did it go? What did you decide?'

- 'Has anyone asked about what you might want in the event of an emergency at school?'

- 'Does the therapy center have a requirement for a resuscitation plan in the event of an emergency?'

Being prepared to talk about options for resuscitation is best. Having a clear and systematic way to document the decisions is essential. Understanding that the early conversations can set the stage for later, more complex discussions is reassuring.

As the intensity in medical care increases and the limits of interventions emerge, or as quality of life declines, the conversation may take on a new dimension. Being open to discussing the options, or helping to connect the family with someone who is skilled with these conversations can be a genuine relief to everyone. Presenting the opportunity to talk through a plan before the crisis arises can help the family feel prepared for something they may have already imagined.

The conversation will often follow the parent's concern for providing the best quality of life, and wanting to be the best parent they can be. Often, there are no clear right and wrong decisions. The question could be asked

- *'Given the events of your last hospitalization, can you tell me what is most important to you right now regarding Julie's care? Having a better understanding of your goals for her will help me to best make recommendations to support you.'*

Focusing on the parent's goals of care and priorities, will guide the discussion. If it becomes clear that the Intensive Care Unit (ICU) and hospitalizations are a significant source of stress, and may not be adding to the child's perceived quality of life, an alternative of staying home with added support can be a natural segue to revisiting the plan for resuscitation and other interventions. In this case, the question could be,

- *'Would you like to talk about other options to hospitalization? One question to consider is whether it is more important to stay at home and focus on comfort or return to the hospital for interventions to support her breathing, like she received last time in the ICU.'*

Moving through the options for increased comfort in the home can help to set the stage for changes in the plan for resuscitation, or for a Do Not Resuscitate (DNR) order. Helping parents to understand that the plan for resuscitation can be changed should circumstances change can also be helpful as they come to their decisions (Wolf et al. 2011).

Mortality risk/life expectancy

Questions of life expectancy may arise as a family begins to prepare for the long-term care of their child. Future financial and legal planning is a real concern and may generate more anxiety than a conversation about a limited lifespan. Being able to offer statistics may prove to be part of a practical and helpful response when questions arise relative to planning for the future (Brooks et al. 2014).

Life expectancy is the average survival time based on calculations of historical and scientific data. Utilizing a number of databases comparing data for similar disabilities, projections are generated that prove similar across data sets. The main factors for estimating life expectancy in cerebral palsy are gross motor function and method of feeding. Fine motor function, cognitive function and epilepsy are less significant factors but if severe may impact survival (see www.lifeexpectancy.org). Other factors of medical severity such as frequency of pneumonia, need for supplemental oxygen or invasive or non-invasive ventilation, need for jejunal feedings and malnutrition may also impact life expectancy.

When discussing life expectancy with families it is important to note that these are statistical measures of average survival and that for any one individual it is difficult to

Table 20.2 Life expectancy: additional years (standard error) for adolescents and adults with cerebral palsy[a]

Sex/age	Cannot lift head			Lifts head or chest			Rolls/sits			Walks unaided[b]	General population
	TF	FBO	SF	TF	FBO	SF	TF	FBO	SF		
Female											
15y	14 (1.0)	18 (1.2)	–	18 (1.5)	23 (1.0)	–	27 (1.8)	37 (1.3)	48 (1.2)	55 (1.0)	66.2
30y	14 (0.9)	19 (1.2)	–	14 (0.8)	23 (1.1)	–	18 (1.8)	32 (1.2)	37 (0.8)	43 (0.7)	51.6
45y	12 (1.0)	14 (1.0)	–	12 (1.0)	17 (1.2)	–	12 (1.5)	21 (1.0)	25 (0.6)	29 (0.6)	37.4
60y	7 (0.8)	10 (1.4)	–	7 (0.8)	10 (1.1)	–	7 (0.8)	10 (0.8)	16 (0.5)	19 (0.7)	24.1
Male											
15y	14 (1.0)	18 (1.2)	–	18 (1.4)	23 (1.0)	–	27 (1.7)	33 (1.1)	45 (1.1)	52 (0.9)	61.4
30y	14 (0.9)	19 (1.2)	–	14 (0.8)	23 (1.1)	–	18 (1.7)	28 (1.1)	33 (0.7)	39 (0.6)	47.4
45y	12 (1.0)	14 (1.0)	–	12 (1.0)	17 (1.1)	–	12 (1.5)	18 (0.9)	22 (0.5)	25 (0.5)	33.5
60y	7 (0.8)	10 (1.4)	–	7 (0.8)	10 (1.1)	–	7 (0.8)	10 (0.8)	12 (0.4)	15 (0.5)	21.1

–, Results not shown because of small sample size. [a]As noted in the text, these life expectancies do not necessarily apply to younger children. [b]Life expectancies for the 'walks unaided' groups assume that individuals in the group will remain ambulatory until at least age 60. FBO, fed orally by others; SF, self–feeds orally; TF, tube fed.

state with certainty actual survival. While being realistic, it is also important to preserve a sense of hope for the family as they manage great uncertainty (Table 20.2). The data from Table 20.2 have been published and widely accepted as reasonable and are from a large database of patients with CP older than 4 years followed through California's Department of Developmental Services between 1983 and 2010.

Conclusion: kindness and compassion

Children with complex CP and their families face significant physical and emotional challenges every day. Coping with challenge becomes part of the fabric of life. It can be stressful, even in the best of times. Getting through the day or week or year takes extra energy, and may be described more as a marathon, than a quick jog. Life with complex CP requires endurance.

So too, life with complex CP requires kindness and compassion. We all know how the smallest, intentional act of kindness is remembered long after the details of a difficult conversation: a cup of tea, a glass of water offered before beginning discussions; a moment of gentle silence to allow for the words and emotion to sink in; a friendly greeting, or a softened tone of voice to ease the conversation along. Or, the proximity and touch that signal our care for the patient. Kindness and compassion are the necessary foundations for difficult conversations. Nurturing those attributes in ourselves will go a long way to providing comfort to our patients and their families as they face the day-to-day challenges of their lives.

Key points

- When it comes to difficult conversations, take your time, take a breath.
- Begin with open-ended questions and use reflective listening.
- Anticipate potential long-term decision making before the decision is required.
- Remember that many complicated decisions evolve over time.
- Shared goal setting can be a routine part of care planning.
- Be prepared before you enter the room.
- Consider rehearsing your opening lines before you use them.
- Stay curious, reflective and empathic.
- It is always helpful to be aware of the defenses being used by the parent.
- Find help, expand the team when you feel overwhelmed.

References

Brooks JC, et al (2014) Recent trends in cerebral palsy survival. Part II: individual survival prognosis. *Dev MedChild Neurol* **56**: 1065–1071.

Feudtner C (2007) Collaborative communication in pediatric palliative care: a foundation for problem-solving and decision-making. *Pediatr Clin North Am* **54**: 583–607.

Friedman SL, Norwood KW (2016) Out-of-home placement for children and adolescents with disabilities – addendum: care options for children and adolescents with disabilities and medical complexity. *Pediatrics* **138**: e20163216.

Grossberg RI (2008) Psychoanalytic contributions to the care of medically fragile children. *J PsychPrac* **14**: 307–311.

Mack JW, Joffe S (2014) Communicating about prognosis: ethical responsibilities of pediatricians and parents. *Pediatrics* **133**: S24–S30.

Whitaker AT, Sharkey M, Diab M (2015) Spinal fusion for scoliosis in patients with globally involved cerebral palsy. *J Bone Joint Surg Am* **97**: 782–787.

Wolfe J, Hinds P, Sourkes B (2011) *Textbook of Interdisciplinary Pediatric Palliative Care: Expert Consult Premium Edition*. Philadelphia: Elsevier Saunders.

Chapter 21

Through the eyes of parents

Michele Shusterman,
Carol Shrader and Jennifer Lyman

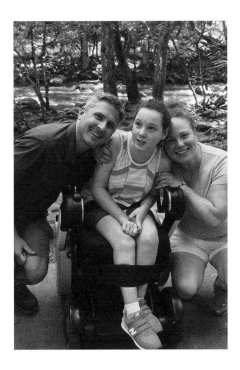

As a pediatrician or family doctor, you may be the medical professional that interacts the most with the family of a child with cerebral palsy (CP). How you relate to the family and the insight and resources you have to offer can make a big difference in how they approach and experience life. This chapter is written by Michele Shusterman, founder of CP NOW a nonprofit organization and CP Daily Living blog, with contributions from Carol Shrader and Jennifer Lyman. Like Michele, Carol and Jennifer are mothers of young people with CP as well as community advocates. Michele is the parent of a 10-year old girl, Jennifer is the parent to a 12-year old boy and Carol is the mother of four children, two of whom are 20-year old young men with CP. We have chosen to compose this chapter as though we were sitting talking to the medical professional about this topic, in a personal, casual and direct manner.

Parenting an infant and young child can be challenging for all caregivers. Adding a complex form of CP to the typical challenges of raising a child makes life even more complicated. When developmental and medical issues first become apparent, at birth or sometime afterward, family members struggle with a wide range of practical, emotional and social problems.

The most important thing you can do as a clinician is to approach the family with a helpful attitude. Physicians and therapists who demonstrate humility, honesty and receptivity to parents' feelings and perspectives empower families to help their child.

First-time, as well as experienced, parents initially feel lost and unprepared to meet the unique physical, emotional and developmental needs of a child who has a diversity of medical conditions. When there are complex medical issues, parents can feel caught in a game of 'whack-a-mole'; as soon one problem is addressed, another critical issue pops up to take its place. Spontaneity is replaced with the need for planning and flexibility, and families are immediately thrown into a world that is unfamiliar and frightening. Parents may be spending most of their time trying to figure out how to meet their child's most basic needs and feeling that they and their child are not making progress. Parents are in a constant state of worry about the child's eating, sleeping, bowel habits and movement. In some cases, the family is doing all they can to avoid another visit to the hospital. They may feel tremendous tension and anxiety trying to meet their existing obligations at work and at home. The parents' own needs often take a back seat.

The combination of emotional, physical, and financial strain can be overwhelming, especially as parents repeatedly adjust different facets of their lives in response to their child's needs. How parents learn to cope with the fact that their child has medical problems impacts not only the child but the whole family.

As their physician, you can acknowledge the difficulty of the situation and help them identify the specific areas of where they are feeling the most pressure and anxiety.

By having this focus, they can begin to strategize and address those areas of concern.

Emotional impact

Grieving the loss of the child they thought they would have is common for parents of a child with CP. Grief takes many forms and is a process that each family member moves through at their own pace. Personal histories, strategies for coping and the support available all affect how someone grieves and how long that grief lasts. Many parents have shared with me that they still grieve from time to time many years out from their child's diagnosis. I include myself as one of them. As a physician, you can help families by letting them know that grieving is normal, takes time, and is part of the journey toward acceptance. By being patient and understanding with parents you will be able to encourage them to understand and deal with their grief.

If you are concerned about how a parent or family member is coping with their grief, or how the grief may be influencing the care of the child, it may be helpful to recommend counseling.

Reassure parents and other family members that there is no shame in seeking guidance and support from a professional counselor or member of their clergy. Approaching the parents with compassion, rather than judgment, is key to getting parents to accept your help.

Considerations to support family life

It is often hard for others to relate to a family who has a child with a complex medical condition. As the parents struggle to cope with the child's care they are likely to be less available for family and friends, often just struggling to keep their heads above water. It is common for others to pull away from the parents. It may be that they do not know how to be helpful or that they feel unsure about how to interact with the family. Families are vulnerable to feeling isolated and unsure about the support available to them as their time becomes more consumed with caring for their child. They are likely to miss out on social events they used to enjoy because they find it too difficult to attend.

The family must figure out how to educate others about their 'new normal' while facing the fact that not everyone will be accepting and supportive. It takes time to navigate these changes in social connections and it may involve working through pain and grief in the process. It may be necessary for the family to transition to a different or more expanded network of friends and people who relate to what they are experiencing. In the interim, parents and siblings will feel vulnerable and may need extra encouragement and support. Single parents have unique challenges and can be particularly at risk for being overwhelmed and isolated.

As a physician, you can help parents understand that family and friend issues are common and that there are ways to deal with them.

Offer families your ear

You can go a long way in helping parents by being a good listener – actively listening without judgment. By inviting parents to share their authentic feelings in a safe place, you may be offering them a rare opportunity to let their guard down. This in itself is a great gift to offer parents and it gives you the opportunity to more clearly identify where the family may need additional support or perhaps counseling. As a clinician, you will not have all the answers to a parent's questions, but you can become a trusted advisor and collaborator dedicated to helping the family organize themselves and their approach to caring for their child. Parenting a child with a disability requires tremendous flexibility with lots of unknown variables. Having a physician who offers consistent support gives parents much needed comfort and stability. This can be a challenge for a busy practice, and takes teamwork on the part the social workers, nursing staff and others, but it is invaluable for these families.

Help parents learn to take care of themselves

Helping parents learn to take care of themselves can be a daunting task. Here is a specific example from my own history:

Ever since my daughter's diagnosis of CP 10 years ago, I have struggled with the ongoing tension between wanting to seize opportunities to encourage her greatest potential and wanting to make our lives about more than just therapy and treatment. When she was very young I kept seeing all of the activities and peer interactions she was missing out on and I felt I needed to fight harder against her CP. I spent most of my day thinking about my daughter and making mental lists of what I needed to do to support her health and development. I thought I had no time to consider and address my own needs. As she got older, however, I had to let go of this thinking as I saw that my daughter continued to get further behind her peers, even as I pushed the daily limits of her energy and the energy of our family to overcome her problems. Her peers began to run and develop fine motor skills when we were still working on crawling.

Once my daughter began kindergarten, my husband and I realized that we needed to change how we approached each day. We did not have nearly as many hours to dedicate to therapy and she was very tired after a full day at school. There were also additional developmental needs that became apparent and required our attention. Some of these problems included addressing a visual processing disorder and figuring out how she could successfully learn in a classroom setting. Ultimately, learning to take care of myself became a process that began with me experiencing the limits of my own power and honoring my daughter's need for fun and relaxation. Embracing her limitations and mine become easier with time, practice and greater acceptance of my daughter's disability. I now spend much less of my time and energy thinking about how to make her symptoms of CP go away. We focus more on helping her plan and achieve her individual goals in a timeline that is best for her and our family.

It's important to realize that simply telling parents that that they must take care of themselves is often ineffective.

Most parents realize they need to take better care of themselves but do not know how to make the time to do it. They often become consumed with their child's daily needs and even when they have a few moments or longer for a break, they may spend that time thinking about their child and family. As a physician, you can recommend parents create a schedule where there is designated time for fun together as a family, as a couple and time alone.

Foster the child's independence

How to foster independence in a child is an issue for all parents. For parents of a child with a disability, it can be especially confusing. How much help should the parent offer the child? Humans are hardwired to respond to an infant as soon as they begin to cry by offering them nourishment, comfort or maybe bringing a toy closer within reach. When a child has experienced medical trauma, or is demonstrating developmental delays, the parent often feels more compelled to cater to the child and help them minimize their frustration and pain. While this perspective is understandable it can also interfere with the child's development and growth. When parents view the child as incompetent or incapable of even trying to do things independently, they stop looking for and creating those opportunities for their child.

Over time this dynamic can lead to learned helplessness where the child responds to the parent by being unable to perceive or work toward her or his own competencies. Even the child with a disability who relies heavily upon a caregiver or technology for navigating her or his day, must be given opportunities and choices to push themselves. It is difficult for parents to figure out how much room to give the child to explore and to experiment. If the child meets with failure, should the parent encourage the struggle or assist and after how long? Parents may need the ongoing assistance of their Early Intervention and therapy team to arrange the child's environment so they can practice working toward mastering tasks that are at their level. These opportunities are unique to the child but they may involve learning to use supportive equipment and devices which improve the child's independent access to the world. Given the appropriate boundaries, parents can foster confidence and competence in their child by giving them the chance to work through aspects of their daily activities on their own.

With my own child, I break down all of her activities of daily living into smaller segments (sometimes even parts of segments) where she can challenge herself while having opportunities to succeed. I have learned over time that by providing ongoing opportunities for my daughter to take responsibility for negotiating as much of her day as possible, I am influencing her personality development. Sometimes this becomes more important than mastering the specific tasks themselves. The alternative to finding ways to foster independence and confidence in the child is to risk having a child grow up expecting everyone around them to cater to their needs (and getting angry when people do not respond as their parents do) rather than taking ownership and responsibility for what they can do.

Tips for Parents of Children with Complex CP

Below are some tips that have helped me free up some of my emotional and mental energy and some of my time. They have acted as guideposts for helping me approach my daily life with the intention of creating more balance.

1. **Pay attention to how much intellectual and personal energy you are giving toward finding answers for your child.** Be sure to carve out times during the day to simply be with your child, other family members, or spouse without thinking about CP and the challenges your child faces.

2. **Don't sacrifice reason and good sense to help your child.** New therapies will constantly be presented as *the* treatment for CP. Before trying a new therapy, make a list of the sacrifices the treatment will require you and your family to make. Weigh the emotional and financial costs and the physical, safety, and unknown risks the treatment will present against the possible benefits for your child. Remember that a treatment without any known risks does not mean it is risk free. Discuss these issues with people you trust and your child's medical team. Set time commitment limits and financial limits and be aware of your expectations about the treatment.

3. **Your child will have his or her own developmental timeline.** When you compare your child to other same aged peers, you may subliminally approach your child with disappointment and he or she may perceive this as something he or she is doing wrong. Focus on the positive points, the things that are working and the small, incremental steps that lead to putting together larger developmental pieces.

4. **Assess and honor your child's physical and cognitive energy limits each day.** These may change daily. You know your child best. Don't be afraid to speak up if you think what is best for your child is different from what the experts advise.

5. **Be aware of what is driving your approach to your child's therapy/developmental support program.** Be honest with yourself and look out for guilt, fear, and hopelessness that are motivating you to push your child and other family members too much. This may be difficult territory to sort through and balance, but is often part of the emotional journey that is a necessary step to accept the CP diagnosis. Remember, it's your child who ultimately has to participate in the therapy and integrate all the information that comes from your therapy planning.

6. **Creating a balanced schedule becomes easier as your child's developmental picture becomes clearer.** Over time, as you and your professional team have had a chance to observe your child, you will have a better understanding of how to focus your time and which therapies and treatments work best for your child. In addition, you child's clinical team may use the Gross Motor Classification System (GMFCS, see Chapter 1) to help guide decision making around goals and treatments.

7. **Focus on what your child does well and what they like.** Integrate interests with opportunities for development. For instance, perhaps a child likes the water. Swimming is an activity that your child can enjoy while also developing their motor skills.

8. **Explore respite resources in your area** including what is offered by local parent-to-parent offices, churches or other religious centers, and state programming that allows for in-home support for your child. Some US states offer programs through Medicaid/TEFRA/Katie Beckett that allow for parents to have respite hours. Additionally, your area may have medical day care centers which offer out-of-home respite programs. Contact your local Health and Human Services Agency for more information.

Support siblings

Carol Shrader

Often the child with a disability is not the only child in the family. Family dynamics are not a benign issue. Parents often struggle to find the balance in caring for their child with special needs in relation to their other children. They can err on the side of ignoring the typically developing child or bounce as far as glorifying the typically developing child while ignoring the child with special needs. Finding the balance is key to successful family dynamics that encourage relationship and compassion on all fronts.

When my triplets – two of whom have cerebral palsy – began preschool, I was stunned at our first parent-teacher meeting. The preschool teachers' faces looked a bit less than inviting as I sat across from them and their tone was serious and commanding of my attention.

'Claire doesn't share.'

I almost choked. Claire, my only daughter? The triplet sibling of two boys with cerebral palsy? A child whose very life has required her to share since the womb. Are you kidding me?

'She sits with her legs in a V-shape in front of Benjamin and Mason. She keeps the toys they want to play with in the V and will not let any other children share them.'

My heart swelled with pride, even as my head wanted to roar. I took a deep breath before saying, 'This is not called "not-sharing". This is called protecting her brothers. Benjamin and Mason cannot get the toys they like or keep them if someone else grabs them. Claire is simply ensuring they have a chance to play also.'

It was the first time I realized educating the world on how siblings of children with special needs behave would be as important as educating the world about my boys.

Encourage the parents of your patients by reminding them that they are not alone in the tug-of-war they are experiencing. Cerebral palsy colors our home life. It colors our family. It colors our life experiences. And likewise, it will color the lives of the families you serve. Often siblings are more mature than their peers, with a level of empathy that is unmatched.

When the triplets were teenagers, one of my sons had a major surgery. As soon as he was released from the hospital, his triplet sister left for a mission trip abroad. Claire struggled with feelings of guilt, of leaving the family when they needed her assistance. We pushed her out the door. She called with a heavy heart:

'Mom, these teenagers want to talk about boys, about clothes and about what kind of car they drive. I want to scream that my brother just had major spine surgery and is fighting to recover!'

Even still, the needs of the sibling are important and can be fairly basic. In a recent panel of now-adult siblings of children with special needs, a facilitator asked my daughter and her peers to name the one thing they wish their parents had known they needed as children. Every single sibling listed the same thing: one-on-one time with the parents.

> *Claire: 'My brothers needed so much undivided attention from my mom, and though I didn't need her to get dressed, I craved that one-on-one time, too,' Most people with at least one other sibling can relate to this, but when your siblings have disabilities, I think this desire for alone time is even stronger. It took so much for my parents to plan time out for just me that every time they did it was as if they were telling me, "You are special. You are valued. You are loved."'*

Often, parents are running from therapy to therapy, doctor to doctor, with educational meetings thrown in. The idea of time alone with one child is a foreign concept. And yet, these siblings are clear with their message.

> *When the triplets were 8, we had another child. Cate was 2-years-old when she climbed down from her high chair and up on the wheel of Benjamin's wheelchair and wiped the dripping ice cream from his chin. She was 4 when I stopped her little fist as it flew toward a little boy's face who had told her that her brother was weird. Cerebral palsy definitely colors her world.*

Encourage your parents to allow the siblings to take some ownership in the disability. Three-year-old Claire knew inherently to form a V-shape with her legs and protect her triplet brothers. When Cate was 4 she knew the same.

When the anxiety level increases in a home – due to therapies, pending surgeries, illnesses – the child with cerebral palsy and the parents are not alone in feeling apprehensive. The siblings feel the stress as well. Younger siblings can benefit from pre-operative appointments with a Child Life Specialist who can help them process the upcoming event. Remind your parents that anxiety can manifest itself in many ways in siblings – anger, sadness, jealousy, and even a seeming lack of compassion.

Finding the balance between caring for the typically developing child and the child with special needs can be a challenge. However, if communication lines are open, if all the children know that home is a safe place for expressing emotions, feelings, fears, then even though the balance might not be any easier to achieve, it is at least less toxic.

Finally, encourage your parents that the life lessons and skills learned in growing up in a family colored by cerebral palsy are priceless.

Claire (to a group of parents): It is because I'm a special needs sibling that I'm most fulfilled when volunteering with children and adults with disabilities. Oh my goodness, I have gotten to know and serve some simply incredible people,' 'It is because I'm a special needs sibling that I'm working towards becoming an occupational therapist to serve these amazing children. And it is because I am a special needs sibling that I understand the challenges, yet also believe that being a member of my amazing family has made me who I am.

Because Cate is younger, because she is not one of the three, and perhaps because we have the advantage of her perspective, we have tried things that forced the boys to watch. She has challenged us to try things outside the wheelchair-accessibility bubble. She has forced us to be creative in including the boys, in trying new things and in realizing it is ok for the boys to occasionally have to sit on the outside looking in. But the main thing she has done is make us realize as a family that the primary focus does not always have to be on the disabilities in our home. Sometimes, the focus can be on softball. Or ballet. Or fishing.

Being the sibling is not painless. Being the sibling is not without cost. Claire, at 17, was still the little girl wanting to sit with her legs in a V-shape in front of her brothers and protect them from those who would steal their toys – or even their joy.

Talk about quality of life

What is quality of life? The World Health Organization defines it as 'an individual's perception of their position in life in the context of the culture and value system in which they live, and in relation to their goals, expectations, standards and concerns' (WHO 1995). Most parents want the highest quality of life possible for their child and therefore the conversation about quality of life is important to have. Supporting a good quality of life for a child with complex CP means different things to different parents and individual children. For some parents these feelings may be tied to what they hear directly from their child about what is important and fulfilling to them. It can be especially challenging when the child is unable to clearly communicate what is important and fulfilling. In addition, parents have their own personal values and expectations about what a good quality of life means for their child. Wherever possible it is important to understand the perspective of the child as well as the parents. There may be cases where what the child wants is different from what the parents want. It is helpful to highlight those dynamics so they can be addressed. If parents and children can agree on goals, moving forward is enhanced.

It was very reassuring to me to hear recently that there have been several studies that repeatedly demonstrate that a child with CP's self-reported quality of life is like that of their peers who do not have CP. According to the SPARCLE study, a large-scale study investigating the quality of life of children and adolescents who have CP, self-reported quality of life does not change with the type of CP or severity when it comes to psychological well-being, self-perception, social support, school environment, financial resources and social acceptance (Colver 2006). The following quote from Albrecht and Devlinger cited in one of the SPARCLE papers particularly struck me:

> Possibly, from the perspective of a non-disabled adult imagining what it would be like to be disabled *would be upsetting* [my emphasis], but probably not from the perspective of a child whose sense of self from birth incorporates their impairment and who embraces the growth, development and living with the same excitement as most children' (Stockman 2009).

Families can find the SPARCLE (2017) study and the papers linked there at http://research.ncl.ac.uk/sparcle/

These results do not mean there are not areas of specific concern for children with CP, but they can bring relief to a worried parent.

> *I never thought about my daughter's quality of life in a broad context. Looking back, I can see that my husband and I instinctively addressed aspects of our daughter's quality of life by considering parts of her day and how much variety she is getting with her activities, interactions and movement. As parents, we have worried about and monitored how much time our daughter spends at home and in the same room and in the same piece of equipment. We balance these concerns with her energy levels, our energy and her requests for what she would like to do with her day.*

> *We periodically sit down together as a family and discuss our daughter's goals and how she feels about school, therapy, time with her friends and family, and what she likes or does not like about her activities. Sometimes we struggle to keep up our physical energy to support our ideas and our daughter's, for what she would like to do with her day. This has led us to purchase different equipment that makes transferring her easier. We have also increased the number of hours we have additional help. It has been very useful for us to identify specific goals around what we all feel constitutes a good quality of life for our daughter and setting up our weekly routine to work toward meeting those goals.*

When discussing quality of life with families, it is important to discuss the child's mental health because children with CP are at higher risk of mental health disorders than their peers without CP.

> *My daughter has struggled through periods of intense anger and anxiety. Thankfully we sought the support and guidance of a psychologist to help us learn how to help her cope with and move through these feelings. Along the way we learned that much of her anger was tied to issues such as insomnia, pain, frustration with feeling different and side effects*

from her epilepsy medication. I have also learned that anxiety, in particular, is common among children with CP. Given how obviously heightened her nervous system responds to noises, crowded areas and new activities, I wonder how her early brain injury may have increased her susceptibility to anxiety and made it more difficult for her to manage her feelings.

Many children with CP may experience these same feelings and issues or they may have secondary conditions, such as communication difficulties, that lead to emotional outbursts. Encourage parents to meet their children where they are and seek the professional support they need when it comes to their emotions, behavior, movement, learning and social skills. If children receive support and acceptance at home and in their community, the emotional difficulties will be easier to manage.

Encourage participation in recreation and leisure activities

Jennifer Lyman

Helping children with complex forms of CP find meaningful recreational and social opportunities often feels like an uphill battle for parents. Traditional childhood activities and programs aren't usually geared toward including those with significant disabilities, especially physical ones. There are frequently issues with physical access to activities (i.e. the terrain, inaccessible bathroom facilities, etc.) and it can sometimes be difficult to adjust the pace and nature of an activity to facilitate a child's participation. There can also be problems with how program directors and other families and children relate to kids with significant disabilities. Despite these challenges, there are successful programs and there are also strategies for establishing inclusive programming and fostering social interaction. When the child feels strongly about being included in an activity, a family's efforts to facilitate that inclusion can feel well worth the time and energy. At the same time, there is also the opportunity to rethink what constitutes participation and recreation for the child.

If a family or individual child is trying to find a way to include their child in a program or activity it is often very helpful to look at successful existing programs, even outside of the local area. It is not always necessary to re-invent the wheel – parents or interested program directors can benefit from others' ideas about successfully adapting a program and including a child with complex physical disabilities. An example of an existing program is the *Ballet for All* program that was developed in Syracuse, New York by Dr. Nienke Dosa, Dr. Lisa Neville and their team (see Sports, recreation and leisure in the Information and resources section for more information). They developed a manual for facilitating the participation of kids with CP in dance programs, including wheelchair users. Another example is Miracle League, a popular adaptive sports program available in many places in the US.

At the same time, while structured activities and adaptive sports may appeal to some children with CP it may not appeal to others. My son participated in an adaptive baseball and a ballet program but he didn't like either one. I realized that just like any other child, some things he liked and some things he didn't.

Just because it was an activity designed for children with disabilities, it didn't mean that my son would want to be a part of it. If a family needs ideas for creating opportunities for recreation you, as the primary medical provider, can help them by guiding them to consider what the family enjoys doing together and what is fun and fulfilling for the individual child.

Social media also offers a wealth of information. Through social media, parents can discover successful programs and approaches that can be used to create a local program or provide insight about including a child in an existing program.

Parents can benefit from trying to find a balance between advocating for their child to be included, and identifying and celebrating the many ways their child is participating already. Both families and physicians often adopt the mindset of trying to find activities that mimic or are a variation of what a typically developing child would be experiencing. Participation and recreation is approached through the lens of seeing how closely the child with disabilities can come to experiencing an activity or social interaction the way their peers do. Thinking about participation and recreation in this way is a natural tendency and it makes sense in some situations, but it can be frustrating when the gaps are too big. It is helpful to encourage parents to embrace the idea that the child with complex physical limitations will experience life in their own unique way and at their own pace. This acceptance requires a shift in the parents' thinking and can be very painful territory. Parents may need help in navigating this new way of thinking.

Our family has learned that it is important to slow down and appreciate what we can do together. If parents are spending significant time and energy fighting for accommodations so their child can participate, the result may ultimately be unfulfilling, exhausting, or worse, cause their child anger and resentment, especially if the child was never interested in participating in the first place.

You may be surprised to hear that some families and children, like ours, may find joy in things like simply hanging out together and listening to music or cooking. By helping the family identify their collective and individual interests, you can help them decide how to approach their free time, rather than becoming lost in someone else's ideas of what recreation and leisure should like for them. Some families may feel relieved to hear that it is OK to slow down rather than trying to look like other families.

For our family, before our son was born, we were avid whitewater kayakers, mountain bikers and skiers. We enjoyed camping and going on long hikes. After he was born and after the first few years of addressing his complex medical needs, we knew that the activities we enjoyed likely wouldn't be activities that he could do with us on a regular basis. We had to redefine what 'meaningful opportunities' looked like, and identify the best opportunities to enjoy ourselves. If we didn't take this approach we would constantly feel like we were coming up short. Families of children with disabilities benefit from seeing their child and their experiences on their own merit and not compared to what other families experience.

We still offer our son opportunities that are adventurous and fun. He participates in an adaptive skiing program, he attends overnight CP camp each summer and some day we will take him whitewater rafting, but these are all events, not the day-to-day activities that he enjoys and that sustain him. Instead, we as a family go downtown and listen to music or walk around, we hang out, relax and he rides his trike and we go swimming, an activity that is relatively barrier free. We go for drives and go fishing. He is on the school soccer team. His classmates push him on the field and he loves cheering for them from the sidelines. These are all meaningful activities for him and us.

I have learned to carve out specific time for participation and recreation for my son aside from his exercise and therapy time. Some families may find ways of combining the two that are satisfying, but we prefer to separate them. My son still has 'therapy' and I still make sure that he gets his strength and cardio activity whether it be from tricycle riding during physical education at school, using his gait trainer or having him practice his swim skills before he can play. But when it comes time to family time, we prefer to slow down.

I have worked with his therapists and his physicians to find equipment that will allow him to participate in ways that are comfortable and that he enjoys. He has a camp chair that we take almost everywhere so he can get out of his wheelchair and hang out with us. He uses water wings or a life vest in the pool so he can swim independently. He began using powered mobility at an early age to help him learn to develop the skills necessary to get to where *he* wants to be. If he wants to ride his tricycle, I am always happy to go for a long, slow walk while he rides. Often, we find ourselves chatting with friends and neighbors who we don't get to see and this gives my son an opportunity to meet new people. These are all examples of how we have facilitated my son's participation in recreation and leisure activities. He finds these opportunities fulfilling and they make him happy.

Recreation and leisure time for people with complex CP is a tricky endeavor, but with an open mind, creativity, persistence and a generous perspective, it can be a source of great pleasure and satisfaction for the whole family.

Plan for the future

Thinking about the future of a child with CP can be confusing and worrisome to parents. It is a complicated topic involving the person's unique abilities and limitations, family dynamics, financial resources and community resources.

Making predictions

Countless parents have told me that their child's doctor or therapist said their child would *never* speak, stand, learn, use a power chair, feed themselves, walk, or have meaningful relationships. But then the child accomplished what the parents were told the child would never do. When parents hear what their child cannot or will not ever be able to do, they can easily lose hope for their child's future. There are so many variables that contribute to what a child with CP can learn, that it is impossible to know for certain what can be achieved.

As a medical professional it is important that you encourage parents to be open about the future. Do not make specific and absolute predictions about a child's development.

Start with the child's interests

One of the most helpful pieces of advice we received as parents of a child with CP came from a developmental pediatrician who saw our daughter when she was 3 years old. He asked us to begin exploring and focusing on what *interested* our daughter. Was there an area of interest or a talent we could help her develop? This guidance was invaluable for many reasons, including helping us to shift our vision toward what was working for our daughter instead of what was working against her. It forced me to approach my daughter with curiosity rather than worry which was a different experience for me. It did not take me long to identify that she loved music.

> We have continued to surround my daughter with music. She doesn't go anywhere without her wireless headphones and she uses music throughout her day as a way of entertaining herself, relaxing and making her therapy and exercise routines fun. Last year we asked her if she would like to take music lessons. She immediately said she wanted to learn to play the piano. Truthfully, with her limited fine motor skills I was doubtful we could make it work. But, I have learned to expect to be surprised and to set her up for success as best as I can. There is no harm in trying a new activity. Often this means rethinking conventional ways of participating and breaking down movements until she can comfortably work through them at her own pace. Even if we try an activity and it ends up not working out, we usually learn something helpful in the process about what kinds of support and technology she needs or what activities are more easily adaptable for her. Once in a while we all decide it is best to let something go, but if our daughter is very persistent we will keep trying to facilitate her participation.

Fortunately, her school's music instructor had a background in special education and was eager to teach our daughter. The first time I sat in on one of her lessons I was in shock. It was beautiful to watch. Despite how hard she had to work to coordinate her vision and hand movements (with arm support from me and hand support from her instructor), she loved it. She has continued to improve and looks forward to her weekly lesson.

For me, it doesn't matter if piano becomes a part of my daughter's future. What matters is that facilitating her participation in something that interests her has allowed her to have a creative outlet that brings her great joy. Surprisingly, it also improved her fine motor skills. I share this example because parents need to be open to creating opportunities to develop their child's interests. By doing this, parents help their child learn to establish a lifelong habit of goal setting and learning about what kind of support they need to meet those goals. It also gives a message that, despite the child's limitations, meaningful goals can be achieved. Experiences like this enhance a positive, forward-looking attitude in the child.

Anticipate transition to adulthood

As a medical professional, you can help the parents, with the input of the individual with CP, to consider the future when the time is right. As the child gets older, this discussion becomes more pertinent (see Chapter 18 Transition). The timing of the conversation depends on the family, the child, and resources available in the community. When discussing the future, you may find that some parents unload a host of concerns whereas other parents may ask to delay the conversation until a later time. Whenever possible make sure you invite the perspective of the individual who has CP, as appropriate. Practical considerations play a role in when you choose to have these discussions especially when time is needed to arrange transitions for housing, adult medical care, education and vocational training.

Children with CP, like other children often have ideas about their own future. Check in with the person periodically to see how their goals are developing and changing. At the age of 10 my daughter already has some clear goals and ideas for herself. She wants to live in her own apartment with assistance, in a nearby city and go to college to become a doctor like her father. Her ideas and goals may change over time and whether or not she can achieve them depends in part on what support is available to help her. As she gets older, our family will need support from professionals who have guided families before us as well as from families who have already been through this transition.

People with complex CP have different impairments and barriers to employment and participation in life activities. Some parents of young children may already be concerned about what kind of future their child will have and what choices are available to them. Will they need to live at home? Will they want to? If so, what does that mean about the larger family's future and needs? If they live in a group setting who will take care of their medical needs? What kind of financial plans does the family need to arrange for the future? You can help families by connecting them with information about options available for housing and medical care in your community.

There is a nonprofit organization in Australia called Fighting Chance that was started by Laura and Jordan O'Reilly, the siblings of a young man who passed away from complications related to CP (http://fightingchance.org.au). Laura was frustrated with the lack of vocational opportunities available to her brother Shane after he finished high school. Together she and her brother Jordan started Fighting Chance. Fighting Chance provides opportunities for meaningful social participation, employment, work experience and skill development to young people with the most significant disabilities in their community. This is an example of how families can advocate for change and how communities can develop programs that provide meaningful opportunities for people with significant disabilities.

Conclusion

There are many examples of adults with complex forms of CP who have created meaningful lives for themselves with the help of technology, social and community support. As described in the example above, advocacy for people with disabilities is changing the way society thinks about and supports people with CP. The result is exciting new possibilities that will help those with complex CP lead fulfilling lives. As a provider you help families evaluate the various options that become available for their loved one and encourage or even partner with caregivers to continue to advocate for more so that each individual with complex CP can live up to their potential with whatever supports they may need.

Key Points

- As a clinician, you will not have all the answers to a parent's questions, but you can become a trusted advisor and collaborator dedicated to helping the family organize themselves and their approach to caring for their child.

- Support families in their unique grieving, including accepting changes in their expectations about parenting, social life and daily routines.

- Most parents realize they need to take better care of themselves but do not know how to make the time to do it. Here you will find strategies for guiding families to create more balance in their daily life.

- How to foster independence in a child is an issue for all parents. For parents of a child with a disability, it can be especially confusing with an ongoing tension of empowering the child versus not frustrating them too much.

- Finding the balance between supporting the typically developing child as well as the child with CP is key to successful family dynamics that encourage relationship and compassion on all fronts.

- Supporting a good quality of life for a child with complex CP means different things to different parents and individual children. If a family needs ideas for creating opportunities for recreation have them consider what the family enjoys doing together and what is fun and fulfilling for the individual child.

- Thinking about the future of a child with CP can be confusing and worrisome to parents. It is a complicated topic involving the person's unique abilities and limitations, family dynamics, financial resources and community resources.

Information and resources

It is important to have a wide range of reliable information to offer parents about many topics related to CP. However, parents vary in how they handle information about CP. Some parents want lots of information and articles to review; others want to know as little as possible. It can be helpful to check in with parents to see where they are and how they are most comfortable receiving information. Some families may wish to have you point out or provide resources to read about a condition on their own and then discuss it with you later. Others may want to discuss their concerns (and yours) in depth. And for some families it may be helpful to let them know in advance about a discussion you would like to have. Keep in mind there will be some parents who react with anger at the information you provide. This could reflect an inability to deal with the pain associated with their child's problems.

The resources below can both educate parents and reassure them that other parents have successfully navigated the same issues they are facing.

CP Tool Kit, https://cpnowfoundation.org, is a comprehensive diagnosis resource guide for parents and caregivers.

CP Daily Living, http://cpdailyliving.com, is a comprehensive resource website and blog created to share information and resources about CP. It also documents our journey as a family and share how we navigate difficult issues our daughter faces and that we face as a family. The CP Daily Living website includes a support resource section that includes online and local resources for families based in the US: www.cpdailyliving.com/disability-information-by-state/.

Inspire, https://www.inspire.com, is a popular online health community network with individual pages dedicated to specific conditions.

Hope for HIE, http://www.hopeforhie.org, is US-based and offers education and support resources for families whose children have been diagnosed with hypoxic ischemic encephalopathy. They also have a Facebook page where families can interact with one another.

Mommies of Miracles, www.facebook.com/MommiesofMiracles/, is a popular Facebook page for families who have children with complex medical needs. They also have local online discussion groups throughout the world.

Preemie World, http://preemieworld.com, has books, videos, and other products and tools to help families adjust to life beyond the neonatal intensive care unit NICU (neonatal intensive care unit). They write newsletters for professionals and families, publish an international directory of support groups and preemie resources, and run an online preemie support forum through *Inspire*.

The Four Walls of My Freedom: Lessons I've Learned from a Life of Caregiving, by Donna Thompson. http://www.donnathomson.com. Donna is the parent and caregiver of her adult son who has a very complex form of cerebral palsy, and is also the primary caregiver to her mother who is living with Alzheimer's. She also hosts a popular blog and Facebook page called, 'The Caregiver's Living Room'.

The Six F-words Framework Poster, https://worldcpday.org/wp-content/uploads/2016/06/WCPD_2016_Six_F-Words_for_Cerebral_Palsy_Poster.pdf, is a very helpful visual guide to have in your office and to hand out to parents to refer to in order to assess how parents are balancing life for their child and family. The six 'F-words' for cerebral palsy are Function, Family, Fitness, Friends, Fun and Future.

How to Make and Keep Friends™ book series by Donna Shea and Nadine Briggs. http://www.howtomakeandkeepfriends.com. These books provide quick, easy tips to help kids manage their feelings. The series was created as a resource to support the social success of children at home, at school and on the playground.

Respite

In the US, free respite may only be available through state-based Medicaid Waiver programs. Parents will need to apply and qualify for respite care, so keeping a list of local phone numbers and websites related to accessing respite services is invaluable to families.

TEFRA/Katie Beckett Medicaid Programs, http://cahpp.org/project/the-catalyst-center/financing-strategy/tefra/.

Home and community-based services, https://www.medicaid.gov/medicaid/hcbs/authorities/1915-c/index.html. States can develop home and community-based services waivers (HCBS Waivers) to meet the needs of people who prefer to get long-term care services and supports in their home or community, rather than in an institutional setting. These programs often include respite services.

United States Department of Labor – Disability resources, https://www.dol.gov/odep/topics/disability.htm. In the US you can find information and links to many local services and agencies on this website.

Siblings

ForeverSibs, https://www.facebook.com/pg/ForeverSibs/about/, is a nonprofit whose mission is to 'honor and recognize the unique role of brothers and sisters with rare diseases/disorders and autism through social support and education, thereby decreasing their anxiety and isolation'. It offers sibling support on Facebook, twitter and by mail for siblings of people with cerebral palsy and other conditions.

Sibshops, https://www.siblingsupport.org/sibshops, is a US-based program offering online, print, workshops and state, by state-based support to siblings of individuals with special needs.

Sports, recreation and leisure

Here are some resources for adaptive sports and recreation programs as well as examples of programming supporting the participation and inclusion of people with physical disabilities.

Ballet for All is a ballet dance program for children with cerebral palsy developed by developmental pediatrician Dr. Nienke Dosa and occupational therapist and dancer Lisa Neville. They offer a resource guide for dance assistants to understand cerebral palsy and how to work with children to include them in a ballet class. You can find their resource guide for dance assistants here: http://bbi.syr.edu/projects/Fit-In/docs/BalletForAll_Web_Tagged.2015.pdf.

Best Day Foundation, https://bestdayfoundation.org, is a US-based nonprofit dedicated to providing safe, fun adventure activities, like surfing, sea kayaking, snowboarding and more, to children with special needs.

Blaze Sports America, http://blazesports.org, is an international organization offering a variety of camp, recreation and adapted sport activities, including golf, fencing, swimming, and more, for children with disabilities and veterans.

Challenged Athletes Foundation, http://www.challengedathletes.org/resources/, offers a comprehensive state, by state adaptive sport guide.

CP Daily Living, http://cpdailyliving.com/activities/, has a recreation resource section with links to many programs, organizations and other lists that families may find helpful.

Miracle League, http://www.themiracleleague.net, offers adaptive baseball, soccer, basketball and other league programming throughout the US.

Serious Fun Network, https://www.seriousfunnetwork.org, actor Paul Newman has sponsored camps throughout the world that include and focus on the needs of children with cerebral palsy and other disabilities or illnesses.

Tri My Best Triathlon, trimybesttriathalon@gmail.com, is a community-based physical fitness opportunity run by volunteers for individuals with developmental disabilities. There are several locations throughout the US that offer this program. For more information, send an email to the address listed above.

Variety Children's Charity, https://www.varietypittsburgh.org, Variety's signature program is the 'My Bike' Program, which provides adaptive bikes individually customized to eligible children with disabilities.

Very Special Camps, http://www.veryspecialcamps.com, is a specialized directory dedicated exclusively to camps that serve individuals with one or more of a wide range of special needs.

Transition

Fighting Chance, http://fightingchance.org.au, is an Australian nonprofit founded by Laura and Jordan O'Reilly, the siblings of a young man who passed away from complications related to cerebral palsy. The organization works to create comprehensive and meaningful employment, social, educational, and community-based opportunities for individuals with disabilities.

Got Transition, http://www.gottransition.org, seeks to empower patients, families and health care providers through comprehensive resource and training programs designed to assist with the transition from pediatric health care to adult health care for individuals with disabilities.

References

Colver A (2006) Study protocol: SPARCLE – a multi-centre European study of the relationship of environment to participation and quality of life in children with cerebral palsy. *BMC Public Health* 6: 105.

SPARCLE (2017) SPARCLE study of participation and quality of life of children with cerebral palsy. Available from: http://research.ncl.ac.uk/sparcle/

Stockman JA (2009) Self-reported quality of life of 8–12-year-old children with cerebral palsy: a cross-sectional European study. *Yearbook of Pediatrics* 2009: 404–405.

World Health Organization (1995) The World Health Organization quality of life assessment (WHOQOL): Position paper from the World Health Organization. *Social Science & Medicine* 41: 1403–1409.

Chapter 22

Growing up, growing well with cerebral palsy

Jaylan Norfleet, Benjamin Shrader,
Andrew J. Smith, Chelsea Strawser and Garey Noritz

Introduction

This chapter is written by adolescents and adults with (CP) and edited by a physician who practices adult and pediatric neurodevelopmental medicine. Our purpose is to look back at a childhood and young adulthood lived with CP to provide the patient's perspective. It is imperative that successful care of individuals with CP be designed to care for all facets of their lives, not just their physical disability.

The stories below, authored by individuals with a range of functional abilities, represent personal perspectives on living with CP.

In creating this chapter, the editor presented each contributor with a series of questions. The authors responded in a written format and the editor then arranged responses thematically. The questions included the following:

- When and how did you first realize you had CP, and had differences from other kids?

- Did you think your parents treated you differently from other kids? Did you see this as good or bad?

- What was it like to try and make friends as a child (first elementary school, then later on in school)?

- What kind of differences do you see in your doctors and therapists now, versus when you were a kid? What do you wish your doctors and therapists knew about cerebral palsy?

- What are your challenges in terms of trying to be independent? Do you have trouble living independently?

- Have you had difficulty making and sustaining close friendships, including romantic relationships?

- If you could give advice to yourself as a young child, what would it be?

Realizing differences

Jaylan: When I was 5 or 6, I realized I could not do some of the things my friends could. Some of the differences were that during recess time when they were throwing a ball I couldn't; they could run and stand on their own and I couldn't.

Andrew: I think the first time I realized that I had CP and was different from other kids was when I was hit by a car when I was five years old. I remember all the different things that had to be done because of my CP as opposed to others and I was well aware of the different surgeries I would have to go through as a result of not just being hit by a car, but because of my CP. I can remember being in third and fourth grade and having to be pushed around in a wheelchair for a large portion of the year because of leg surgeries that I had to have done as a result of my CP.

I got a lot of comments from the third grade onward about how I walked. I got called a lot of names as a kid and a lot of kids would exclude me from things like kick-ball during recess because I had difficulty kicking the ball at times.

Chelsea: CP is something I have had my entire life, and I can't recall a defining moment of realizing this is something I had, it was just part of my everyday life from the start. I was reminded that I was different with every physical activity I did.

I have an identical twin sister who does not have cerebral palsy. Some people couldn't tell us apart if we were sitting down. Physically though, it was night and day. She pushed me to keep up with her, and because of her I saw what I should be doing so I would try my hardest to keep up. One thing I learned very quickly in life is to adapt and go with it. I would almost always do all the same activities. My mom was a stay at home mom so she did a lot for us both, never more for one than the other. We would go to an amusement park and I would walk the same amount as my family, no excuses! I was expected to get good grades and behave in school.

Benjamin: I am a triplet. My brother has CP and my sister does not. I think because of our sister, I always knew that my brother and I were different and I always understood the nature of CP. Had I not had her around I don't know that I would have understood so quickly.

Parental relationships

Jaylan: I don't think my parents treat me differently because of my CP; they just give me a little more attention to see if I need help with anything. I see this as good because it shows me that they care about me.

Chelsea: My parents were hard on me and pushed me to work hard. They refused to let me say I couldn't do something. They still won't let me say that today. Sometimes, I could get over on my dad a little, but that was because I was his little girl, not because I had CP.

Once I remember crying about not wanting to have surgery and that I was scared. Mostly it was because I knew that I would spend most of my summer in bed, and what was left in recovery. My grandmother told me 'Chelsea, you have a choice to make here. You can look at all the blessings you have in life or you can cry about the bad things. I know it won't always be fun but we will make the best of it!' She then promised me things like movie dates and trips to the zoo, things I could do in my wheelchair.

Andrew: I wouldn't say that my parents or grandparents treated me differently than other kids apart from letting me know early on what things I could and could not do because of CP. My mother and other family members always told me that I could do anything within my limitations as long as I worked hard and set my mind to it, and that's what I have always tried to do.

There were times when teachers and schools would tell my mother that I needed to be put in special classrooms and that I needed to be separated from other kids and she refused to allow them to do that. I think that I am where I am today in part because my mother fought so hard for me to be treated the same as the other kids. There were times when I would be told by doctors that I would never be able to do certain things and told by teachers that I wasn't smart enough to go to college, or that I needed some special form of teaching and this drove me to not only prove all of them wrong, but to set a precedent so that other kids in my same position could see that it is possible. I wanted all those other kids that were in the CP clinic with me when I was little to see that it could be done and to never give up no matter how hard things got. My parents allowed me to set my own limits and figure out for myself where those limitations lie.

Benjamin: Being a triplet, I was never isolated. I didn't feel like I had received any special treatment from my parents because on the one end there was another child with CP and on the other there was an able-bodied child. I think this allowed us to form a unique relationship with our parents and also taught us what unity looked like.

Making friends

Chelsea: I remember hearing my parents talking with their friends about how they were worried that I would have no friends and I could never understand why – inside I felt like every other kid. If anything, I think this pushed me to make more friends. I was lucky and blessed to attend a small town elementary school. This gave me the chance to make some friends that I still have to this day. I would say my social life has always been pretty active.

In high school and in college I attended all the events and had just as many friends as anyone else. I had normal high school and college experiences compared to everyone I knew. My friends tell me all the time they don't even see my CP after a while.

I always jokingly say I have to be outgoing and don't know a stranger, because sometimes you have to ask a stranger to help you up the stairs when there is no ramp. That is actually the way I met one of my friends and I ended up in her wedding!

Andrew: It was very difficult making friends growing up. A lot of the kids could see that I was treated different than others and they could all notice the way I walked and the fact that I wore thick glasses. Many kids didn't want anything to do with me because they found me strange. They didn't want to be made fun of for associating with me and so they avoided me when they had the chance. I would often sit alone away from other kids at school during lunch and recess, not entirely by choice, but because each time I would sit next to someone at lunch they would choose to move away from me. Many students would play pranks on me in school and there were times that kids would push me or trip me to make me fall. This was made worse by the fact that a student from class in elementary would be assigned to help me do certain things in my wheelchair. There were a few times during recess that I would be left outside without any help from the person assigned to assist me and I would have to wheel myself back inside through grass. At the time I had a good idea why they did these things and I never really fully blamed them for that because I understood how other kids could be towards them.

As I got older things got even more difficult because my medical issues started to cause more problems and I wasn't able to do the things that most kids my age were able to do. In middle school I did have a close group of a few friends and formed a bond with one another due to the fact that we were all picked on by others for various reasons, but they weren't with me in high school.

I couldn't get into any sports during high school because of my physical limitations and so that didn't give me the chance to perhaps change the image that a lot of people had about me and my condition. I was shoved into lockers, tripped and had things stolen from me regularly during my high school years. The few friends that I did have during high school I later found out were not my real friends at all and that they were simply hanging around me out of pity. Despite all the name calling and all of the bad things that were being done I still wanted to help those same people when they needed it and I still wanted to be nice to everyone because I felt that doing mean things back to them would not solve the problem and it would not change their mindset at all.

It was very hard to convince myself that someone really could be my friend. Going to college, I had some of those same problems, but I think that in a lot of cases once people learned a bit more about my condition and understood it they had a completely different outlook on the whole situation. I can't really remember any truly negative experiences while I was in college and for the most part people treated me the same as everyone else, but there would be times where you would hear people say and do things and make a joke here and there, but I still get that today from time to time and I think that it is something that is going to happen no matter what a person does. I can say that in terms of school, college was the best experience I had with making friends and getting to know new people. I think that was in large part because assignments allowed us to break barriers and I think it was also due to the fact that professors treated everyone exactly the same.

Benjamin: In elementary school, I had a group of three friends. On the surface, all three showed some level of interest in me, but over time it became clear that really only one of them was interested in our friendship. The other two were very protective of the third friend, steering him away from me at recess. As I look back, I am not sure if this was direct bigotry or a juvenile selfishness but it certainly felt as if I was being excluded because of my disability. I very much wanted to be part of their group – the fourth member in a sense – but they did not seem to want that. This illustrated for me the 'filter effect' of CP for the first time. There would be people that wouldn't appreciate and value me as a member of their circle but when friends came along that did, it made it all the more special.

This filter left only the really good friends. I knew that one had to be a very special person to embrace my differences so I was kind of able to use it to my advantage.

As I have grown up, the situation has stayed mostly the same. Obviously, I have more than a couple of friends, but CP still functions as a filter.

Jaylan: Making friends when I was younger in elementary school was a lot easier because I didn't know what I had and people would ask less questions. In middle school it's a little different because there are awkward teenage feelings that make you wonder if people like you for you or are friendly because of my disability, but I do have a lot of friends.

Doctors and therapists – now and then

Jaylan: I wish doctors and therapists knew that sometimes it's hard for me mentally because I'm constantly asked to do things, and even if I don't feel like it, I still have to do it. I see that they talk to me more than they did from when I was younger to ask how I feel about certain things and they expect more responsibility from me now as I advocate for myself.

Benjamin: I wish they talked to me directly instead of just my parents. Until relatively recently, I always felt like a fly on the wall at my own appointments or therapy sessions. I felt sometimes that doctors or therapists merely engaged me as a case rather than who I was. I wish, even at a young age, people had talked directly to me. As I transition into adulthood, they are beginning to ask me what I want. This allows me to take responsibility for my own care.

When I was six years old I was about to have a major surgery. My brother had actually had the same operation the previous year. I remembered talking to him on the phone when he was in the hospital and the ghostly quietness in his voice as he tried to talk back. One thing you should know about me is that what I lack in physical ability, I try to make up for in talkativeness, so I was afraid the same would happen to me. When I asked, the doctor didn't seem to take my concerns seriously, flippantly reminding me that the surgery had nothing to do with my vocal cords. I wasn't entirely convinced but I took him at his word. But sure enough, when I woke from the operation I had difficulty talking. The difficulty was so great that I panicked and began vomiting. At which point, the nurses sedated me. When I woke up the same thing happened again, they sedated me. When the cycle repeated itself a third time, my mom finally spoke up and said it was because I couldn't talk that I was getting so upset. She suggested they give me time to wake up so I could see that I could talk. She was right.

My physical therapist through my teen years urged me to take control of my own care. She reminded me that it was my body after all and that I was in charge. This has really helped me as I transition into adulthood and try to gain increasing independence. I am very grateful for her.

Andrew: As a kid many doctors would say that they had done all they could do and that I was as good as I was going to get and so there was no need to come back. Many doctors would attribute issues that I had to a side effect of my CP before even doing an examination and they would not listen to my explanations as to why I believed that it was something else unrelated to my CP. There would be many times when my pain would get worse or I would notice changes and they would simply tell me that there was nothing that they could do to help.

The doctors I have now are far and above different compared to those that I had as a kid. For the most part, doctors now are listening a lot more and they are allowing me to talk and explain differences to them. They are asking questions to better understand the condition itself not just for me, but for their other patients with CP. They want to understand and they want to help and they are more up front and honest about either not knowing a lot about CP or telling me what they do know and asking me what may be right or different about my case. I'm able to talk to my doctors a lot more easily. I also think that the fact that doctors are talking to each other more is also a nice change

I want doctors to know that it's very hard to answer questions about pain and how I am feeling in terms of pain. I learned to deal with the day to day pain and just accept it and sort of push it out of my mind without the use of pain medication. I got used to the pain and limitations and so it's very hard at times to convey to doctors that I am in pain. I think that for the most part many doctors and therapists are starting to understand CP overall and things that were a constant problem no longer seem that way.

Living independently

Chelsea: Now that I am 25 and have established myself into a career I have been looking for houses. Living alone scares me, to be honest. I think it scares most women, but my added fears are ice on the driveway and water on the floor. I wonder what life will be like living alone.

Benjamin: I have difficulties ranging from eating to dressing myself to typing. Although this may sound like an oxymoron, I feel that in order to be as independent as I can be I must accept the help others graciously offer me in doing these tasks. In doing so, I maintain an active relationship with my caregivers and I allow them to understand the things I want to do.

Andrew: As I got older I started to have more and more problems that I never used to have and as a result I have not been able to use my degree to its full potential to get a good enough job to live fully independently. I always have that fear in the back of my mind that something is going to go medically wrong, and I can see how things like going up and down the stairs or putting on socks and shoes are reverting back to the difficulties I had when I was little.

It scares me at times because I am unsure how these things will pan out and I can feel the pain and the limitations it is causing. I can't stand for long periods of time and I am not able to carry heavy things like I used to when I was working during the summer while in college. I notice a lot more how I run out of energy quickly when doing anything physical and how there are days when I don't want to do anything but rest or sleep.

This set of unknowns coupled with my known limitations make it hard for me to get hired at a job. I know that I need to rest a lot when standing or doing physical work and even typing on a keyboard can be unpredictable at times with one day being fine and another day very difficult. I share these limitations with employers because I want them to understand and I want to be placed in a position where I can be effective despite my limitations. The problem is that a lot of employers are unwilling or unable to accommodate me. I am now working online as a contractor at a job where I can set my own hours and take breaks, but I don't make enough to truly live independently on my own.

Adult friendships, romantic relationships

Jaylan: I don't have a girlfriend yet but that's because I am more interested in my school work.

Chelsea: I have a lot of friendships and close friends that are amazing. I can confidently say with friendships I have no issues making and sustaining lasting relationships.

Dating is another story. (I have tried to write my answer to this question three times and stopped when I start crying.) I would say this would be the one reason I wish I didn't have CP because I let it affect my dating life and always have. I have dated some in the past years, mostly in college. However, I have a huge complex about the way I look and the way I walk when it comes to dating. I always say it will take a special heart to love me and I hope I find that one day. When you're picking the one person to spend the rest of your life with, I have always wondered if a man will ever pick the girl that is damaged. I hate saying this because it is contradictory to my other statements and beliefs!

Andrew: A lot of my close friendships did not last because of my medical issues and because of pressure from those outside. My medical issues didn't allow me to do a lot of things that my close friends wanted to do and as a result we grew apart from one another.

As far as romantic relationships I haven't really had too many to speak of. The main problem was that during school people didn't see me in that way and all the other preconceived notions made it next to impossible to try to start a romantic relationship with someone regardless of how much I wanted to. There were no girls who wanted to date someone with my condition and when I finally did get to a point where that might be a possibility, other things would prevent it from happening.

I think the biggest issue when it comes to romantic relationships is the medical issues and the financial problems that it causes. I always grew up wanting to make my own way. The stress of not being able to work a regular job and the fact that my finances were not all that great prevented me from even pursuing the issue, and when I finally was financially stable enough to maybe give it a chance the medical issues would get in the way. The last thing I wanted was to become a burden to my romantic partner either because of financial or medical problems. I worry about my financial stability and about my future health and until I get to a point where I am at the very least financially stable and independent I don't think that a romantic relationship is a possibility. When you spend a large part of your life being dependent on doctors and others for help the last thing you want is to be in a relationship where you feel a lot of the same things. Right or wrong I felt like a burden a lot growing up and it drove me to want to be truly independent and to make my own way.

Benjamin: With regard to friendships, I again say that my CP works as something of a filter, only allowing truly special people in.

I may not be the best person to talk about romantic relationships since I haven't had one (yet), but I will give it my best shot. I believe the filter effect is also true of romantic relationships but with one added component, when we look at romantic relationships we see that all of us –including me – have a sort of predetermined view in our minds of what that sort of thing looks like. Often that view does not include a wheelchair. I believe this is in part due to a cultural perception that we must change. I believe the way we do that is by fostering these relationships over long periods of time. For example, at first, a parent simply can't see themselves having a child with a disability but eventually come to love the child. This is the approach that those of us with disabilities must take regarding romantic relationships. We must first foster friendships in which we become someone's friend, not their friend with a disability.

If you could give advice to yourself as a young child, what would it be?

Jaylan: The advice I would give to my young self would be to never give up, always be optimistic, remember it's okay to take a break when things get hard, don't be afraid to try new things and always ask for advice when you need it.

Andrew: It would have been to use all the extra time I had to write more. I always wanted to earn enough money through writing that I could help people in need and it's still a goal of mine to do that and I think that if I had been able to give that advice to myself as a child I would have already been at that point today. As a child I felt that I would have plenty of time to do it and before I knew it I was grown up and that large amount of free time was gone. I would also tell myself to spend that time learning different languages because I think that had I started at a young age it would have given me some extra tools that I could have used later in life to perhaps get different types of jobs that required that sort of thing.

Benjamin: For many years I downplayed my disability to myself and was not actively involved in the fight for disability rights. I would tell my younger self to embrace his diversity and use it to fight to ensure everyone has the opportunities that I have had.

Chelsea: I would say smile at those people that stared at you, they didn't realize it made you cry! To the comments that hurt your feelings, one day you'll realize they made you stronger.

To the friends willing to lend a helping hand, hold onto them! Cherish them like gold. Thank them for including you in everything, even if it takes longer to get somewhere. Realize that they enjoy your company and they don't mind helping you. Take a look at the group of friends you have because they are a blessing. Thank the strangers that help you when it's icy, thank let them know you're happy that they were there.

You're going to fall. Actually, you're going to fall a lot! Don't cry; unless it's from laughing too hard. Trust me, those moments make for good stories with your best friend later. You will encounter more good people than bad ones! Count your blessings, learn from your failures, and thank your friends and family again and again! The people that doubted you, thank them most of all!!

Discussion

In editing this chapter, I was struck by several of the themes that ring true for everyone who has grown through the adolescent phase of alienation, with a disability or not.

The young people credit much of their success in life to the attitudes and attachment to their parents, who were loving and supportive. At home, they did not feel as if they were treated differently because of their CP, though their childhoods were filled with doctor's appointments, therapy sessions, and surgeries. At school, there was a varying sense of being set apart because of the CP. This illustrates the challenges we have to fully integrate people with disabilities, which is society's problem to solve collectively, not the individuals'.

As young adults, my coauthors continue to strive for more independence and to establish themselves in life. Their accomplishments so far can provide lessons to parents and other young people with CP as to the kinds of attitudes and actions that lead to success.

Chapter 23

Care tools for clinical practice

Laurie J. Glader, Darcy Fehlings, Jonathan Greenwood, Christopher D. Lunsford, Kerim M. Munir, Garey Noritz, Jim Plews-Ogan, Michele Shusterman, Benjamin Shore, Jilda N. Vargus-Adams and Richard D. Stevenson

In this chapter we offer some clinical tools that we hope will facilitate and organize encounters with children with complex cerebral palsy. Given broad practice variation across the world and the fact that so many providers and clinics have embraced electronic medical records, we have kept these worksheets fairly basic in the hope that they could be adapted to fit most systems. We offer three different tools: a Health review for children (Table 23.1), an Equipment, Supplies and Supports Checklist (Table 23.2), and an International Classification of Functioning, Disability and Health (ICF)-based care: goals and management form (Table 23.3). These forms are not intended to represent true Care Maps as those already exist at some institutions (see Chapter 2 for an example) and are beyond the scope of this manual. Rather they are offered as tools to help provide a framework to organize data gathering, goal setting, decision-making, and management plans during clinical encounters.

Comprehensive guidelines of care for children with complex cerebral palsy are needed and currently do not exist. Their need has been highlighted recently in an international forum. Some focused guidelines on aspects of diagnosis and treatment (such as the care pathways by the American Academy of Cerebral Palsy and Developmental Medicine) have been developed, and they have been referenced throughout this book where appropriate.

The three tools are intended for use as follows:

1) The **Health Review for children** (Table 23.1) is intended to help trigger questions relevant to the medical care of children with complex cerebral palsy, and is to be used collaboratively by the provider and the family. It can be used similarly to the traditional 'Review of systems' and is organized with most common issues

at the top and less common at the bottom. The medication section is not meant to represent a comprehensive medication reconciliation but rather to highlight important concerns or questions relating to a child's medication management.

2) The **Equipment, supplies and supports** (Table 23.2) is intended as a concise way to summarize equipment and services that the child utilizes and to identify areas of unmet need. It also provides opportunity to note concerns or needs relating to any of the items on the checklist. The form could potentially be provided to families to fill out prior to an appointment.

3) The **ICF-based care: goals and management form** (Table 23.3) provides a framework to ensure that a thorough review is conducted and plan created at a comprehensive visit for a child with complex cerebral palsy. In essence, it assists in keeping all items of importance or concern 'on the radar screen.' Our goal is to foster integration of ICF concepts into clinical care. The scope of review may be conducted by a single provider but it is broad and may best be divided amongst clinicians of different expertise. We have grounded this form in the original five components of the ICF (body structure and function, activities, participation, environment and personal factors). Additionally, we have added three areas which merit their own recognition given the frequency with which they arise in caring for children with complex cerebral palsy: medical technology and devices, family systems, and team management (Glader et al. 2016). The last, team management, deserves significant consideration, as the teams caring for this population of children are often quite large and delegation of tasks is integral to ensuring that tasks are indeed completed. Team management might include identification of key personnel responsible for the issue outlined, necessary communication between team members (which may include community entities such as home nursing and school therapists), and required documentation, such as orders for school, emergency or sick plans. This information can be articulated in the last column of the ICF-based care: goals and management form. Of note, the Health review for children relates neatly to the body structure and function component of the ICF-based care: goals and management form, while the Equipment, supplies and supports checklist spans multiple components.

The final section of the ICF-based care: goals and management form includes personal goals. Goal-based care is a central element of crafting a meaningful plan with individuals and families. In the end, this form could be used as a contractual agreement between providers and an individual with cerebral palsy, or the caregivers who make medical decisions on their behalf. It offers a clear reminder of goals as well as roles and responsibilities in reaching those goals.

These tools are intended for providers of many backgrounds and may be used individually or in any combination, as clinical venues vary widely. Their scope is broad, reflecting the breadth of knowledge and expertise required to care for children with complex cerebral palsy. They provide a framework for much of the 'stuff' of this manual, incorporating everything from the nuts and bolts of medical care, to functional concerns and person-centered goals. We hope you find them useful.

Resources

Cerebral Palsy Foundation: yourcpf.org
CP Channel – CP NOW: https://**cpnow**foundation.org

References

Glader L, Plews-Ogan J, Agrawal R (2016) Children with medical complexity: creating a framework for care based on the International Classification of Functioning, Disability and Health. *Dev Med Child Neurol* 58(11): 1116–23.

The Care Tools found in this chapter are available to download at http://www.mackeith.co.uk/shop/complex-cerebral-palsy-care-and-management/

Table 23.1 Health review for children

System	Concerns	Plans
General 'What's going well?' Interim changes Caregiver concerns Pain		
Medications Recent changes or additions Concern for side effects		
Development Gross motor Fine motor Communication Cognition Feeding Toileting		
Musculoskeletal Equipment needs Therapeutic needs Surgical history/plans Caregiver challenges Most recent X-ray results		

Neurology
Tone management
Sleep
Seizures
Neuroimaging
Baseline temperature
Causation of cerebral palsy:
    Neuroimaging
    Genetic concerns
    Loss of milestones?		

Sensory Hearing status Visual concerns		

Table 23.1 (Continued)

System	Concerns	Plans

FEN/GI
Nutrition
Growth trajectory
Constipation
GERD symptoms
Abdominal discomfort
Feeding route:
   Oral/Gtube/GJtube
Diet:
   Table food: yes/no
   Modified texture: yes/no
Formula type _____
Feeding schedule
 	
_____		

Mental/Behavioral Health Mood Challenging behaviors Psychosocial concerns Abuse screening as indicated		
Ear, nose and throat/dental Sialorrhea OSA Oral health issues		
Pulmonary Chronic cough/congestion Reactive airway disease H/O pneumonia Concerns for aspiration Oxygen requirement		
Endocrine Bone health Fracture history Pubertal development/concerns		

Table 23.1 (Continued)

System	Concerns	Plans
Cardiology Congenital defect/surgery Baseline HR Baseline BP		
Renal/urology UTI history Urinary retention Vesicoureteral reflux Kidney stones Continence		
Hematology Anemia Neutropenia Thrombocytopenia		
Allergy/immunology Seasonal allergies Food allergies		
Infectious disease Colonization Recurrent infections		
Dermatology Eczema Pressure ulcers		

FEN: fluids, electrolytes and nutrition; GI: Gastrointestinal; OSA: Obstructive sleep apnea; H/O: history of; HR: heart rate; BP: blood pressure; UTI: urinary tract infection.

Table 23.2 Equipment, supplies and supports checklist

Please review the following list which might include items or therapies related to your child. Check off those that your child has/uses and please list any concerns or needs you may have related to those items.

Medical technology and devices	

Concerns/needs:
 	
_____
_____
_____
	☐ Enteral tube
	    Type_____ size_____
	    Managed by _____
	☐ Tracheostomy
	    Type_____ size_____
	    Managed by _____
	    Ostomy
	    Type_____
	    Managed by _____
	☐ Baclofen pump
	    Type_____ size_____
	    Managed by _____
	    Port for access
	    Type_____
	☐ VP Shunt
	    Managed by _____
	    Hearing devices
	    Type_____
	☐ Glasses/contacts
	☐ Durable medical equipment (DME)
	    ○ Feeding pump
	    ○ Nebulizer
	    ○ Oximeter
	    ○ Bottled oxygen
	    ○ Oxygen compressor
	    ○ CPAP/BiPAP
	    ○ Ventilator
	    ○ Chest PT vest
	    ○ Cough assist
	☐ Other _____

Table 23.2 (Continued)

Medical technology and devices	
Orthoses, mobility and positioning devices	
Concerns/needs: _____ _____ _____	☐ Wheelchair ☐ Adaptive stroller ☐ Stander ☐ Gait trainer/walker ☐ Canes/crutches ☐ Bath seat ☐ Specialized bed Type _____ ☐ Lift ☐ AFOs ☐ Wrist splints ☐ TLSO/trunk support ☐ Other _____
Communication	
Concerns/needs: _____ _____ _____	☐ Communication device Type: _____ ☐ Switches ☐ Picture system
School services	
Concerns/needs: _____ _____ _____	☐ Name of school/Early intervention _____ ☐ Grade _____ ☐ Classroom type _____ ☐ IEP ☐ Where does your child receive therapies? _____ ☐ PT frequency: _____ Focus of therapy_____ ☐ OT frequency: _____ Focus of therapy_____ ☐ Speech frequency: _____ Focus of therapy_____ ☐ Vision frequency: _____ Focus of therapy_____

Table 23.2 (Continued)

Medical technology and devices	
	☐ Feeding frequency: _____
	Focus of therapy_____
	☐ ABA frequency: _____
	Focus of therapy_____
	☐ Behavior frequency: _____
	Focus of therapy_____
	☐ Other_____
	_____
Home/community supports	
Concerns/needs:	Personal care attendant
_____	Number of hours: _____
_____	☐ Home nursing
_____	Number of hours: _____
	Name of agency: _____
	☐ In home services
	Type: _____
	☐ Respite
	Facility: _____
	☐ Community agency affiliations
	_____
	_____
	☐ Counseling/behavioral support
	☐ Additional support
	_____
	☐ Recent changes at home
	_____
	☐ Financial concerns
	_____

CPAP: continuous positive airway pressure; BiPAP: BiLevel positive airway pressure; PT: physical therapy; AFO: ankle foot orthosis; TLSO: Thoraco-lumbar scoliosis orthosis; IFP: Individualized Family Plan; PT: physical therapy; OT: occupational therapy; ABA: applied behavioral analysis.

Table 23.3 ICF-based care: goals and management

Components	Priorities	Notes	Goals and management
Structure and function	Health issues		
Medical technology and devices	Identified areas of need		
Activities	Communication		
	Sitting and mobility		
	Feeding/eating		
	Self-care		
	Therapies		
Participation	Family		
	Friends		
	School		
	Community		
Environment and adaptive technology	Mobility devices and orthoses		
	Communication aids		
	Physical environment		
	Attitudinal milieu		

Family system	Family education
	Cerebral palsy resources
	Cerebral Palsy Foundation
	• CP Channel app
	• CP NOW (cerebral palsy Toolkit)
	• Siblings
	Family health and supports
	Research participation
	Issues related to age
Personal factors	Transition
	Early Intervention to school
	• High school
	• Graduation
	• Adult services
	• Guardianship
	Sex/Sexuality
	Goals of care
	• Functional
	• Social
	• Medical (health care proxy, DNR/DNI)

Index

NOTE: Figures, boxes, tables and appendices are denoted by an italic, lower case *f, b, t* and *app* respectively. "Cerebral Palsy" is abbreviated to "CP" in subheadings throughout.